The Rhetoric of Food

Routledge Studies in Rhetoric and Communication

The Rhetoric of Food

Discourse, Materiality, and Power

Edited by Joshua J. Frye
and Michael S. Bruner

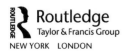
Routledge
Taylor & Francis Group

NEW YORK   LONDON

First published 2012
by Routledge
711 Third Avenue, New York, NY 10017

Simultaneously published in the UK
by Routledge
2 Park Square, Milton Park, Abingdon, Oxon OX14 4RN

*Routledge is an imprint of the Taylor & Francis Group,
an informa business*

Library of Congress Cataloging-in-Publication Data
The rhetoric of food : discourse, materiality, and power / edited by
Joshua J. Frye and Michael S. Bruner.
    p. cm. — (Routledge studies in rhetoric and communication ; 9)
    Includes bibliographical references and index.
 1. Food—Social aspects.   2. Food—Moral and ethical aspects.
3. Communication and culture.   4. Rhetoric—Political aspects.
I. Frye, Joshua.   II. Bruner, Michael S.
    GN407.R48 2012
    394.1'2—dc23
    2011050772

ISBN13: 978-0-415-72756-3 (pbk)

First issued in paperback 2013

Typeset in Sabon
by IBT Global

To all those who hunger for an end to starvation, injustice, malnutrition, unsustainable food systems, and cruelty to our planet and all its inhabitants.

Contents

Figures

Foreword

Raymie E. McKerrow

As the editors of this volume—Joshua J. Frye and Michael S. Bruner—indicate, "food interactions are central to humankind." As they also note, this edited collection of essays arrives as interest in the symbolic meanings associated with food in all its guises is growing exponentially. What prompts this interest? It may well be a natural reaction to the pervasive nature of discourses about food and its relation to a healthy lifestyle. In 1940, the nutritionist Victor Hugo Landlahr published a book with a title that reflects the relationship between self and food: *You Are What You Eat* (1940, National Nutrition Society). That phrase did not start the preoccupation with food, but it symbolizes what has become a commonplace notion: our interactions with others are impacted in manifold ways, often unconsciously, by our eating habits. For example, within the American environment, fast food chains offer choices that are quick and easy to obtain and consume, while doing little to abate a growing concern with obesity, among children as well as adults. Diet fads proclaim easy and painless ways to achieve healthier living. Communities engage citizens in campaigns to lose weight. Reality TV showcases obese individuals who compete to lose more than the other contestants. "Wellness" becomes the new catch phrase in re-titling fitness centers in communities to highlight the advantages of a healthy lifestyle. Hotels now routinely offer workout spaces, while college campuses build and name new "gyms" as "wellness centers." We are a nation that makes fun of those who have ignored the deleterious effects of food intake, while reveling in the struggles of "the biggest loser" (and that can be taken in more ways than one) on a reality TV show.

As the editors and authors of the essays in this volume illustrate, the obsession with weight is only one of the myriad ways in which food impacts our lives. Issues of race, sex, gender, and class all interact in producing particular relations with the importance (or lack thereof) of how our food practices, from growing to consumption, foster or inhibit personal, community, and societal decisions. My purpose in this foreword is to set a general context for the practice of applying rhetorical concepts to food. After all, from one perspective, food is simply food—that which we might plant, harvest, mill, form into edible products, purchase, and consume (to chronicle just one of many types of food we might ingest).

As a Montana farm boy, I recall sifting the chaff and bugs from a handful of wheat grabbed from the truck as the combine unloaded it, and chewing it to make wheat gum. Ironically, I now am prohibited from eating any wheat-based products due to a disease known as celiac sprue. In restaurants, I rarely ever suggest, however, that "I have a disease; I can't eat wheat (or barley or rye)." Instead, I indicate I have an "allergy" to wheat. This is a simple example of the power of language—to announce a "disease" is to engender the possibility of creating dis-ease in the person being informed. On other occasions, I may say "I'm allergic to gluten"—in this instance, the term used requires that the person I am informing understands it. Even then, I may get the response, "Well, since you can't have the bun, how about pasta?" In other words, translating "He can't eat a bun made of wheat" into "that means he can't eat any wheat-based products, of which pasta is a key one" requires making connections beyond those presented. This is not intended as a complaint about dense servers in a restaurant—it is, rather, intended to suggest that communicative interactions are never as simple as one might suppose. A visit to small towns in southern Ireland serves as a counter to these experiences. In place after place, I started to mention my food restriction, only to be met with "You have Celiac, eh? Here's what we can do." Familiarity with the disease is part of their daily life. Celiac sprue and gluten, as a named disease or a protein product, are not, in themselves, rhetorical.

How we entertain these labels, the attitudes we attribute to them, and the choices we make on hearing them all represent functions that are based in the language we use. Words do matter—the old saying that "sticks and stones may break my bones, but words will never harm me" is a lie—words of praise and blame are so-called because they have impacts on how we think about ourselves, what we think of those using them, and how we then react, physically, nonverbally, or with passionate expression (or all three at some point). Thus, how we frame our conversations about food in particular ("dried cow pies would taste better"; "that is an elegant presentation—so artistic and aesthetically pleasing that I dare not eat it") conveys a wealth of information about who we are, how we are willing to interact with others (presuming the first example is rude, and the second not so much), and what we are thinking at a given moment. We speak ourselves, just as the food we eat is us. And, in the same way, the food speaks for us as well. We need to be careful here, as what is "spoken" by food may not always be precise. A person who announces she is a "meat-eater" may not consume certain meats, just as person who acknowledges being a "vegan" covers a multitude of very different orders of choice with respect to what he will and won't consume in living a specific vegan lifestyle.

The critical task, in recognizing the complex ways in which rhetoric functions in relation to objects and events, is to be clear about what is happening within the social, political, and economic context in which discourses abound. Asking "Who is empowered to speak to whom with what effect?" is one entry-point into a more critical analysis that uncovers relations of power. Other questions include: What language resonates within the culture and what terms live for a moment and then fade away (language never quite goes away; there are always traces that may be picked up in a later time and become salient once more)? If rhetoric is considered not simply associated with material artifacts, but materially forceful in its own right, how does this merger of a "material rhetoric" influence the way in which we talk about the impact of symbols? Food is not a language in the sense of speaking its own words; rather, its impact exists in and through the language we use to describe it. It can function symbolically as a powerful weapon—withholding it from the hungry further empowers those in control of the distribution system while diminishing the social others from whom it is withheld; conversely, shipping tons of food to a famine-ravaged land conveys meanings of charity and selflessness in the face of another's tragedy. As suggested earlier, these meanings do not reside in the food as such; they are creations of the moment in providing a rhetorical frame within which we hope to convey intentions. They can be misread just as easily as they can be received as presented.

The further task of a critic is one that goes beyond reflection on what is to a more evocative framing of what should be. It is one thing to note the power of language to frame food in positive or negative ways; it is another to suggest ways in which language might be re-made, that terms might increase or decrease their salience in particular ways in order to create a new matrix of power relations within or across a community or culture. Or, at the very least, the critic may outline those spaces where intervention by those most impacted by the existing power relations may find a way to go beyond the current relations into a new, as yet uncharted space.

In various ways, the essays in this volume testify to a fulfillment of this obligation—charging the existing frame within which food discourses operate with conduct that does not represent the best that we can be, or otherwise noting the ethical lapse that is represented by a particular configuration of power or its expression. In doing so, they bring theoretical sophistication to the fore in utilizing the voices of Butler, Burke, Derrida, Foucault, Fraser, Kierkegaard, and Rancière, to name a few, as part of their critique. The themes undertaken range widely, but the "center that holds" across these contributions is a sensitivity to the power of food as rhetoric, and of naming that food in ways that create a powerful social narrative. While the editors have dealt with the essays in more detail, it remains valuable to underscore the themes that are addressed in the text. Whether referencing the soil (and the Montana farm boy in me returns to the soil as a means of nourishing the soul), dietary choices, food packaging, representations of the obese body, the salience of "eating organic" over and against that afforded "eating vegan," standardizing food discourse as a grammar, explicating the meaning of suicide as a protest against the power of economic forces that diminish the power of small farmers, interrogating the symbolic power of a presidential ritual in pardoning a turkey, unpacking the role of space in relation to its use in agriculture or in the sale of farm products, examining the First Lady's role in promoting a healthy lifestyle, critiquing an effort to reform school-based food, challenging the rhetorical choices offered via the fast-food industry, delineating the power of food producers in managing the discourse of what counts as healthy food, or articulating the change in attitudes toward cannibalism, the essays in this volume constitute a major advance in our understanding of food as rhetoric.

Acknowledgments

The editors would like to thank the following individuals and organizations: the Public Address Division of the National Communication Association, Professor Kirt Wilson (Vice Chair), and the reviewers, for sponsoring our panel at the 2010 annual convention from which this book grew; Elizabeth Levine, for seeing the potential of this project and being our advocate at Routledge; our families, for their patience, support, feedback, and space/time granted during the many long months and late nights of working on this book; the anonymous external reviewers, for their insightful recommendations during the planning process for *The Rhetoric of Food*; Josh's faculty colleagues and students at the State University of New York, for understanding the time and energy necessary to successfully fulfill a book project; Humboldt State University, for its support of Michael's Fall 2010 sabbatical leave as a visiting scholar at the University of California, Berkeley; Jun Virola of the Asian Farmers Association for Sustainable Rural Development, for his generosity in sharing the image of Lee Kyung Hae's Memorial Hall; Crystal Fraioli, for her able assistance with the compilation and organization of the index; Jim Greenberg at the Teaching, Learning, and Technology Center at the State University of New York, for his expertise with locating, scanning, and converting texts and images; all of the authors, for contributing their original scholarship to this book; the University Press of Kentucky, for granting us copyright permissions to reprint Sir Albert Howard's classic essay on *The Operations of Nature* (originally published in 1947 by the Devin-Adair Company); Action Against Hunger, for its willingness to grant copyright permissions for the photographic images in Chapter 2; Raymie McKerrow, for his willingness to share his expertise in rhetorical theory and his wise words in the foreword. All of the blame in fact or judgment is ours. All of the praise goes to those for whom we write.

Introduction

Joshua J. Frye and Michael S. Bruner

[T]he relationship between the material and the discursive is one of mutual entailment. Neither is articulated/articulable in the absence of the other; matter and meaning are mutually articulated. Neither discursive practices nor material phenomena are ontologically or epistemologically prior. Neither can be explained in terms of the other. Neither has privileged status in determining the other.[1]

Discourse. Materiality. Power. These are the sinews that connect rhetoric to food. Food is central to humankind. It is a requirement for survival, but also functions as a defining element of human culture and identity. Modes of producing, distributing, consuming, and marketing food have socioecological, socioeconomic, and sociopolitical motives and consequences. Throughout time, agricultural practices have facilitated a fundamental re-organization of human-nature relationships, discourses, and power structures. From the ability to live a sedentary life and support dense population centers to contributing to the decline and fall of civilizations, food has always been a preoccupation of the symbol-using human animal. Aside from these sweeping sociobiological evolutionary roles, food rhetoric is increasingly dominant discourse and suffuses co-cultures, popular culture, countercultures, global economics, and environmental policies. Contemporary food rhetoric instantiations appear as: Food System; Food Shed; Food Deserts; Local Food; Fast Food; Slow Food; Food Network; Food First; Food Not Bombs; GM Food; Organic Food; Functional Food; Whole Food; Food, Inc.; Food Banks; Food Riots; Food Sovereignty; Food Security; Food Insecurity; Real Food; Snack Food; Food Scare; Food Channel, and so forth. Food rhetoric is expanding our lexicon, revising our attitudes toward food, and re-organizing relationships with our earth and our bodies.

The Rhetoric of Food: Discourse, Materiality, and Power takes food, material conditions of all sorts, and power seriously, but is firmly grounded in a rhetorical perspective. This book, then, tries to hold food, discourse, materiality, and power together—to acknowledge and honor all the connections and tensions—while using rhetorical analyses to help explain the dynamics and the consequences.

What is rhetoric? In this book, we are guided by three perspectives on rhetoric. From Kenneth Burke, we take the direct definition that rhetoric is symbolism designed to "form attitudes or to induce actions in other human agents."[2] From Aristotle, we borrow the notion that rhetoric is "the power to observe the persuasiveness of which any particular matter admits."[3] Third, with post-modern scholars, (a) we understand that rhetoric is multi-directional and multi-level and (b) we agree that, to be useful, rhetorical studies must take a critical stance (address issues of power, privilege, identity, culture, and control) and must offer alternatives through the auspices of imagination, message (de/re)construction, representation, (re)constitution, policy critique, ideological framing, evaluation of values, metaphors, narratives, rituals, land-use, everyday practices, claimed materiality, privilege, image, and oppression. These three perspectives undergird this collection of essays. In the end, however, we openly relinquish whatever forms of privilege that we might claim as critics. Further, we openly acknowledge that this book is a form of rhetoric. If rhetoric is the graveyard of all human reality as well as the midwife of discourse, our hope is to intervene in the flow of living discourse in order to reflect it, illuminate it, and possibly even focus it as a magnifying glass to set fire to our assumptions, norms, biases, practices, policies, and values so they may rise again from the ashes, reborn. This book—as rhetoric—must also be judged as persuasive or not, and as useful or not, in the ongoing conversations that are addressing the significant issues of our day.

The editors and authors recognize with deep appreciation the work of other writers who address food-in-public-discourse. There are too many individuals and groups working in this broad area to mention separately, but we will list three: (1) Popular books, such as *Bottomfeeder: How to Eat Ethically in a World of Vanishing Seafood* (Taras Grescoe) and *The Omnivore's Dilemma* (Michael Pollan), have done a great deal to make food a central topic in public discourse; (2) The collections of essays in *Edible Ideologies* (2008), edited by Kathleen LeBesco and Peter Maccardo, and in *Food as Communication: Communication as Food* (2011), edited by Janet Cramer, Carlnita Greene, and Lynn Walters, have helped to delineate a communication perspective on food studies; (3) Oppositional rhetoric, that might criticize a discursive approach to food studies, has helped to keep the discussion interesting and honest. In this regard, we mention *Agrarian Dreams: The Paradox of Organic Farming in California* (2004), by Julie Guthman.

What follows in this volume are fifteen diverse essays that take various rhetorical approaches to analyzing *The Rhetoric of Food*. The reader will note both the breadth of subjects and the breadth of rhetorical topics in these essays, such as co-optation, framing, green-washing, homologies, justice, neoliberal individualism, propaganda, protest rhetoric, the public screen, resignification, structuralism, tropes, and visual rhetoric. The chapters included in this collection engage salient contemporary issues from novel and eclectic theoretical frameworks. The authors, too, are diverse—women, men, well-known, less well-known, national, international, more traditional, more radical. As editors, it is our hope that *The Rhetoric of Food* will be readable and stimulating. We hope that this book will play a part in the important, ongoing conversations about rhetoric and food and re-frame or extend readers' understanding of the role of rhetoric in mediating our perceptions of why discourse, materiality, and power are interwoven as well as the prospect for imagining reconstituted relations with the earth, each other, culture, power, and ourselves—through food. In short, we trust that these essays offer cogent critiques and suggest alternatives.

This volume of collected essays begins, appropriately, with "The Operations of Nature," by Sir Albert Howard, published originally in 1947 as Chapter 2 in Howard's book *The Soil and Health: A Study of Organic Agriculture*. The soil is an appropriate starting point, because the soil is the basis of agriculture, agriculture provides much of our food, and food is necessary for life. Furthermore, Howard was one of the early leaders in the alternative agriculture social movement in the processes of frame adoption and diffusion in Western civilization. Howard's perspective on the soil is an appropriate starting point for the current volume, because Howard captures the connections and tensions between soil-as-living-matter and bio-chemical processes, on the one hand, and the rhetorical, mythological, and ideological dimensions of "the living soil," on the other hand. The advocacy in Howard's ode to the soil is obvious when he promotes organic agriculture. What may be less obvious is how discourse, materiality, and power are woven through his text, "The Operations of Nature."

"Visual rhetoric" is one of the most dynamic areas of inquiry in contemporary rhetorical criticism. Jean Retzinger's chapter is grounded in the work of Kevin DeLuca (*Image Politics*) and DeLuca and Jennifer Peeples (the "Public Screen"). Retzinger analyzes representations of the hungry body and the obese body, through a careful study of websites for hunger and relief organizations, including over six hundred photographs. Using both content and semiotic analysis, and touching on issues such as "the gaze" and audience emotional response, Retzinger provides considerable insight into food politics today. Moving beyond insight and critique, Retzinger also offers alternatives. She suggests that images of empowerment and food production might be more useful in addressing the issues of hunger and obesity.

The central question in the chapter by Laura K. Hahn and Michael S. Bruner is: Why has the vegetarian/vegan movement failed to achieve the same rhetorical traction in contemporary public discourse as the organic movement? At first, the authors seem to answer the question through social movement theory. Later in the chapter, it becomes clear that Hahn and Bruner are offering a rhetorical analysis, instead, of the symbolic dynamics of "co-optation," "sacrifice," "the Market," and "visual rhetoric" in mass media. Two of the chapter's case studies are particularly stimulating. In the Alar case study, Hahn and Bruner point out that "oppositional rhetoric"

is one of the key ingredients in the success of the organic movement. In the
case study of the PETA "Thanksgiving Prayer," Hahn and Bruner address
the issue of "animal rights," and touch on how veganism's "do no harm"
credo goes beyond "dietary veganism."

John Thompson grounds his chapter, "'Food Talk': Bridging Power in
a Globalizing World," in rhetorical concepts developed by Kenneth Burke,
Roderick Hart, and Barry Brummett. For example, Thompson speaks of
"tropes" and "grammar" (Burke), "rhetorical homologies" (Brummett),
and an "inventory of meanings" (Hart), in advancing his argument that
"food talk" today is evolving to take on the same proportions and significance that "rights talk" held in the twentieth century. Thompson's work is
relevant to contemporary rhetorical studies, because he links "food talk"
to negotiating power in a globalized world. The nation-state, according
to Thompson, no longer provides adequate rhetorical resources for the
twenty-first century. Former "citizens" now seek a new grammar in "food
talk" and fresh meanings/identity in "eating."

Alison Henderson and Vanessa Johnson explore, document, and explain
the rhetoric of an international functional food manufacturing organization. As the intersections of medicine and food blur with the advent of new
technologies, what constitutes "healthy" and "nutritious" food is negotiated
among food producers, medical professionals, regulatory authorities, and
consumers. Through semi-structured interviews with research & development and marketing staff, as well as analysis of organizational documents
and marketing materials, Henderson and Johnson adeptly discuss how the
myriad tensions stemming from the need of food-producing organizations
to identify with diverse stakeholders result in rhetorical challenges and
questions as to who will control the future discourse of "healthy" food.

In his chapter, "Parsing Poverty," Maxwell Schnurer addresses broader
issues of justice and power through an analysis of advocacy for food subsidies. Focusing his attention on the American Farmland Trust, Schnurer
demonstrates how the positive emotional resonance of "the family farm,"
for example, can be turned rhetorically into support for something alto-
gether different. This form of advocacy, which Schnurer calls "propaganda," has some of the same characteristics as covert forms of persuasion
known as "green-washing" or "astro-turfing." The main point is that discourse may lead to dire material consequences around the globe.

The ritual of the "presidential pardon of the Thanksgiving turkey"
hardly seems like serious news in the US. Nevertheless, co-authors Carrie
Packwood Freeman and Oana Leventi-Perez see in the satirical pardon "an
antagonism," one that represents an opening between the vegan advocacy
of animal rights rhetoric and the advertising rhetoric of the meat industry.
In their analysis of news stories over a period of twenty years about the pardon, Packwood Freeman and Leventi-Perez shine a rhetorical searchlight on
the use of the comic frame. Their analysis includes a discussion of ethics in
journalism and an exploration of alternatives, such as free-range farming.

The 2008 documentary film *The Garden* (directed by Scott Hamilton Kennedy) portrays how a large community garden grew out of the ashes of the riots in Los Angeles. In her chapter, Natasha Seegert describes and analyzes another urban garden, "The People's Portable Garden," in Salt Lake City. Both the film and the essay address: (a) space and the possible and (b) the transformation of urban landscapes. But Seegert's analysis is rhetorical, through and through, when she discusses resignification.

Suicide as a form of protest rhetoric in a social movement (social movement self-sacrifice) is Joshua Frye's topic in Chapter 9. Frye takes a close look at the rhetorical aspects of the suicide of Lee Kyung-Hae, a South Korean farmer-leader, who killed himself outside the September 2003 meeting of the World Trade Organization Ministerial. According to Frye, "Viewing the phenomenon of taking one's own life from a rhetorical vantage has a somewhat different frame than the social scientific and establishment media perspectives. Social movement self-sacrifice is a bodily performance and a rhetoric of resistance." What links Lee Kyung-Hae's sacrifice to the present volume is the link between his death and the global food system.

Michelle Obama has a significant presence in popular media and in contemporary public discourse. For example, numerous magazines have featured Michelle Obama in a cover photo, including *Ebony*, *Essence*, *Ladies Home Journal*, *People*, and *Time*. It is especially noteworthy that *Children's Health* magazine and *Prevention* magazine linked the First Lady to health and nutrition issues. In her analysis of Michelle Obama's health rhetoric, Abigail Seiler draws upon Michel Foucault and Pierre Bourdieu to make the distinction between approaches to obesity based on individualism and approaches based on systemic changes. Seiler concludes that Michelle Obama occasionally addresses systemic issues and the need for structural change, but often relies upon the vocabulary and concepts of neoliberal individualism.

Justin Eckstein and Donovan Conley argue that Denver's Cherry Creek Farmers Market (CCFM) is a space where semiotics and somatics fuse into a novel rhetorical form in which private pleasure and public morality meet. Eckstein and Conley focus on the under-attended material aspects (smell, sound, taste) of a humanly constructed symbolic space to eloquently articulate how the affective dimensions of a community farmers' market enable a relational training forum for potentially new political values, such as community.

With 50 percent of its adult citizens classified as "obese," Huntington, West Virginia (and surrounding area) was declared, in 2006, to be the most unhealthy city in the US. Chef Jamie Oliver noticed this problem and made Huntington a project for his reality TV show, *Food Revolution*. Oliver adopted school food as the primary focus of the intervention to address obesity. He quickly discovered that one of the major barriers to change was the US Department of Agriculture's program that provided low-cost food to schools. In his chapter on Oliver versus unhealthy school food, Garrett Broad analyzes the rhetorical and material tensions situated in systemic problems. As his analysis indicates, to move toward healthy food and healthy eating in our schools, we must challenge the status quo at the individual, family, community, and national levels.

"Cannibalism" is not a typical topic in the literature on the rhetoric of food, but in his chapter, "Eating the Other," Alexander V. Kozin makes a case for examining cannibalism as a complex social phenomenon. As an international author, grounded in Freud and Husserl, Kozin makes his analysis accessible to a wide audience through the case studies drawn from popular literature: *Robinson Crusoe* by Daniel Defoe and the *Hannibal* trilogy by Thomas Harris.

Food is not a problem! That insight is one clear message from those who would point us toward a more healthy relationship with food. In May of 2010, Oprah Winfrey introduced her newest guru, an author by the name of Geneen Roth, who is attempting to raise the nation's collective consciousness about eating more slowly, more responsibly, more conscientiously, and more intuitively. In addressing the topic of a healthier relationship with food, Kara Shultz grounds her chapter in Heidegger's concept of mindfulness. It is a testament to the sweeping purview and relevance of rhetoric that Shultz can move from Heidegger to Oprah to four books that urge readers to develop a more authentic relationship with food.

Mohan J. Dutta ruptures the hegemonic meta-narrative of the neoliberal monologue by co-constructing alternative narratives from voices at the margins of poverty in the global south. Specifically, Mohan Dutta explicates the complex structural strands of the neoliberal economic order and exposes the faulty assumptions and false promises that institutions such as the World Bank, International Monetary Fund, and the World Trade Organization impose on rural communities and individuals in Northern India through trade-related intellectual property rights policies and structural adjustment programs. Dutta empowers subaltern and marginalized West Bengali residents through participatory fieldwork aimed at resisting the veneer of economic progress in India and co-constructing an alternative narrative: a narrative of piracy, deception, exploitation, and hunger.

NOTES

1. Karen Barad, "Posthumanist Performativity: Toward an Understanding of How Matter Comes to Matter," *Signs: Journal of Women in Culture and Society* 28 (2003): 822.
2. Kenneth Burke, *A Rhetoric of Motives* (Berkeley: University of California Press, 1969), 41.
3. Aristotle, *The Art of Rhetoric*, trans. Hugh Lawson-Tancred (New York, NY: Penguin Books, 1991), 73.

1   The Operations of Nature

Sir Albert Howard

The introduction to this book describes an adventure in agricultural research and records the conclusions reached. If the somewhat unorthodox views set out are sound, they will not stand alone but will be supported and confirmed in a number of directions—by the farming experience of the past and above all by the way Nature, the supreme farmer, manages her kingdom. In this chapter the manner in which she conducts her various agricultural operations will be briefly reviewed. In surveying the significant characteristics of the life—vegetable and animal—met with in Nature particular attention will be paid to the importance of fertility in the soil and to the occurrence and elimination of disease in plants and animals.

What is the character of life on this planet? What are its great qualities? The answer is simple: The outstanding characteristics of Nature are variety and stability.

The variety of the natural life around us is such as to strike even the child's imagination, who sees in the fields and copses near his home, in the ponds and streams and seaside pools around which he plays, or, if being city-born he be deprived of these delightful playgrounds, even in his poor back-garden or in the neighbouring park, an infinite choice of different flowers and plants and trees, coupled with an animal world full of rich changes and surprises, in fact, a plenitude of the forms of living things constituting the first and probably the most powerful introduction he will ever receive into the nature of the universe of which he is himself a part.

The infinite variety of forms visible to the naked eye is carried much farther by the microscope. When, for example, the green slime in stagnant water is examined, a new world is disclosed—a multitude of simple flowerless plants—the blue-green and the green algae—always accompanied by the lower forms of animal life. We shall see in a later chapter that on the operations of these green algae the well-being of the rice crop, which

Editors' note: When Albert Howard refers to "introduction," "volume," and "chapter," he is referring to his book, *The Soil and Health*, in which "The Operations of Nature" originally appeared.

nourishes countless millions of the human race, depends. If a fragment of mouldy bread is suitably magnified, members of still another group of flowerless plants, made up of fine, transparent threads entirely devoid of green colouring matter, come into view. These belong to the fungi, a large section of the vegetable kingdom, which are of supreme importance in farming and gardening.

It needs a more refined perception to recognize throughout this stupendous wealth of varying shapes and forms the principle of stability. Yet this principle dominates. It dominates by means of an ever-recurring cycle, a cycle which, repeating itself silently and ceaselessly, ensures the continuation of living matter. This cycle is constituted of the successive and repeated processes of birth, growth, maturity, death, and decay.

An eastern religion calls this cycle the Wheel of Life and no better name could be given to it. The revolutions of this Wheel never falter and are perfect. Death supersedes life and life rises again from what is dead and decayed.

Because we are ourselves alive we are much more conscious of the processes of growth than we are of the processes involved in death and decay. This is perfectly natural and justifiable. Indeed, it is a very powerful instinct in us and a healthy one. Yet, if we are fully grown human beings, our education should have developed in our minds so much of knowledge and reflection as to enable us to grasp intelligently the vast role played in the universe by the processes making up the other or more hidden half of the Wheel. In this respect, however, our general education in the past has been gravely defective partly because science itself has so sadly misled us. Those branches of knowledge dealing with the vegetable and animal kingdoms—botany and zoology—have confined themselves almost entirely to a study of *living* things and have given little or no attention to what happens to these units of the universe when they die and to the way in which their waste products and remains affect the general environment on which both the plant and animal world depend. When science itself is unbalanced, how can we blame education for omitting in her teaching one of the things that really matter?

For though the phases which are preparatory to life are, as a rule, less obvious than the phases associated with the moment of birth and the periods of growth, they are not less important. If once we can grasp this and think in terms of ever-repeated advance and recession, recession and advance, we have a truer view of the universe than if we define death merely as an ending of what has been alive.

Nature herself is never satisfied except by an even balancing of her processes—growth and decay. It is precisely this even balancing which gives her unchallengeable stability. That stability is rock-like. Indeed, this figure of speech is a poor one, for the stability of Nature is far more permanent than anything we can call a rock—rocks being creations which themselves are subject to the great stream of dissolution and rebirth, seeing that they suffer from weathering and are formed again, that they can be changed into other substances and caught up in the grand process of living: they too, as we shall see, are part of the Wheel of Life. However, we may at a first glance omit the changes which affect the inert masses of this planet, petrological and mineralogical: though very soon we shall realize how intimate is the connection even between these and what is, in the common parlance, alive. There is a direct bridge between things inorganic and things organic and this too is part of the Wheel.

But before we start on our examination of that part of the great process which now concerns us—namely, plant and animal life and the use man makes of them—there is one further idea which we must master. It is this: The stability of Nature is secured not only by means of a very even balancing of her Wheel, by a perfect timing, so to say, of her mechanisms, but also rests on a basis of enormous reserves. Nature is never a hand-to-mouth practitioner. She is often called lavish and wasteful, and at first sight one can be bewildered and astonished at the apparent waste and extravagance which accompany the carrying on of vegetable and animal existence. Yet a more exact examination shows her working with an assured background of accumulated reserves, which are stupendous and also essential. The least depletion in these reserves induces vast changes and not until she has built them up again does she resume the particular process on which she was engaged. A realization of this principle of reserves is thus a further necessary item in a wide view of natural law. Anyone who has recovered from a serious illness, during which the human body lives partly on its own reserves, will realize how Nature afterwards deals with such situations. During the period of convalescence the patient appears to make little progress till suddenly he resumes his old-time activities. During this waiting period the reserves used up during illness are being replenished.

THE LIFE OF THE PLANT

A survey of the Wheel of Nature will best start from that rather rapid series of processes which cause what we commonly call living matter to come into active existence; that is, in fact, from the point where life most obviously, to our eyes, begins. The section of the Wheel embracing these processes is studied in physiology from the Greek word φύσις , the root Φύω meaning to bring to life, to grow.

But how does life begin on this planet? We can only say this: that the prime agency in carrying it on is sunlight, because it is the source of energy, and that the instrument for intercepting this energy and turning it to account is the green leaf.

This wonderful little example of Nature's invention is a battery of intricate mechanisms. Each cell in the interior of a green leaf contains minute specks of a substance called chlorophyll and it is this chlorophyll which enables the plant to grow. Growth implies a continuous supply of

nourishment. Now plants do not merely collect their food: they manufacture it before they can feed. In this they differ from animals and man,
who search for what they can pass through their stomachs and alimentary
systems, but cannot do more; if they are unable to find what is suitable to
their natures and ready for them, they perish. A plant is, in a way, a more
wonderful instrument. It is an actual food factory, making what it requires
before it begins the processes of feeding and digestion. The chlorophyll in
the green leaf, with its capacity for intercepting the energy of the sun, is
the power unit that, so to say, runs the machine. The green leaf enables the
plant to draw simple raw materials from diverse sources and to work them
up into complex combinations.

Thus from the air it absorbs carbon-dioxide (a compound of two parts
of oxygen to one of carbon), which is combined with more oxygen from the
atmosphere and with other substances, both living and inert, drawn from
the soil and from the water which permeates the soil. All these raw materials
are then assimilated in the plant and made into food. They become organic
compounds, i.e. compounds of carbon, classified conveniently into groups
known as carbohydrates, proteins, and fats; together with an enormous volume of water (often over 90 per cent of the whole plant) and interspersed
with small quantities of chemical salts which have not yet been converted
into the organic phase, they make up the whole structure of the plant—root,
stem, leaf, flower, and seed. This structure includes a big food reserve. The
life principle, the nature of which evades us and in all probability always
will, resides in the proteins looked at in the mass. These proteins carry on
their work in a cellulose framework made up of cells protected by an outer
integument and supported by a set of structures known as the vascular bun-
dles, which also conduct the sap from the roots to the leaves and distribute
the food manufactured there to the various centres of growth. The whole of
the plant structures are kept turgid by means of water.

The green leaf, with its chlorophyll battery, is therefore a perfectly
adapted agency for continuing life. It is, speaking plainly, the only agency
that can do this and is unique. Its efficiency is of supreme importance.
Because animals, including man, feed eventually on green vegetation, either
directly or through the bodies of other animals, it is our sole final source of
nutriment. There is no alternative supply. Without sunlight and the capacity of the earth's green carpet to intercept its energy for us, our industries,
our trade, and our possessions would soon be useless. It follows therefore
that everything on this planet must depend on the way mankind makes use
of this green carpet, in other words on its efficiency.

The green leaf does not, however, work by itself. It is only a part of the
plant. It is curious how easy it is to forget that normally we see only one-
half of each flowering plant, shrub, or tree: the rest is buried in the ground.
Yet the dying down of the visible growth of many plants in the winter,
their quick reappearance in the spring, should teach us how essential and
important a portion of all vegetation lives out of our sight; it is evident

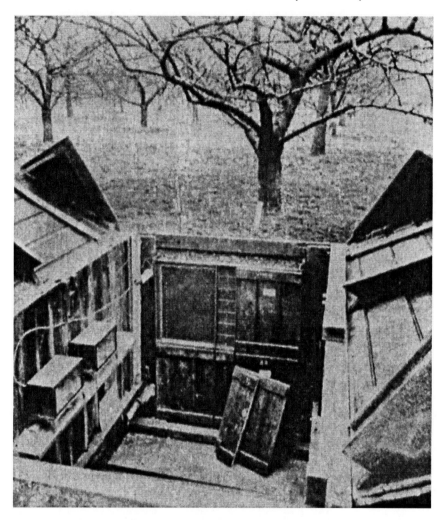

Figure 1.1 Observation chamber for root studies at East Malling.

that the root system, buried in the ground, also holds the life of the plant in its grasp. It is therefore not surprising to find that leaves and roots work together, forming a partnership which must be put into fresh working order each season if the plant is to live and grow.

If the function of the green leaf armed with its chlorophyll is to manufacture the food the plant needs, the purpose of the roots is to obtain the water and most of the raw materials required—the sap of the plant being the medium by which these raw materials (collected from the soil by the roots) are moved to the leaf. The work of the leaf we found to be intricate:

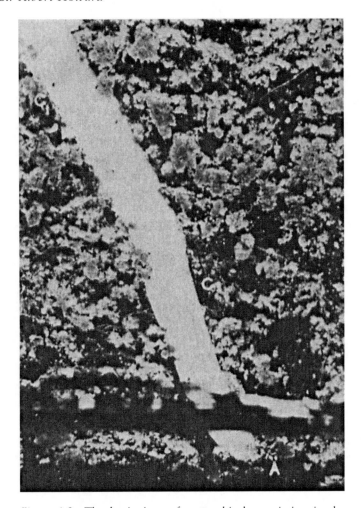

Figure 1.2 The beginnings of mycorrhizal association in the apple. Root-tip (x 12) of *Lane's Prince Albert* on root-stock M XVI at sixteen inches below the surface, showing root-cap (A), young root hairs (C), and older root hairs with drops of exudate (C₁). The cobweb-like mycelial strands are well seen approaching the rootlet in the region marked (C).

that of the roots is not less so. What is surprising is to come upon two quite distinct ways in which the roots set about collecting the materials which it is their business to supply to the leaf; these two methods are carried on simultaneously. We can make a very shrewd guess at the master principle which has put the second method along-side the first: it is again the principle of providing a reserve—this time of the vital proteins.

None of the materials that reach the green leaf by whatever method is food: it is only the raw stuff from which food can be manufactured. By the first method, which is the most obvious one, the root hairs search out and pass into the transpiration current of the plant dissolved substances which they find in the thin films of water spread between and around each particle of earth; this film is known as the soil solution. The substances dissolved in it include gases (mainly carbon dioxide and oxygen) and a series of other substances known as chemical salts like nitrates, compounds of potassium and phosphorus, and so forth, all obtained by the breaking down of organic matter or from the destruction of the mineral portions of the soil. In this breaking down of organic matter we see in operation the reverse of the building-up process which takes place in the leaf. Organic matter is continuously reverting to the inorganic state: it becomes mineralized: nitrates are one form of the outcome. It is the business of the root hairs to absorb these substances from the soil solution and to pass them into the sap, so that the new life-building process can start up again. In a soil in good heart the soil solution will be well supplied with these salts. Incidentally, we may note that it has been the proved existence of these mineral chemical constituents in the soil which, since the time of Liebig, has focused attention on soil chemistry and has emphasized the passage of chemical food materials from soil to plant to the neglect of other considerations.

But the earth's green carpet is not confined to its remarkable power of transforming the inert nitrates and mineral contents of the soil into an active organic phase: it is utilized by Nature to establish for itself, in addition, a direct connection, a kind of living bridge, between its own life and the living portion of the soil. This is the second method by which plants feed themselves. The importance of this process, physiological in nature and not merely chemical, cannot be over-emphasized and some description of it will now be attempted.

THE LIVING SOIL

The soil is, as a matter of fact, full of live organisms. It is essential to conceive of it as something pulsating with life, not as a dead or inert mass. There could be no greater misconception than to regard the earth as dead: a handful of soil is teeming with life. The living fungi, bacteria, and protozoa, invisibly present in the soil complex, are known as the soil population. This population of millions and millions of minute existences, quite invisible to our eyes of course, pursue their own lives. They come into being, grow, work, and die: they sometimes fight each other, win victories, or perish; for they are divided into groups and families fitted to exist under all sorts of conditions. The state of a soil will change with the victories won or the losses sustained; and in one or other soil, or at one or other moment, different groups will predominate.

This lively and exciting life of the soil is the first thing that sets in motion the great Wheel of Life. Not without truth have poets and priests paid worship to "Mother Earth," the source of our being. What poetry or religion have vaguely celebrated, science has minutely examined, and very complete descriptions now exist of the character and nature of the soil population, the various species of which have been classified, labelled, and carefully observed. It is this life which is continually being passed into the plant.

The process can actually be followed under the microscope. Some of the individuals belonging to one of the most important groups in this mixed population—the soil fungi—can be seen functioning. If we arrange a vertical darkened glass window on the side of a deep pit in an orchard, it is not difficult to see with the help of a good lens or a low-power horizontal microscope (arranged to travel up and down a vertical fixed rod) some of these soil fungi at work. They are visible in the interstices of the soil as glistening white branching threads, reminiscent of cobwebs. In Dr. Rogers's interesting experiments on the root systems of fruit trees at East Malling Research Station, where this method of observing them was initiated and demonstrated to me, these fungous threads could be seen approaching the young apple roots in the absorbing region (just behind the advancing root tips) on which the root hairs are to be found. Dr. Rogers very kindly presented me with two excellent photographs—one showing the general arrangement of his observation chamber (Plate I), the other, taken on 6th July 1933, of a root tip (magnified by about twelve) of *Lane's Prince Albert* (grafted on root stock XVI) at sixteen inches below the surface, showing abundant fungous strands running in the soil and coming into direct contact with the growing root (Plate II).

But this is only the beginning of the story. When a suitable section of one of these young apple roots, growing in fertile soil and bearing active root hairs, is examined, it will be found that these fine fungous threads actually invade the cells of the root, where they can easily be observed passing from one cell to another. But they do not remain there very long. After a time the apple roots absorb these threads. All stages of the actual digestion can be seen.

The significance of this process needs no argument. Here we have a simple arrangement on the part of Nature by which the soil material on which these fungi feed can be joined up, as it were, with the sap of the tree. These fungous threads are very rich in protein and may contain as much as 10 per cent of organic nitrogen; this protein is easily digested by the ferments (enzymes) in the cells of the root; the resulting nitrogen complexes, which are readily soluble, are then passed into the sap current and so into the green leaf. An easy passage, as it were, has been provided for food material to move from soil to plant in the form of proteins and their digestion products, which latter in due course reach the green leaf. The marriage of a fertile soil and the tree it nourishes is thus arranged. Science calls these fungous threads *mycelium* (again from a Greek word, μύκης), and as the

Greek for root is ρίζα *(rhiza,* cf. rhizome), the whole process is known as the *mycorrhizal association*.[1] This partnership is universal in the forest and is general throughout the vegetable kingdom. A few exceptions, however, exist which will be referred to in the next paragraph.

Among the plants in which this mycorrhizal association has hitherto not been observed are the tomato and certain cultivated members of the cabbage family, many of which possess a very diffuse root system and exceptionally elongated root hairs. Nevertheless, all these examples respond very markedly to the condition of the soil in which they are grown and if fed with dressings of humus will prosper. The question naturally arises: Exactly how does this take place? What is the alternative mechanism that replaces the absent mycorrhizal association?A simple explanation would appear to be this. Fertile soils invariably contain a greatly enhanced bacterial population whose dead remains must be profusely scattered in the water films which bathe the compound soil particles and the root hairs of the crops themselves; these specks of dead organic matter, rich in protein, are finally mineralized into simple salts like nitrates. We have already mentioned this breaking-down process of the soil population. What is here to be noted is that it is no sudden transformation, but takes place in stages. May not, therefore, some at least of the first-formed nitrogen complexes, which result from this breaking down, be absorbed by the root hairs and so added to the sap current? That is to say that the non-mycorrhiza-forming plants, not drawing on the soil fungi, do compensate themselves by absorbing organic nitrogen in this form—they catch the bacterial soil population, as it were, before it has been reduced to an entirely inert phase and so have their link also with the biological life of the soil. That there must be some such passage of matter on a biological basis is suggested by the fact that only in fertile soil, i.e. in soils teeming with bacteria, do these non-mycorrhiza formers reveal resistance to disease and high quality in the produce, which means that only in these soils are they really properly fed.

This would be a third method used by plants for feeding themselves, a sort of half-way method between the absorption powers exercised by the root hairs and the direct digestive capacity of the roots: as the mechanism used in this method is presumably the root hairs, the diffuseness of the root system of plants of the cabbage family would be explained. It is possible that even mycorrhiza formers use this alternative passage for organic nitrogen. There seems no reason at all why this should not be so.

But how do the various agencies concerned in these intricate operations manage to carry on their work, buried as they are away from the light and thus unable to derive anything from the source of energy, the sun? How do they do their initial work at all until they can hand over to the green leaf? They derive their energy by oxidising (i.e. burning up) the stores of organic matter in the soil. As in an ordinary fire, this process of oxidation releases energy. The oxygen needed for this slow combustion is drawn from the air, in part washed down by the rain, which dissolves it from the atmosphere in its descent. Incidentally this explains why rain is so superior as a moistening agency for plants to any form of watering from a can: incidentally, again, we can understand the need for cultivating the soil and keeping it open, so that the drawing in of oxygen, or the respiration of the soil, can proceed and the excess carbon dioxide can be expelled into the atmosphere.

Humus is the Latin word for soil or earth. But as used by the husbandman humus nowadays does not mean just earth in general, but indicates that undecayed residue of vegetable and animal waste lying on the surface, combined with the dead bodies of these bacteria and fungi themselves when they have done their work, the whole being a highly complex and somewhat varying substance which is, so to say, the mine or store or bank from which the organisms of the soil and then, in direct succession, the plant, the tree, and thereafter the animal, draw what they need for their existence. This store is all important.

The Significance of Humus

Humus is the most significant of all Nature's reserves and as such deserves a detailed examination.

A very perfect example of the methods by which Nature makes humus and thus initiates the turning of her Wheel is afforded by the floor of the forest. Dig down idly with a stick under any forest tree: first there will be a rich, loose accumulation of litter made up of dead leaves, flowers, twigs, fragments of bark, bits of decaying wood, and so forth, passing gradually as the material becomes more tightly packed into rich, moist, sweet-smelling earth, which continues downwards for some inches and which, when disturbed, reveals many forms of tiny insect and animal life. We have been given here a glimpse of the way Nature makes humus—the source from which the trunk of the tree has drawn its resisting strength, its leaves their glittering beauty.

Throughout the year, endlessly and continuously, though faster at some seasons than at others, the wastes of the forest thus accumulate and at once undergo transformation. These wastes are of many kinds and mix as they fall; for leaf mingles with twig and stem, flower with moss, and bark with seed-coats. Moreover, vegetable mingles with animal. Let us beware of the false idea that the forest is a part of the vegetable kingdom only. Millions of animal existences are housed in it; mammals and birds are everywhere and can be seen with the naked eye. The lower forms of animal life—the invertebrates—are even more numerous. Insects, earthworms, and so forth are obvious: the microscope reveals new worlds of animal life down to simple protozoa. The excreta of these animals while living and their dead bodies constitute an important component of what lies on the forest floor; even the bodies of insects form in the mass a constituent element not without importance, so that in the end the two sources of waste are completely represented and are, above all, completely mingled. But the volume of the vegetable wastes is several times greater than that of the animal residues.

These wastes lie gently, only disturbed by wind or by the foot of a passing animal. The top layer is thus very loose; ample air circulates for several inches downwards: the conditions for the fermentation by the moulds and microbes (which feed on the litter) are, as the scientist would say, *aerobic*. But partly by pressure from above and partly as the result of fermentation the lower layers are forced to pack more closely and the final manufacture of humus goes on without much air: the conditions are now *anaerobic*. This is a succession of two modes of manufacture which we shall do well to remember, as in our practical work it has to be imitated.

This mass of accumulated wastes is acted on by the sunlight and the rain; both are dispersed and fragmented by the leaf canopy of the trees, and undergrowth. The sunlight warms the litter; the rain keeps it moist. The rain does not reach the litter as a driving sheet, but is split up into, small drops the impetus of whose fall is well broken. Nor does the sunlight burn without shade; it is tempered. Finally, though air circulates freely, there is perfect protection from the cooling and drying effects of strong wind.

With abundant air, warmth, and water at their disposal the fungi and bacteria, with which, as we have already noted, the soil is teeming, do their work. The fallen mixed wastes are broken up; some passes through the bodies of earthworms and insects: all is imperceptibly crumbled and changed until it decomposes into that rich mass of dark colour and earthy smell which is so characteristic of the forest floor and which holds such a wealth of potential plant nourishment.

The process that takes place in a prairie, a meadow, or a steppe is similar; perhaps slower, and the richness of the layer of humus will depend on a good many factors. One, in particular, has an obvious effect, namely, the supply of air. If, for some reason, this is cut off, the formation of humus is greatly impeded. Areas, therefore, that are partly or completely waterlogged will not form humus as the forest does: the upper portion of the soil will not have access to sufficient free oxygen, nor will there be much oxygen in the standing water. In the first case a moor will result; in the second a bog or morass will be formed. In both these the conditions are anaerobic: the organisms derive their oxygen not from the air but from the vegetable and animal residues including the proteins. In this fermentation nitrogen is always lost and the resulting low-quality humus is known as peat.

But the forest, the prairie, the moor, and the bog are not the only areas where humus formation is in progress. It is constantly going on in the most unlikely places—on exposed rock surfaces, on old walls, on the trunks and branches of trees, and indeed wherever the lower forms of plant life—algae, lichens, mosses, and liverworts—can live and then slowly build up a small store of humus.

Nature, in fact, conforming to that principle of reserves, does not attempt to create the higher forms of plant life until she has secured a good store of humus. Watch how the small bits of decayed vegetation fall into some crack in the rock and decompose: here is the little fern, the tiny flower, secure of its supply of food and well able to look after itself, as it thrusts its roots down into the rich pocket of nourishment. Nature adapts her flora very carefully to her varying supplies of humus. The plant above is the indicator of what the soil below is like, and a trained observer, sweeping his eye over the countryside, will be able to read it like the pages of a book and to tell without troubling to cross a valley exactly where the ground is waterlogged, where it is accumulating humus, where it is being eroded. He looks at the kind and type of plant, and infers from their species and condition the nature of the soil which they at once cover and reveal.

But we are not at the end of the mechanisms employed by Nature to get her great Wheel to revolve with smooth efficiency. The humus that lies on the surface must be distributed and made accessible to the roots of plants and especially to the absorbing portions of the roots and their tiny prolongations known as root hairs—for it is these which do the delicate work of absorption. How can this be done? Nature has, perforce, laid her accumulation on the surface of the soil. But she has no fork or spade: she cannot dig a trench and lay the food materials at the bottom where the plant root can strike down and get them. It seems an impasse, but the solution is again curiously simple and complete. Nature has her own labour force—ants, termites, and above all earthworms. These carry the humus down to the required deeper levels where the thrusting roots can have access to it. This distribution process goes on continually, varying in intensity with night and day, with wetness or dryness, heat or cold, which alternately brings the worms to the surface for fresh supplies or sends them down many feet. It is interesting to note how a little heap of leaves in the garden disappears in the course of a night or two when the earthworms are actively at work. The mechanism of humus distribution is a give and take, for where a root has died the earthworm or the termite will often follow the minute channel thus created a long way.

Actually the earthworm eats of the humus and of the soil and passes them through its body, leaving behind the casts which are really enriched earth—perfectly conditioned for the use of plants. Analyses of these casts show that they are some 40 per cent richer in humus than the surface soil, but very much richer in such essential food materials as combined nitrogen, phosphate, and potash. Recent results obtained by Lunt and Jacobson of the Connecticut Experiment Station show that the casts of earthworms are five times richer in combined nitrogen, seven times richer in available phosphate, and eleven times richer in potash than the upper six inches of soil.

It is estimated that on each acre of fertile land no less than twenty-five tons of fresh worm casts are deposited each year. Besides this the dead bodies of the earthworms must make an appreciable contribution to the supply of manure. In these ways Nature in her farming has arranged that the earth itself shall be her manure factory.

As the humus is continually being created, so it is continually being used up. Not more than a certain depth accumulates on the surface, normally anything from a few inches to two or three feet. For after a time the process ceases to be additive and becomes simply continuous: the growing plants use up the product at a rate equaling the rate of manufacture—the even turning of the Wheel of Life—the perfect example of balanced manuring. A reserve, however, is at all times present, and on virgin and undisturbed land it may be very great indeed. This is an important asset in man's husbandry; we shall later see how important.

The Importance of Minerals

Is the humus the only source from which the plant draws its nourishment? That is not so. The subsoil, i.e. that part of the soil derived from the decay of rocks, which lies below the layer of humus, also has its part to play. The subsoil is, as it were, a depository of raw material. It may be of many types, clay, sand, etc.; the geological formation will vary widely. It always includes a mineral content—potash, phosphates, and many rarer elements.

Now these minerals play an important part in the life of living things. They have to be conveyed to us in our food in an organic form, and it is from the plant, which transforms them into an organic phase and holds them thus, that we and the other animals derive them for our well-being.

How does the plant obtain them? We have seen that there is a power in the roots of all plants, even the tiniest, of absorbing them from the soil solution. But how is the soil solution itself impregnated with these substances? Mainly through the dissolving power of the soil water, which contains carbon dioxide in solution and so acts as a weak solvent. It would appear that the roots of trees, which thrust down into the subsoil, draw on the dissolved mineral wealth there stored and absorb this wealth into their structure. In tapping the lower levels of water present in the subsoil—for trees are like great pumps drawing at a deep well—they also tap the minerals dissolved therein. These minerals are then passed into all parts of the tree, including the foliage. When in the autumn the foliage decays and falls, the stored minerals, now in an organic phase, are dropped too and become available on the top layers of the soil: they become incorporated in the humus. This explains the importance of the leaf-fall in preserving the land in good heart and incidentally is one reason why gardeners love to accumulate leaf-mould. By this means they feed their vegetables, fruit, and flowers with the minerals they need.

The tree has acted as a great circulatory system, and its importance in this direction is to be stressed. The destruction of trees and forests is therefore most injurious to the land, for not only are the physical effects harmful—the anchoring roots and the sheltering leaf canopy being alike removed—but the necessary circulation of minerals is put out of action. It is at least possible that the present mineral poverty of certain tracts of the earth's surface, e.g. on the South African veldt, is due to the destruction over wide areas and for long periods of all forest growth, both by the wasteful practices of indigenous tribes and latterly sometimes by exploiting Western interests.

SUMMARY

Before we turn to consider the ways in which man has delved and dug into all these riches and disturbed them for his own benefit, let us sum up with one final glance at the operations of Nature. Perhaps one fact will strike us as symptomatic of what we have been reviewing, namely, the enormous care bestowed by Nature on the processes both of destruction and of storage. She is as minute and careful, as generous in her intentions, and as lavish in breaking down what she has created as she was originally in building it up. The subsoil is called upon for some of its water and minerals, the leaf has to decay and fall, the twig is snapped by the wind, the very stem of the tree must break, lie, and gradually be eaten away by minute vegetable or animal agents; these in turn die, their bodies are acted on by quite invisible fungi and bacteria; these also die, they are added to all the other wastes, and the earthworm or ant begins to carry this—accumulated reserve of all earthly decay away. This accumulated reserve—humus—is the very beginning of vegetable life and therefore of animal life and of our own being. Such care, such intricate arrangements are surely worth studying, as they are the basis of all Nature's farming and can be summed up in a phrase— the Law of Return.

We have thus seen that one of the outstanding features of Nature's farming is the care devoted to the manufacture of humus and to the building up of a reserve. What does she do to control such things as insect, fungous, and virus diseases in plants and the various afflictions of her animal kingdom? What provision is to be found for plant protection or for checking the diseases of animals? How is the work of mycologists, entomologists, and veterinarians done by Mother Earth? Is there any special method of dealing with diseased material such as destruction by fire? For many years I have diligently searched for some answer to these questions, or for some light on these matters. My quest has produced only negative evidence. There appears to be no special natural provision for controlling pests, for the destruction of diseased material, or for protecting plants and animals against infection. All manner of pests and diseases can be found here and there in any wood or forest; the disease-infected wastes find their way into the litter and are duly converted into humus. Methods designed for the protection of plants and animals against infection do not appear to have been provided. It would seem that the provision of humus is all that Nature needs to protect her vegetation; and, nourished by the food thus grown, in due course the animals look after themselves.

In their survey of world agriculture—past and present—the various schools of agricultural science might be expected to include these operations of Nature in their teaching. But when we examine the syllabuses of these schools, we find hardly any references to this subject and nothing whatever about the great Law of Return. The great principle underlying Nature's farming has been ignored. Nay more, it has been flouted and the cheapest method of transferring the reserves of humus (left by the prairie and the forest) to the profit and loss account of *homo sapiens* has been stressed instead. Surely there must be something wrong somewhere with our agricultural education.

NOTES

1. The reader who wishes to delve into the technical details relating to the mycorrhizal association and its bearing on forestry and agriculture should consult the following works:
    1. Rayner, M. C. and Neilson-Jones, W.—*Problems in Tree Nutrition*, Faber & Faber, London, 1944.
    2. Balfour, Lady Eve—*The Living Soil*, Faber & Faber, London, 1944.
    3. Howard, Sir Albert—*An Agricultural Testament*, Oxford University Press, London, 1940.
    4. Rodale, J. I.—*Pay Dirt*, The Devin-Adair Company, New York, 1945.

2 Empty Bellies/Empty Calories
Representing Hunger and Obesity

Jean Retzinger

Over the past decade, dietary choices and food politics (the production, regulation, and distribution of food) along with their health and environmental consequences have garnered considerable attention in both news and entertainment media while simultaneously finding further expression in the everyday practices of material culture. Buzzwords and calories abound. Locavores mingle with global fair trade advocates in cityscapes dotted with fast-food restaurants, farmers' markets, and upscale food boutiques. Food packaging displays an ever-increasing array of signs and signifiers with organic, fair-trade, and GMO-free certifications taking their place alongside calorie counts, nutrition facts, and health claims. Pro-ana images circulate in cyberspace alongside statistics on America's obesity epidemic, while the bodies of celebrities, supermodels, *Biggest Loser* contestants, and the "People of Walmart" all serve as spectacle for the viewing public. Amidst this surfeit of body image and food discourse, hunger, too, has begun to attract media attention. Marion Nestle has listed hunger as the most important food issue for the coming decade.[1]

In October 2009, the UN Food and Agriculture Organization released a report stating that a record one billion people, or about one-sixth of the world's population, suffer from hunger.[2] The global dimensions of the problem leave few, if any, nations unaffected—including the United States. Hundreds of organizations (NPOs and NGOs) have launched campaigns to feed the hungry, both locally and abroad, in response to natural disasters and environmental crises as well as the daily grind of poverty.

This chapter examines contemporary visual and verbal discourses of hunger found on websites and in other promotional materials for both domestic and international food relief organizations. Although I pay some attention to the causes of hunger and proposed solutions, my primary interest lies in how hunger is depicted (or given a "face") in contemporary campaigns—and, in the process, how the hungry body is represented and exposed. To further this analysis, I also examine other discourses and spectacles of the body, specifically the obese body. Images and other representations of both the hungry body and the obese body navigate a complex and contradictory terrain. Both bodies share the commonality of malnutrition and are subjected to the same surveilling and subordinating gaze, but each is framed differently, thus encouraging divergent judgments and responses: innocence or culpability, pity or condemnation.

LITERATURE REVIEW

Marita Sturken and Lisa Cartwright sound a familiar theme in their introduction to visual culture. In discussing "the gaze and the exotic," they note, "the photographic gaze thus helps to establish relationships of power. The person with the camera looks at a person, event, place, or object. The act of looking is commonly thought of as awarding more power to the person who is looking than to the person who is the object of the look."[3] Photographs thus function in varying degrees to "represent codes of dominance and subjugation, difference and otherness."[4]

In a chapter on the images of blacks in advertising, Jan Pieterse offers a similar argument specifically in relation to fund-raising campaigns for African relief aid. Such campaigns, he notes, often recycle stereotypes. "The appeal of children and victim imagery are clichés of the genre, a matrix exploited by organizations ranging from Oxfam to the Leprosy Foundation, and well-entrenched in popular media."[5] In discussing the selection of images most often employed, Pieterse writes that camera angles position viewers so that we are "literally looking down on people, which reinforces the impression of their passivity and, on the part of the viewer, the sensation of power and control."[6] "Fund-raising for famine relief in Africa," Pieterse asserts, "over and over again shows people starving, down to the flies in their eyes."[7] He offers a forceful argument as to the consequences of this imagery:

> The macabre reverse effect of this imagery is that while it shows 'the Third World' in a state of utter destitution, thus instilling a false sense of a gulf yawning between North and South, it nourishes the complacency and narcissism of the West. Rather than producing human solidarity this kind of imagery tends to foster estrangement.[8]

Pieterse's argument was echoed in the phrase "compassion fatigue," coined that same year (1992) in an article by Carla Joinson. Originally referencing secondary traumatic stress disorder experienced by nurses, the phrase quickly caught on to describe a more widespread apathy provoked by "over-exposure" to images of suffering in the media.[9]

In the interim, other scholars have also explored photographs of suffering. Arthur and Joan Kleinman examine the use of such images not for fund-raising but as emotional appeals exploited to gain market share among media audiences. They write, "This globalization of suffering is one of the more troubling signs of the cultural transformations of the current era: troubling because experience is being used as a commodity, and through this cultural representation of suffering, experience is being remade, thinned out, and distorted."[10] Kleinman and Kleinman devote considerable attention to a single image: Kevin Carter's photograph of a vulture perched near a tiny Sudanese child who has collapsed from hunger. The photograph was published in the *New York Times* in March 1993 and became, as the authors note, "an icon of starvation."[11] Kevin Carter committed suicide the following year, a few months after the *New York Times* won a Pulitzer Prize for publishing his work. The Kleinmans' analysis links the photograph to "an almost neocolonial ideology of failure, inadequacy, passivity, fatalism, and inevitability."[12] They continue:

> Suffering is presented as if it existed free of local people and local worlds. The child is alone. This, of course, is not the way that disasters, illnesses, and deaths are usually dealt with in African or other non-Western societies, or, for that matter, in the West. Yet, the image of famine is culturally represented in an ideologically Western mode: it becomes the experience of the lone individual.[13]

The ideological emphasis on the individual extends to our own viewing experience. We stare at the image in private on digital screens or in the pages of mass media publications that arrive at our door.

Susan Sontag's most recent investigation of photography examines images of pain and suffering, particularly in connection with war photography. "There are," she notes, "innumerable opportunities a modern life supplies for regarding—at a distance, through the medium of photography—other people's pain."[14] But photography, in Sontag's analysis, maintains rather than bridges that distance. Sontag argues, "Thus postcolonial Africa exists in the consciousness of the general public in the rich world—besides through its sexy music—mainly as a succession of unforgettable photographs of large-eyed victims, starting with figures in the famine lands of Biafra in the late 1960s."[15] These images simultaneously convey two different messages. "They show a suffering that is outrageous, unjust, and should be repaired. They confirm that this is the sort of thing which happens in that place"— and thus "nourish belief in the inevitability of tragedy in the benighted or backward—that is, poor—parts of the world."[16] Sympathy may be readily won through images of suffering, but to inspire action, images must first overcome a sense of futility, fostering instead a belief that change is possible.

A more recent examination of charity campaigns by John Hutnyk also links geo-politics and Western imperialism to images of poverty. In their effort to stimulate sympathy, images of children often serve as the primary form of currency for relief agencies. Unlike Pieterse, who focused on images displaying abject poverty and suffering, Hutnyk instead critiques "the myriad pictures of cute children—what I will call the archive of photogenic poverty,"[17] which feature smiling faces, happy countenances that "beam out at the beneficence of the aid workers and their undemocratic but morally righteous self-appointed 'humanitarian' interventions on behalf of us all."[18] For Hutnyk, the danger of such campaigns is that they promote infantilism—the infantilism of the viewer. Emotions rather than reason are enlisted. Viewers are encouraged to believe that by sending even a few coins lives will be improved—but these appeals leave unacknowledged the more complex social, political, and economic structures that remain in place and thus serve to perpetuate poverty and global inequities.

Thus images of the poor and hungry, whether they are shown suffering or smiling, seem to be denounced by scholars as destructive, exploitative, and imperialistic. One experimental study by Deborah Small and Nicole Verrochi put such distinctions to a test, devising a series of lab experiments in which subjects viewed sets of charity ads containing both happy and sad facial expressions.[19] Building on "recent consumer behavior research in domains outside charitable giving that emphasizes the crucial distinction between 'heart and mind' thought processes,"[20] the authors devised a series of experiments that tested levels of sympathy generated by the images alone and images paired with verbal descriptions of the child's plight. Among other findings, the study concludes that a "sad expression enhances sympathy and giving"[21] and the authors challenge charities to engage in a direct market test of images.

Pieterse's response to such research (offered actually seventeen years in advance of the study by Small and Verrochi) might be as follows:

> The images of Africa that are most effective and lucrative from the point of view of the fundraising organizations are not necessarily the right ones. The bureaucracy and the rhetoric of aid and relief stand in the way of solidarity and empowerment, or rather, channel them in a single direction and in the process promote a reverse empowerment, the empowerment of the West. The agency that comes off best in this kind of advertising is the relief agency itself—catering to Western stereotypes. And recycling the imagery of blind passivity.[22]

I quote Pieterse at length because in large measure his work served as the impetus for my own investigation. Although his critique emphasizes the need to examine images of hunger, it does not point to solutions. Hunger persists. The need to address it remains pressing.

This chapter examines ten top-rated hunger relief websites, five with an international focus and five with a domestic focus, attending to both their verbal and visual content.[23] Words anchor and give meaning to images;[24] together they help expose the extent and the causes of hunger and suggest solutions. In emphasizing the pictorial representation of hunger, my aim is not to simply add further denunciation of the imagery employed. If, as Kevin DeLuca and Jennifer Peeples argue, images broadcast across the public screen can serve activists, the photographic image should also be capable of offering new visions rather than simply recycling tired stereotypes and destructive attitudes.[25] But I begin with words and numbers.

REPRESENTING HUNGER: BY THE NUMBERS

The enormous growth of the World Wide Web in the past two decades has created new means of raising funds—along with awareness—of a myriad of social and political issues, including hunger. No longer restricted to the space of a single-page print advertisement or even a fund-raising letter, relief charities with a web presence have far more extensive tools at their disposal for capturing attention and encouraging contributions.

Each of the websites examined offers at least some statistical data on hunger, although such accounts vary both in terms of their prominence within the various websites as well as the specificity of the information given. On some sites detailed information can be found in the form of technical reports available as PDFs. For example, the Action Against Hunger website contains links to twenty-three such reports, allowing interested individuals to delve more deeply into some of the factors contributing to hunger across the globe.

On the international sites, both the numbers presented and the rhetorical strategies employed to describe the extent of hunger and malnutrition across the globe vary somewhat. At the low end of the scale, Food for the Hungry claims "an estimated 854 million people in the developing world currently do not consume enough calories to sustain healthy bodies."[26] In contrast, both the Freedom from Hunger and The Hunger Project websites claim hunger affected 1.02 billion people in the year 2009.[27] The Hunger Project website adds that although that number "has decreased to 925 million in 2010, the figures are still devastating."[28]

The sheer enormity of the problem—and its corresponding numerical descriptor—are likely to be abstract to many readers. Some sites attempt to make these figures more meaningful by breaking them down into smaller units, often by focusing on one particular demographic group: children. Another strategy entails sliding up and down a numerical scale to present the same information in multiple ways. Thus, the Food for the Hungry website asks:

> Did you know every day **25,000 people die** from hunger and hunger-related causes? Of those, 18,000 are children. One person dies of hunger every 3.6 seconds. That is more than 17 people each minute; 1,042 each hour; which translates into 9,125,000 every single year! One in six people on the planet is hungry.[29]

Although such numbers may be daunting (perhaps helping to explain their unobtrusive presence on some sites), the assurances that every contribution (or even prayer) will help alleviate hunger are far more visible.

The domestic websites describe the problem of hunger on national, state, and local levels. Links to the USDA's "Hunger in America Report 2010" were found on four food bank sites, offering an overview of the scope of the problem. Feeding America, the self-described "leading domestic hunger-relief charity" in the nation with a network of over two hundred food banks, claims that "each year, the Feeding America network provides food to more than 37 million low-income people facing hunger in the United States, including 14 million children and nearly 3 million seniors."[30] Elsewhere on the site, the simple ratio "**one in eight Americans now rely on Feeding America** for food and groceries"[31] offers a starker and perhaps more effective description of the problem.

Smaller domestic organizations reference the larger problem, but focus, as would be expected, on its local impact. A report entitled "Hunger: The Faces and the Facts, 2010" available on the Alameda County Community Food Bank website opens with the statement, "In Alameda County [CA], 1 in 6 residents visits at least one of the Food Bank's 275 soup kitchens, food pantries, after-school programs, senior centers, shelters, or other community agencies annually—the vast majority on a repeated basis. There is hunger in virtually every neighborhood."[32] Similarly, the Food Bank for New York City states in bold font, "**In New York City, one of the richest cities in the world, food poverty is around every corner.** Throughout the five boroughs, approximately 1.4 million people—mainly women, children, seniors, the working poor and people with disabilities—rely on soup kitchens and food pantries."[33] Both of these sites offer statistics on each of these vulnerable demographic groups coupled with first-person accounts from representative food bank clients.

One other rhetorical strategy for describing the extent of hunger in America emphasizes the food itself rather than its recipients. The website for a Washington, DC food bank notes that "volunteers working at Martha's Table and at their churches, synagogues and work places prepare at least 1200 sandwiches, 65 gallons of soups and 65 gallons of beverages daily."[34] The Food Depot of New Mexico states that each month it "distributes an average of 300,000 pounds of food and household products, providing 400,000 meals through its partner agencies in nine Northern New Mexico counties."[35]

Given the scope of the problem—internationally and domestically—hunger relief organizations must also offer an explanation for it. Each site identifies broad sociopolitical forces as the culprits. The real cause of hunger, argues the Food for the Hungry website, is not world population—"contrary to what some might believe. The real reason nearly one billion of the planet's 6.7 billion people are undernourished is because of food-distribution problems, natural disasters, government policies, civil unrest, inequitable trade policies, lack of knowledge and greed."[36] The Freedom from Hunger site lists five factors contributing to hunger: poverty, armed conflict, environmental overload, discrimination, and "lack of clout." "In the final analysis," the site argues, "chronic hunger is caused by powerlessness. People who don't have power to protect their own interests are hungry. The burden of this condition falls most acutely on children, women and elderly people."[37] Domestic sites like the Alameda County Food Bank also point to poverty as the underlying cause and identify a failure in public policies to fully address wages, work opportunities, education, affordable housing, unemployment benefits, healthcare, and food stamp and child nutrition programs.

In recognition of the complex and deep-seated causes responsible for hunger, relief organizations align along a continuum of those focused more on immediate aid and those working to offer long-term solutions. The latter approach usually involves agricultural improvements and small business opportunities that can empower individuals and communities to ultimately help themselves. Yet regardless of an organization's aims, it emphasizes the dignity and value of every life affected by hunger. This focus on individuals serves both to tug at emotions and encourage a belief that despite the enormity of the problem, lives can be saved and conditions improved. Domestic sites, in particular, explicitly call attention to "the faces of hunger." In this task, images, rather than words or numbers, play a pivotal role.

ADDING IMAGES: FACES AND BODIES

Photographs occupy a prominent place on hunger relief websites. Banners across the home page present photographs of the hungry, automatically refreshing on most sites so that visitors are greeted by multiple images. Virtually every link on every site leads the viewer to yet more photographs. The discursive attention to children on these sites—and in previous scholarship—makes those images and their compositional details of particular interest.

Images of children on both the international and domestic sites take a variety of forms. Most prominent are close-up portraits with both sad and smiling expressions of one or more children. In some the camera pulls back, showing the child alone or with other children, but with no adults in view. Others capture children in the company of adults, whether a mother, a father, both parents, or a medical worker. In just a handful of images, a child's body serves as the focal point, encouraging the viewer to gaze at and examine the physical markers of malnutrition.

The close-up portraits of children seem, at least initially, to avoid the fiercest criticisms directed at charity images by scholars. There are, at the very least, no images of abject suffering; the "flies in their eyes" are absent. Children's faces in particular are often framed with exceptionally tight shots in which the tops of their head or even their chins are cut off at the photograph's edge. The close-up format itself helps mitigate against the charge that the children are alone. The framing is evident; viewers readily understand that the vast scope of the scene occurs beyond the borders of the photograph. The children stare soberly at the camera, and thus at the viewer. The prominence of their eyes, in fact, becomes the unifying and most powerful feature of these images.Their gaze registers agency, but it is also easy to interpret such looks as imploring or even accusatory. Such expressions appear infrequently in a parent's collection of photographs of his or her own child. Nor are these expressions typically found in advertising, in which youthful faces convey almost relentless joy and exuberance, modeling, as Raymond Williams notes, "the mimed celebration of other people's choices."[38] In their departure from these photographic norms, photographs of sad faces call attention to themselves. Rather than inspiring a sense of solidarity or shared "universality," though, they may be more likely to elicit a sense that one is viewing the "other." To the extent this occurs, these portraits may indeed perpetuate the hierarchies of "First World" imperialism and the dominance of the West and North, able to offer aid to the needy.

In the portraits of smiling children, the signs of subordination are far more legible. These images are littered with the nonverbal cues that Erving Goffman, in analyzing gender display in contemporary advertising, terms the "ritualization of subordination."[39] Such cues of inequality are arguably relevant in the context of hungry children as well. Their heads are frequently tilted or canted and, among those who are standing, their bodies occasionally adopt a canted pose as well. Those who are seated, most often on the ground itself, betray in Goffman terms "a classic stereotype of deference."[40] Their large, bright smiles function, according to Goffman, as "ritualistic mollifiers, signaling that nothing antagonistic is intended or invited."[41] Positioning the hands over the face, and particularly placing the hands or a finger over the mouth serve in Goffman's view as a "maladaptive response" or a form of "licensed withdrawal" leaving one "dependent on the protectiveness and goodwill of others."[42] Arguably, hands or fingers over the mouth also serve as a sign that an individual is willingly silencing him or herself, a sign of passivity and submission.

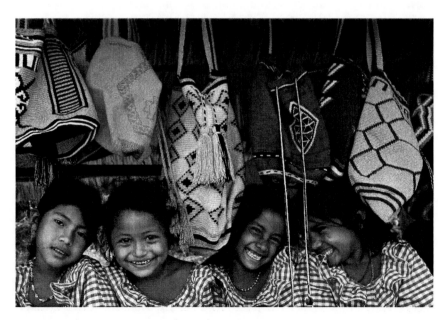

Figure 2.1 Action against Hunger—Colombia, Susana Vera.

The culturally established signs of subordination visible within these portraits may well be the very features that most contribute to the perception of these children as cute or photogenic, even in their poverty. Their subordinated status is recognizable and familiar; their attractiveness is partially a function of that familiarity. If so, such images might ironically be more adept at bridging East and West or North and South, while simultaneously reproducing and reinforcing differences based on power and inequity.

Those images of children alone in a landscape provoke two different criticisms. On the one hand, their strong compositional details aestheticize poverty. In some the children blend into the landscape, with the colors or even the cut of their clothing echoing the scene at large. In others, they (or the colors they wear) are the one detail that stands out against an otherwise dull backdrop. In either case, the surroundings amplify their isolation. Even in pairs or in small groups, the children appear alone and vulnerable, lacking adult care or community, adrift in a bleak, inscrutable, and sometimes dangerous landscape. In writing about racial representation in US advertising, Ellen Seiter argues that "African-American children never appear in the space of domestic fantasies, never share in these utopian visions of 'home.'"[43] Instead, she notes, they are most often shown "out-of-doors, on city streets, or in the negative space of a photography studio set. Thus Black children—the most visible minorities on television commercials—are permanently outside of the golden, homey glow of television's fantasy of safety and love."[44] Many of these images seem to go one step further. Not only are the children excluded from a warm and nurturing home, but also the home itself (seen from without) is condemned as neither safe nor inviting.

The one element shared among these images is the portrayal of children as innocent and thus "worthy" victims, due to their age, their isolation, and the markers of poverty that surround them. Even children shown with parents retain their status as innocent victims, yet these photographs help defuse the fiercest criticisms leveled by scholars. Such parent-child portraits bring adults quite literally into the picture, and with them recognition of the systems of care already in place even within the most devastated of locales. These photographs also seem to me the ones most able to escape the "othering" or exoticizing gaze. The gestures they capture are recognizable but not as markers of subordination. Instead they evoke universal human values: love, comfort, and courage, even in the face of tragedy. Such gestures bind the subjects to each other—and, in doing so, to the viewer as well. A mother or father or grandparent holds a child close, the adult hands often visible, offering firm support or a gentle caress. Two women sit side by side, each with a child at her breast. A mother kisses a crying child's cheek. A mother cooks a meal with her child clinging tightly to her side. A father wraps a blanket around himself and his son, creating a warm cocoon against a backdrop of refugee tents. There are few smiles here.

My memory of hunger relief ads from the 1960s and 1970s is of those depicting a child's emaciated body, skeletally thin arms and legs, and a

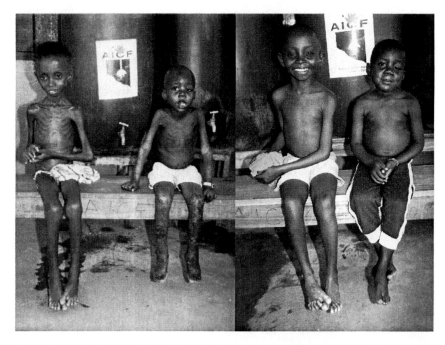

Figure 2.2   "Before and after" shot depicts David and Kaisha at an ACF Stabilization Center. Action Against Hunger—Sierra Leone, ACF-Sierra Leone.

belly swollen from hunger and malnutrition. Whereas contemporary examples of such images can readily be found on the Internet, they appear only infrequently—albeit prominently—on some hunger relief websites. Action Against Hunger also sends out one of these images—a paired set of black and white photographs of two young boys in "before" and "after" shots—in their mailings. The captions accompanying these photographs read:

> **This first photo** shows Kaifa (left) and David, refugee boys from Sierra Leone, when they entered our program. As you can see, they were badly malnourished and in serious medical jeopardy.

> **This second photo** shows the boys 30 days later, after receiving medical treatment and a diet of life-saving formula. What is equally amazing is that we were able to bring these two youngsters back from the brink of death for *little more than two dollars a day!*[45]

Food for the Hungry features a similar before and after photographic pairing on its website, one that is meant to serve as testimony to the effects of deworming. Other photographs document medical personnel weighing one child, measuring the circumference of another's arm, and monitoring yet another child's heartbeat. The bodies on display serve as documentary evidence, a visual record to corroborate the numbers gleaned from these procedures. Both, then, are delivered to website visitors as incontrovertible proof—both of need and of success—and we are actively encouraged to gaze upon, scrutinize, and judge these bodies without fear of discovery or repercussion. The children's benign smiles seem to endorse such behavior on our part. The body shown in such extreme conditions becomes abject, the object of pity, but not necessarily of recognition.

This treatment of the hungry body as spectacle parallels, I believe, contemporary media treatment of the obese body. Yet whereas audiences are encouraged to gaze—undetected—at both, the gaze itself is shifted somewhat, thus altering the response each image is meant to elicit. The similarities as well as differences in the representation of the hungry and obese body thus deserve some attention, for they help clarify the significance of photographic images overall.

Comparing the hungry and the obese body may be justified on another level as well. The Alameda County Community Food Bank's report, "Hunger: The Faces and the Facts 2010," directly addresses the links between obesity and food insecurity, noting that the "lack of access to nutritious foods and safe areas for play have created a counter-intuitive scenario among low-income children, who increasingly suffer from both hunger and obesity."[46] The study notes that "Americans in poverty-struck areas have a higher likelihood of suffering from low-food security and are more likely to be overweight or obese. This paradox is explained, in part, by the types of foods that are readily available to low-income communities."[47] The report singles out fast-food restaurants and convenience stores as unhealthy options for eating, yet notes that twice as many of these establishments are located in low-income communities than in more affluent neighborhoods. The *Atlas of World Hunger* also reports a strong association between obesity and low-income levels in the US.[48]

The hungry body and the obese body are thus paired as signifiers of malnutrition. Whereas hunger may be hidden, particularly within the US, the obese body suffers the reverse, an inescapable visibility. Although rates of obesity seem to be increasing across the globe, the US exhibits one of the highest rates of adult obesity worldwide, making Americans, in Greg Critser's words, "the fattest people on the face of the earth."[49] Thus examining the surfeit of media coverage in the US surrounding an "obesity epidemic"— along with the images accompanying such stories—is of particular interest.[50]

THE OBESE BODY

Like discourses surrounding hunger, media coverage of obesity typically attempts first to describe its prevalence within the US and then offer explanations of its cause. Two organizations at the forefront of obesity education, research, and advocacy are the Obesity Action Coalition (OAC) and the Obesity Society, both of which maintain a web presence. Central to their goals, in the words of the Obesity Society, is a pledge to uphold "compassion: for the lives and situations of those living with obesity" and "respect: for each other and all who are touched by obesity."[51]

The discussion of obesity found on these two websites, though, echoes that found in popular press coverage. "Obesity is a serious and rising health epidemic in our country," notes the OAC in its "Overview" statement. "You are not alone in this fight. It is estimated that nearly 93 million Americans are obese and that number is predicted to climb to 120 million within the next five years."[52] The very language of an "epidemic" suggests the largely medical perspective taken by many experts. Media reports often feature statistics on obesity (like those just mentioned) linked to a lengthy list of medical conditions and health complications.[53] A further set of numbers details the "cost" to society arising from medical expenses and lost productivity. Although a controversial label, the OAC, in its advocacy role, states outright on its website that "obesity is a complex disease."[54] In the view of many scholars, labeling obesity as a disease increases rather than reduces the likelihood of turning fatness "into a deeply stigmatized physical characteristic."[55] Darlene McNaughton borrows from Foucault's *The Birth of the Clinic* to analyze the repercussions of such discourse. "Presenting obesity as a serious health 'threat' of epidemic proportions is, among other things," she writes, "an exercise in power, disciplining and surveillance,"[56] encouraging those who fall outside the "norm" to experience shame and remorse.

If the term "epidemic" implies a disease, popular discourse in news and entertainment alike presents it as a disease brought on almost solely by personal failings: lack of self-control or willpower.[57] Most explanations for the rise of obesity and the concomitant advice for alleviating it, note Irmgard Tischner and Helen Malson, point to the individual and "lifestyle choices, with an emphasis on 'eat less!' and 'move more!'—an approach that fails to take into account the fact that most diets fail in the long term."[58] The language of personal responsibility turns the individuals who suffer from obesity into "culpable victims,"[59] or perhaps, more accurately, culpable collaborators.

Whereas lists of contributing social, political, economic, and structural causes at the societal or even community level are prominent on hunger relief websites, such lists are less readily found in most media discussions or media advocacy websites. The opposite is also true: The hungry are rarely met with the language of "personal responsibility" or culpability for their condition. Solutions to hunger encourage structural changes that will lead to "personal empowerment." Solutions to obesity demand "personal responsibility" up front from those deemed obese. Meanwhile, as Deborah Morrison Thomson points out, such rhetorical sleights of hand shield segments of the food industry from charges of corporate responsibility.[60]

Not only is the obese body chastised and censured in verbal discourse, but also the images accompanying stories on obesity enact a form of violence on the body. Video footage airing in news programs about obesity features images of adults and children taken in public spaces, either photographed from the neck down or from behind.[61] Unlike the hunger relief websites, neither the Obesity Action Coalition website nor the Obesity Society website includes images of obese individuals or of any individuals at all (save for attendees at the most recent Obesity Society conference). A content analysis of the thumbnail images accompanying articles on obesity found on the *Time* magazine website underscored this pattern, however. Of the fifty-four images of people used to illustrate 161 stories on obesity published since the year 2000, twenty-three depict an obese body in which the person's face was cropped off, blurred, or turned away from the camera. Among the twelve overweight or obese individuals whose faces were visible, three were celebrities (Oliver Hardy, a *Biggest Loser* contestant, and a professional baseball player) and three were the same photo of a woman preparing to undergo gastric bypass surgery.[62] Whereas hunger relief organizations actively work to give a "face" to hunger, media representations of obesity deliberately excise the face from the obese body.

This photographic framing renders the obese not simply anonymous (as is the evident intent, at least in part to avoid libel charges), but without agency. They are not permitted to gaze back at the camera, to register their expressions. To borrow Sontag's words, such images suggest an individual "is regarded only as someone to be seen, not someone (like us) who also sees."[63] Thomson, borrowing from Foucault, terms the practice "spectacular decapitation," and argues that it more readily allows the assigning of blame within a "shaming etiology."[64] The body without a face possesses neither an opposing perspective nor a voice. In an effort to correct this tendency and to explore "the subjective experience of being 'large' in contemporary society" Tischner and Malson conducted a series of interviews with eighteen women and three men who either "self-identified being 'large', or thought that others considered them 'large.'"[65] Although the interviews revealed some ability to negotiate their subject positions, for the most part, in their daily lives, these individuals found themselves targeted by the gaze of others, a form of surveillance experienced as oppressive and controlling. Tischner and Malson, like Foucault, conclude that for the most part, "visibility is a trap."[66]

Foucault has noted that our bodies are "molded by a great many distinct regimes,"[67] among them food and the complex codes of behavior associated with eating. The penalties for not disciplining our bodies to conform to normative ideals can be significant—and are imposed with seeming impunity. If fat was once viewed in the West as a signifier of wealth and status, by the late nineteenth century it had lost that connotation, even within the middle class.[68] As Cecilia Hartley argues, 'Fat-phobia is one of the few acceptable forms of prejudice left."[69] Fat now more readily inspires fear and revulsion, all the while attracting morbid fascination.

The obese body as spectacle has persisted in popular culture from circus freak shows in the late nineteenth and early twentieth centuries to contemporary televisual fodder in programs like *The Biggest Loser*.[70] If the bodies of the hungry are relatively rarely put on display, the obese body, by contrast, betrays a long history of being weighed and measured, examined and assessed by experts and authorities (or drummers and salesmen), with viewers invited to witness the proceedings. Derogatory comments directed at the obese have been integral to the exhibition.[71] Photographic images carry traces of this same behavior and attitude. Seven of the images found on the *Time* magazine website depict a headless torso encircled by a tape measure, with the numbers on the tape clearly legible to the viewer. Another image shows a man grasping both ends of a belt that no longer reaches around his waist. The *Biggest Loser* contestant is photographed standing on the scale, his previous weight of 304 in bold numbers projected on the screen beside him while he awaits the latest figure. The male torsos on display within this set of images are often shirtless, bare skin bulging over waistbands. Women's breasts, hips, and bellies strain against snug fabrics. These signs and symbols emphasize deviation from the norm. The body is made monstrous and grotesque, bloated by "empty calories." If photogenic poverty ("cuteness") captures our attention, horror holds it. In being subjected both to medical intervention as well as viewers' unabashed and sustained gaze, the obese body is ultimately made docile, a term that for Foucault joins "the analyzable body to the manipulable body."[72] Looking is paired with the goal of disciplining, dominating, and ultimately re-fashioning the human being at the center of the spectacle. But spectacle provides entertainment more than understanding.

If children occupy a prominent space in the discourse surrounding hunger, they are similarly isolated for specific attention in discussions of obesity. Over a fourth of the *Time* magazine stories on obesity addressed childhood obesity and eleven of the thirty-five photographs of overweight or obese bodies depicted children.[73] Although the bodies of obese children suffer scrutiny, youth is often afforded the protective cloak of "innocence." Still, apparently some blame must be meted out. Because many socializing disciplines begin within the home, parents—or more specifically women— are often held accountable for children's failure to conform to body ideals. Natalie Boero argues that "mother blame" lies just below the surface in much contemporary discourse concerning childhood obesity.[74] McNaughton traces this blame game back to the womb.[75]

News reports are careful to employ the gender-neutral term "parents" in discussing behaviors believed responsible for the increased rates of overweight and obesity in children. Yet as Boero points out, in phrases such as "when both parents work," it is implied that "it is mothers, whose paid work is often seen as unnecessary, who are to blame."[76] Even Michelle Obama's "Let's Move!" campaign, launched in February 2010 to help solve "the challenge of childhood obesity" and raise "a healthier generation of kids,"[77] addresses parents as its primary audience, although it also lists schools, community leaders, chefs, elected officials, and kids themselves as sharing responsibility for both creating and helping to solve the problem. In asking "How did we get here?" the Let's Move website argues,

> Thirty years ago, most people led lives that kept them at a healthy weight. . . . Meals were home-cooked with reasonable portion sizes and there was always a vegetable on the plate. Eating fast food was rare and snacking between meals was an occasional treat.
>
> Today, children experience a very different lifestyle. . . . Parents are busier than ever and families eat fewer home-cooked meals. Snacking between meals is now commonplace.[78]

In referencing a seemingly utopian past, nostalgia, as evidenced here, invariably belies a gender- and class-based bias. Whereas such discourse reveals, as Boero notes, our "social anxieties regarding the changing role of women,"[79] it simultaneously conceals many of the social, political, and economic conditions that lie behind the changes described: falling real wages, higher levels of education, subsidies for agro-industry commodities, and intensified marketing in the food sector among them.

Boero concludes her essay by noting that, "Like the social construction of the 'obesity epidemic' in general, the blaming of mothers for their kids' 'excess' weight draws attention away from very real structural inequities in health care, education, and employment that are often felt hardest by women and minorities."[80] Mothers are found guilty in their neglect and absence, their poor consumer choices, "for passing on poor eating habits,"[81] or even for their "poor awareness" of their child's weight status[82]—in short, for not directing a censoring gaze at their own children's bodies. If children escape some of the blame for their excess weight, mothers shoulder far more than their fair share of the burden.

Yet ironically, if working mothers are viewed as one of the causes of poor childhood nutrition (obesity) within developed nations, in developing nations putting women to work is presented as a solution to malnutrition (hunger). The Hunger Project explicitly states that it "seeks to end hunger and poverty by empowering people to lead lives of self-reliance, meet their own basic needs and build better futures for their children."[83] To this end, its microfinance project aims at developing "the economic empowerment of the most important but least supported food producers on the continent— Africa's women."[84] Access to microfinance credit "enables women to engage in income-generating activities to increase their incomes and invest in their businesses."[85] In the West, nostalgia for an elusive past seems to blind us to possibilities for a progressive future for women and their children.

CONCLUSION

Both the hungry body and the obese body are displayed and dissected in public discourse and the endless circulation of images. The one becomes the object of pity; the other the object of scorn. To the extent that the conventions of photography play into either of these responses, they deserve to be examined and critiqued, for neither response is useful in alleviating either of these key issues in food politics. But critiques alone seem insufficient. Scholars need to be just as adept at suggesting alternatives. Some of the images found already on hunger relief websites point in that direction. I don't know that it suffices to simply label a photograph with the words "This is the look of empowerment" as the Hunger Project site does, but as clichéd as the word has become, the discourse of empowerment may be a useful tactic to deploy both rhetorically and politically.

For me, the most compelling images are those that bring food itself into the photographic frame, although not in the form of a foil packet of "Plumpy'nut" or a chubby hand reaching for a cupcake. Rather, the images of agricultural production and harvest (including rooftop gardens in New York City or urban community gardens from Seattle to Sarasota) help make empowerment palpable. They feature action rather than appearance. They turn urban food deserts into green spaces. They emphasize the importance of education in helping create sustainable models of food production and enlightened food consumption—thus addressing both hunger and obesity simultaneously. Such images—and the practices they depict—offer evidence of the possibilities of systemic change and turn the public screen into a sign of hope rather than shame or despair.

ACKNOWLEDGMENTS

The author would like to thank the following individuals for their helpful commentary and suggestions on preliminary drafts of this essay: Joshua Frye, the anonymous reviewers of the book manuscript, Anastasia Sonkin, and Paul Schwochow.

NOTES

1. Marion Nestle, "Food Politics," *San Francisco Chronicle*, January 3, 2010, K2, http://www.foodpolitics.com/2010/01/whats-up-with-food-and-nutrition-in-2010/.
2. Tom Maliti and Ariel David, "A Record 1 Billion People Hungry," *San Francisco Chronicle*, October 15, 2009, A5, http://www.sfgate.com/cgi-bin/article.cgi?f=/c/a/2009/10/14/MNAI1A5NH9.DTL
3. Marita Sturken and Lisa Cartwright, *Practices of Looking: An Introduction to Visual Culture* (Oxford: Oxford University Press, 2001), 100.

4. Ibid.
5. Jan Nederveen Pieterse, *White on Black: Images of Africa and Blacks in Western Popular Culture* (New Haven: Yale University Press, 1992), 208.
6. Ibid.
7. Ibid., 208–9.
8. Ibid., 209.
9. Carla Joinson, "Coping with Compassion Fatigue," *Nursing* 22 (1992): 116–22.
10. Arthur Kleinman and Joan Kleinman, "The Appeal of Experience; the Dismay of Images: Cultural Appropriations of Suffering in Our Times," *Daedalus* 125 (1996): 1.
11. Ibid., 2.
12. Ibid., 7.
13. Ibid.
14. Susan Sontag, *Regarding the Pain of Others* (New York: Farrar, Straus and Giroux, 2003), 13.
15. Ibid., 71.
16. Ibid.
17. John Hutnyk, "Photogenic Poverty: Souvenirs and Infantilism," *Journal of Visual Culture* 3 (2004): 81.
18. Ibid., 87.
19. Deborah A. Small and Nicole M. Verrochi, "The Face of Need: Facial Emotion Expression on Charity Advertisements," *Journal of Marketing Research* XLVI (2009): 777–87.
20. Ibid., 786.
21. Ibid.
22. Pieterse, *White on Black*, 209.
23. The websites chosen included the six top-rated charities for "hunger" (five with a global focus and one local food bank) listed on the CharityWatch.org website: Action Against Hunger, Bread for the World, Food Bank for New York City, Food for the Hungry, Freedom from Hunger, and Global Hunger Project. Feeding America was chosen for its national focus. An additional two regional sites (all given the top four-star rating by the Charity Navigator website) were selected using a random number generator: Food Depot (northern New Mexico), Martha's Table (Washington, DC). The tenth and final website chosen was that of a local food bank in northern California (Alameda County). The study began with a preliminary content analysis of the 632 photographs found on these sites.
24. Justin Lewis, *The Ideological Octopus* (New York: Routledge, 1991).
25. Kevin Michael DeLuca and Jennifer Peeples, "From Public Sphere to Public Screen: Democracy, Activism, and the 'Violence' of Seattle," *Critical Studies in Media Communication* 19 (2002): 125–51.
26. "Hunger Fact Sheet," *Food for the Hungry*, accessed October 15, 2010, http://www.fh.org/learn/resources. This number appears to be based on a 2007 report issued by the UN Food and Agriculture Organization (FAO) from http://www.nutraingredients-usa.com/Industry/Hunger-a-reality-for-854-million.
27. "Hunger Information," *Freedom from Hunger* and "Know Your World: Facts About Hunger and Poverty," *The Hunger Project*, accessed October 15, 2010, http://thp.org/learn_more/issues/know_your_world_facts_about_hunger_and_poverty. This data is attributed to both the World Bank 2010 report "Overview: Understanding, Measuring, Overcoming Poverty" and the FAO 2009 report "The State of Food Insecurity in the World."
28. "Celebrating World Food Day 2010," *The Hunger Project*, accessed October 15, 2010, http://www.thp.org/learn_more/news/latest_news/celebrating_world_food_day_2010.

29. "Hunger Fact Sheet," *Food for the Hungry* (bold font in the original), accessed October 15, 2010, http://www.fh.org/learn/resources.
30. "How We Work," *Feeding America*, accessed October 15, 2010, http://feeding america.org/our-network/how-we-work.aspx.
31. "Hunger Report 2010," *Feeding America*, accessed October 15, 2010, http://feedingamerica.org/faces-of-hunger/hunger-in-america-2010/hunger-report-2010.aspx.
32. "Hunger: The Faces & The Facts," *Alameda County Community Food Bank*, accessed October 15, 2010, http://www.accfb.org/hunger_study.html.
33. "Food Poverty in NYC," *Food Bank NYC*, accessed October 15, 2010, http://www.foodbanknyc.org/go/food-poverty-in-nyc.
34. "Food and Nutrition: How to Help," *Martha's Table*, accessed October 15, 2010, http://www.marthastable.net/mckennas-wagon.html.
35. "Overview, Mission and Strategies," *Food Depot* (NM), accessed October 15, 2010, http://www.thefooddepot.org/~thefoodd/index.php?option=com_con tent&view=article&id=104&Itemid=127. Feeding America also references its work in terms of the volume of food it has distributed. According to its website, "During the past five years, the Feeding America network and our national corporate donors have provided more than 100 million pounds of emergency food and disaster relief supplies to individuals and families affected by disaster." "Disaster Relief," *Feeding America*, accessed October 15, 2010, http://feedingamerica.org/our-network/networkprograms/disaster-relief.aspx.
36. "Hunger Fact Sheet," *Food for the Hungry*.
37. "Hunger Information: What Causes Chronic Hunger?," *Freedom from Hunger*, accessed October 15, 2010, http://www.freedomfromhunger.org/info/.
38. Raymond Williams, "Advertising: The Magic System," in *Problems in Materialism and Culture, Selected Essays* (London: Verso, 1980), 209.
39. Erving Goffman, "Gender Advertisements," *Studies in the Anthropology of Visual Communication* 3 (1976): 92–154. Goffman's analysis of advertising images focuses on adults, noting that women often adopt the poses of children in these ritualizations of subordination. His analysis may be applied to children, though, because he argues that these signs are readily understood by members of a society and are reinforced in the plethora of images that surround us.
40. Ibid., 110.
41. Ibid., 117.
42. Ibid., 127.
43. Ellen Seiter, "Different Children, Different Dreams: Racial Representation in Advertising," in *Gender, Race and Class in Media: A Text-Reader*, ed. Gail Dines and Jean M. Humez (Thousand Oaks, CA: Sage, 1995), 101.
44. Ibid.
45. Action Against Hunger, direct mail fundraising letter. Bolding and italics in the original.
46. "Hunger: The Faces & The Facts," *Alameda County Community Food Bank*, 7.
47. Ibid., 6.
48. Thomas J. Bassett and Alex Winter-Nelson, *The Atlas of World Hunger* (Chicago: University of Chicago Press, 2010), 32–36.
49. Greg Critser, *Fat Land: How Americans Became the Fattest People in the World* (Boston: Houghton Mifflin, 2003), 4. For global comparison of obesity rates, see Bassett and Winter-Nelson, *Atlas of World Hunger*, 19.
50. To illustrate the amount of media attention directed toward this issue, a search on the LexisNexis database for the terms "obesity" and "overweight" under "Healthcare in the news" for the previous six months (March–September 2011) generated 2,543 citations.

51. "Mission and Vision," *Obesity Society*, accessed September 5, 2011,http://www.obesity.org/about-us/mission-and-vision.htm.
52. "All About Obesity: Overview," *Obesity Action Coalition*, accessed September 5, 2011, http://www.obesityaction.org/aboutobesity/overview.php.
53. The Obesity Action Coalition website follows this practice as well. In "All about Obesity: Related Conditions" the website lists eleven separate "obesity-related conditions" ranging from cancer to psychological depression. For scholarly discussion of this tendency, see Darlene McNaughton, "From the Womb to the Tomb: Obesity and Maternal Responsibility," *Critical Public Health* 21 (2011): 179–90. McNaughton, among others, challenges the strength of medical evidence connecting obesity and myriad health problems.
54. "Advocacy," *Obesity Action Coalition*, accessed September 5, 2011, http://www.obesityaction.org/advocacy/overview.php.
55. McNaughton, "From the Womb to the Tomb," 181.
56. Ibid., 180–81. Michel Foucault, *The Birth of the Clinic: An Archeology of Medical Perception* (New York: Vintage, 1994).
57. See, for instance, Susan Bordo, "Reading the Slender Body," in *Unbearable Weight: Feminism, Western Culture, and the Body* (Berkeley: University of California Press, 1993), 185–212. Bordo argues that following this logic, the "healthy" or slim body, in contrast, represents qualities of "detachment, self-containment, self-mastery, control," (209).
58. Irmgard Tischner and Helen Malson, "Exploring the Politics of Women's In/visible 'Large' Bodies," *Feminism & Psychology* 18 (2008): 260–61. The Obesity Society lists lifestyle/behavioral causes of obesity first, but also names environmental, cultural, and genetic causes. "Domain 01: Basic Knowledge," *Obesity Society*, accessed September 5, 2011, http://www.obesity.org/certification/comp-domain-01.
59. Sanna Inthorn and Tammy Boyce, "'It's Disgusting How Much Salt You Eat!': Television Discourses of Obesity, Health and Morality," *International Journal of Cultural Studies* 13 (2010): 83–100. For a discussion on innocent v. culpable victims, see Don Heider and Koji Fuse, "Class and Local TV News," in *Class and News*, ed. Don Heider (Lanham, MD: Rowman and Littlefield: 2004).
60. Deborah Morrison Thomson, "Big Food and the Body Politics of Personal Responsibility," *Southern Communication Journal* 74 (2009): 15; Ross Singer, "Anti-Corporate Argument and the Spectacle of the Grotesque Rhetorical Body in *Super Size Me*," *Critical Studies in Media Communication* 28 (2011): 135–52.
61. See, for example, ABC News' *Nightline* documentary "Critical Condition: America's Obesity Crisis" (2004). This convention is so well understood that Jon Stewart was able to satirize it in a *Daily Show* special report on obesity: "Poll Smoking—Obesity" (May 8, 2006), http://www.thedailyshow.com/watch/mon-may-8–2006/poll-smoking—obesity.
62. The content analysis revealed a total of 105 images. Twenty-six were of the unrelated magazine cover and another twenty-four were of non-human objects (e.g., food, a scale, etc.).
63. Susan Sontag, *Regarding the Pain*, 72.
64. Thomson, "Big Food," 2–17. As evidence, Thomson examines the publicity campaigns created by the Center for Consumer Freedom, consisting in part of two print advertisements condemning obesity lawsuits, both of which feature a naked male torso.
65. Tischner and Malson, "Exploring the Politics," 261.
66. Ibid., 265. See also Michel Foucault, *Discipline and Punish: The Birth of the Prison* (New York: Vintage, 1977), 200.

67. Michel Foucault, *The Foucault Reader*, ed. Paul Rabinow, repr. (New York: Vintage, 1984), 87.
68. Bordo, "Reading the Slender Body," 185.
69. Cecilia Hartley, "Letting Ourselves Go: Making Room for the Fat Body in Feminist Scholarship" in *Bodies Out of Bounds: Fatness and Transgression*, ed. Jana Evans Braziel and Kathleen LeBesco (Berkeley: University of California Press, 2001), 65.
70. David Haslam and Fiona Haslam, *Fat, Gluttony and Sloth: Obesity in Medicine, Art, and Literature* (Liverpool: Liverpool University Press, 2009); Katherine Sender and Margaret Sullivan, "Epidemics of Will, Failures of Self-Esteem: Responding to Fat Bodies in *The Biggest Loser* and *What Not to Wear*," *Continuum: Journal of Media & Cultural Studies* 22 (2008): 573–84.
71. Haslam and Haslam, *Fat, Gluttony and Sloth*, 43.
72. Foucault, *The Foucault Reader*, 136.
73. Six of the eleven images of teens or children also featured body fragments or were taken from behind.
74. Natalie Boero, "Fat Kids, Working Moms, and the 'Epidemic of Obesity': Race Class and Mother Blame," in *The Fat Studies Reader*, ed. Esther Rothblum and Sondra Solovay (New York: New York University Press, 2009), 113–19.
75. McNaughton, "From the Womb to the Tomb," 179–90.
76. Boero, "Fat Kids, Working Moms," 115.
77. "Learn the Facts," *Let's Move*, accessed September 11, 2011, http://www.letsmove.gov/learn-facts/epidemic-childhood-obesity.
78. Ibid.
79. Boero, "Fat Kids, Working Moms," 118.
80. Ibid.
81. Ibid, 116.
82. L. Michele Maynard et al., "Maternal Perceptions of Weight Status of Children," *Pediatrics* 111 (2003): 1226–31; S. Carnell et al., "Parental Perceptions of Overweight in 3–5 y Olds," *International Journal of Obesity* 29 (2005): 353–55.
83. "What We Do: Microfinance Program in Africa," *The Hunger Project*, accessed September 5, 2011, http://www.thp.org/what_we_do/key_initiatives/microfinance/overview.
84. Ibid.
85. Ibid.

3 Politics on Your Plate
Building and Burning Bridges across Organic, Vegetarian, and Vegan Discourse

Laura K. Hahn and Michael S. Bruner

"Eating organic" offers eaters the luxury of affirming, seeing, and tasting their politics on their plate. As Michael Pollan suggests, "Eating organic thus married the personal to the political."[1] The once counterculture ideals of organic food seem to have found their way into the mainstream (e.g., organic lettuce at Costco). Vegetarian lifestyle choices arguably offer the same instant gratification of seeing (or not seeing as in the absence of animal products) one's politics on one's plate. Yet, despite recent trends, vegetarian politics have not found a broader place in public discourse. Why? If contemporary "organic" rhetoric is so strong, then why is "vegetarian" and "vegan" rhetoric comparatively much weaker? Why has the vegetarian movement failed to gain the same traction as the organic movement within the larger discussion—or obsession—that Americans have with their relationship to food? Why has this movement been largely unsuccessful in translating its values, goals, and beliefs to a large public scale?

This chapter addresses these questions and explores some of the apparent contradictions and implications. For example, Thomas Frank suggests that "Consumerism is no longer about 'conformity', but about 'difference'."[2] Our consumer choices function as a vehicle to make our politics public. If "difference" is so important, then it is perplexing that "vegetarian" discourse does not resonate more deeply with nonconformist consumers. To get at these issues we will analyze representative texts from the organic and vegetarian/vegan movements and conclude with a discussion of why the vegetarian movement has gained less traction than its organic counterpart. Two artifacts related to the organic movement and two related to the vegetarian/vegan movements are presented in this chapter. These specific examples, nonetheless, are representative of the broader issues in these social movements. For the organic movement we will examine (1) the Alar Apple Scare of 1989, as fueled by a report on the CBS News program, *60 Minutes* (February 26, 1989) and (2) the website of the Organic Consumers Association (OCA), accessed at www.organicconsumers.org. For the vegan/vegetarian movement we will look at two recent PETA videos,

"Grace: PETA's Thanksgiving Ad" and "Emily Deschanel's Veggie Testimonial," accessed at www.peta.org.

ORGANIC MOVEMENT

Although the values of the "organic movement" and the values of "environmentalism" currently are combined, it required eighty years of social struggle to achieve this consumer reality. According to Joseph Heckman[3] there are five stages through which the organic movement grew: the development of organic concepts and methods, polarization, recognition, accommodation, and finally further extension. The organic movement, presently in the final stage (further extension), finds itself at odds with its ideological origins.

Historically, the concept and practice of growing organic produce stemmed from aspirations for a mutually beneficial relationship between farmers interested in healthier food and sustainable farming practices, government regulation, and the desire of the youth-oriented counterculture hippies to rebel.[4] However, the rise in popularity and sales of organic food depended on retail outlets willing to introduce, market, advertise, and deliver the products to the consumer. For several years, the market for organic products continued to grow at 17–20 percent a year, making it the fastest growing segment of the American food marketplace.[5] By comparison, the conventional food market was growing only at 2–3 percent a year.[6] Compared to 1980, when there were only six natural food stores in the US, in 2003 organic foods were sold in twenty thousand natural food stores and 73 percent of conventional grocery stores.[7] In 2007, "sales of natural products grew to approximately \$62 billion. . . . a 10% increase over the prior year." The growth in popularity of "natural foods" can be attributed to four factors: (1) a heightened awareness of the role that food and nutrition play in long-term health, which has led to healthier eating patterns; (2) a better educated and wealthier population, which can spend more on "natural products"; (3) increasing consumer concern over the purity and safety of food, due to the presence of pesticide residues, growth hormones, artificial ingredients and other chemicals, and genetically engineered ingredients; and (4) environmental concerns due to the degradation of water and soil quality.[8]

The most recent development in the organic movement is the debate between "big organic" and "little organic." Michael Pollan, writing in *The New York Times*, expressed his fear that "the new corporate and government construction of 'organic' leaves out values that were once part and parcel of the word."[9] In other words, Wal-Mart and other giant businesses, seeking to limit costs, may alter the meaning of the word "organic" so much that it may be time "to move beyond organic," according to Pollan. For example, milk cows in large lots could be fed factory-farmed "organic" feed, but never taste a blade of grass.

In summary, the history of the organic food movement reveals how the movement embraced a particular chain of logic. The central arguments are that the soil is critical, industrial chemicals in food are to be avoided, and government must play a large role in guaranteeing food safety. The interplay of these factors has resulted in increased consumer demand and a highly profitable organic industry. There also is the possibility that the "success" of the organic movement contains the seeds of its undoing.

Organic Campaigns

US history contains many famous "hoaxes," such as the radio broadcast of "The War of the Worlds," which listeners believed to be a news report. In the realm of the organic food movement, the *60 Minutes* segment on Alar is a famous, contested site in public discourse. Critics call the segment a scare tactic and a hoax. Advocates claim that CBS was raising the legitimate issue of possible contamination of food and the consequences of that contamination. The segment, in this view, was not sensationalism but a "news report."

60 Minutes is a popular CBS television news and commentary show coming out of the 1960s. It was among the first to use a narrative approach to news (stories) and a confrontational style. The February 1989 broadcast highlighted potential problems with Alar. Alar, properly named daminozide, was a chemical sprayed on fruit, primarily apples, to regulate growth, make harvest easier, and enhance color. *60 Minutes* referred to a study by the Natural Resources Defense Council (NRDC), to the effect that Alar might cause cancer.[10]

In a powerful, if heavy-handed, display of visual rhetoric, the Alar report on CBS utilized a skull and crossbones overlaid on a red apple. The symbol for poison and death was superimposed on a symbol of nutrition and health. As if the general danger of chemical poisoning was not enough, *60 Minutes* intensified their fear appeal by warning that children were most at risk.

The Alar segment on CBS created a furor in public discourse, with a strong backlash from industry and its allies. According to *PRWatch*,

> Porter/Novelli, a leading food-industry PR firm, helped an industry group called the "Center for Produce Quality" distribute more than twenty thousand "resource kits" to food retailers which scoffed at the scientific data presented on *60 Minutes*. Industry-funded organizations such as the Advancement of Sound Science Coalition and the American Council on Science and Health hammered home the argument that the "Alar scare" was an irrational episode of public hysteria produced by unscrupulous manipulators of media sensationalism.[11]

Overall, the controversy "cost the agriculture industry over 100 million dollars."[12] The agriculture and chemical industries launched a counterattack, pitting industry scientists against the NRDC. The *60 Minutes* report was ridiculed as an unethical use of fear tactics, and anti-Alar activists were mocked for inciting "hysteria."[13] CBS subsequently broadcast a second segment on Alar, giving the industry an opportunity to state its position. In the end, however, the Environmental Protection Agency expressed concern and the manufacturer voluntarily withdrew Alar from the market. The controversy left ripples in public discourse for many months.

Two important rhetorical themes in the Alar controversy are (1) Science as authority, including how to process opposing views of scientists; and (2) What roles do media play in addressing food issues? Where are the lines between education, news, entertainment, and sensationalism? Is the backlash more important than the original artifact in shaping public opinion?

The second text from the organic movement is the website of the Organic Consumers Association, www.organicconsumers.org. Representing itself as "an online and grassroots community," the OCA claims to represent "over 850,000 members, subscribers, and volunteers." The OCA also claims to "promote the views and interests of the nation's estimated 50 million organic and socially responsible consumers." If that figure is accurate, then the OCA speaks for approximately one out of seven Americans.

Looking at the website, the viewer notices that the color green—associated with the earth, plants, and the organic movement—is displayed prominently. The home page has many logos of sponsors as well as pastoral images, such as photos of canned peaches. The top banner articulates an ideology in its choice of terms, including "health," "justice," "sustainability," "peace," and "democracy." Through the use of these iconic terms the discussion of organic food takes on epic proportions.

The website's layout resembles a newspaper. The home page features four major "columns": OCA News Sections; OCA Campaigns; Today's Stories; and OCA Network. In red letters, a featured alert is situated above the third column, Today's Stories. In addition, the home page offers many buttons and links. At first, the website seems "too busy." The amount of information is a bit overwhelming. However, the website provides each user with opportunities to personalize the browsing experience. On the top left, a "Choose Your State" pull-down list enables the user to examine local issues. The linked page for each state reports local news/issues and provides contacts for legislators from that state.

The viewer is challenged with several calls to action. The tone of the website suggests urgency—unless organic consumers are vigilant and active, something will be lost. The website provides opportunities to provide one's zip code, to donate to the OCA, to interact through Facebook, Twitter, and You Tube, and to read in greater depth.

VEGETARIAN/VEGAN MOVEMENT

Next we will offer a brief description of the vegetarian/vegan movement and examine two representative texts. When referring to animals we will invoke the term *non-human animals (NHA)* for several reasons. As many people do not see themselves as animals, the use of the terms *human* and *animal* reinforces a false distinction and allows the doctrine of speciesism— "a prejudice or attitude of bias toward the interests of members of one's own species and against those of members of other species"[14] to come into play. As Carrie Freeman notes, " . . . the hegemonic distinction between human and animal serves as a primary boundary that constrains and impedes an average American's consideration of animal rights as a valid ethical position."[15] We wish to remind readers that we are indeed animals and disrupt a speciest hierarchy.

Welfare v. Rights v. Liberation

Supporters of an animal *welfare* position believe that human animals have the right to use non-human animals for food, as pets, and as exhibits in zoos, but must treat NHA humanely. A welfare position generally supports and reifies the values and institutions of the status quo and does not offer an ideological shift. Animal *rights* supporters, on the other hand, believe that NHA have inherent rights apart from their value to human animals. Animal rights supporters believe that NHA should NOT! be used for food, entertainment, or as subjects of medical and cosmetic testing. As Gary Francione asserts, the goal of the movement should be to "abolish all institutional exploitation" of animals.[16] This position is a direct challenge to economic establishments, as well as to sociocultural traditions. The largest animal rights organization, People for the Ethical Treatment of Animals (PETA), encourages educational outreach, fosters direct action, and produces media campaigns.

Carrying the position that NHA should be freed from exploitation to its logical conclusion, members of animal *liberation* groups, such as the Animal Liberation Front (ALF), break into research facilities that utilize NHA to destroy equipment and free the NHA into private adoptive homes or sanctuaries. Operations of this sort are necessarily covert and membership lists are not available. The ALF website nevertheless contains a guestbook where supporters can offer comments and in many cases names and emails. As of June 2010, there were 10,016,624 entries in the guestbook.

Our main interest here will be diet—vegetarianism and veganism. A vegetarian is a person who abstains from eating NHA flesh of any kind. A vegan goes further, abstaining from eating anything made from NHA. Thus, a vegan does not consume eggs and dairy foods. Going beyond dietary veganism, "lifestyle" vegans also refrain from using leather, wool, or any NHA-derived ingredient.

We have chosen to focus on diet for two reasons. First, as we are interested in comparing organic movement rhetoric with vegetarian/vegan movement rhetoric, a focus on food allows for a consistent, logical frame for comparing dietary messages and appeals. Second, of all the issues of concern for animal activists, a focus on animals used for food arguably should be primary, because the torture and ultimate death of food animals comprises 97 percent of animal deaths caused by humans.[17]

Vegetarian/Vegan Campaigns

Turning to vegetarian/vegan campaigns, we discuss two recent PETA videos. As testament to the organization's growth, the original PETA has launched three new websites designed to target various age groups: PETA KIDS for the elementary school set; PETA2 for teens; and PETA Prime for mature adults. In December 2011, PETA plans to launch a pornographic version of their website, PETA.xxx. Under the xxx domain PETA will showcase its sexy campaign ads and videos.[18] PETA's main website, www. peta.org, hosts sixteen "channels" on PETA TV. These include a range of animal rights topics and, of most relevance here, "Vegetarianism." The "Vegetarian" channel is further divided into four video search and organizational schemes. We primarily are interested in the "Most Popular" category and will focus on the top two videos: "Grace: PETA's Thanksgiving Ad" and "Emily Deschanel's Veggie Testimonial."

In "Grace," the Thanksgiving scene is set when a middle-class, white, three-generational family hug one another as they take their seats at the dining room table. The youngest girl is asked if she would like to say grace. The family members close their eyes, fold their hands in prayer, and lean toward the table. The young, innocent girl begins her prayer:

> Dear God, thank you for the turkey we're about to eat and for the turkey farms where they pack them into dark tiny little sheds for their whole lives. Thank you for when they burn their feathers off while they are still alive and for when turkey gets kicked around like a football and killed by people who think it's fun to stomp on their little turkey heads. And special thanks for all the chemicals and dirt and poop that's in the turkey we're about to eat.

At this point the camera focuses on the turkey on the table with the text, "This Thanksgiving be thankful you're not a turkey." The young girl concludes the prayer: "And oh yeah, thank you for rainbows. Amen. Let's eat." By this point the family members have opened their eyes, unclasped their hands, and sat erect in their chairs, while regarding one another in confusion, shock, and disgust. In the final scene as the girl says, "Amen. Let's eat," the text, "Go Veg. PETA," appears on screen. Noticeably, the girl is the only one who reaches for a serving of food; the rest of the family looks away from the table with ruined appetites.

In the number two spot of PETA's most popular videos is "Emily Deschanel's Vegetarian Testimonial." With a smoggy urban landscape (presumably Los Angeles) behind her, Emily Deschanel delivers her message:

There is no such thing as a meat eating environmentalist. Nowadays being green is very fashionable, especially in Hollywood. While I think it is terrific to recycle and drive a hybrid, you can have an even greater impact on the environment by making one simple choice: don't eat meat. According to a recent UN report on climate change, the meat industry is the largest producer of green house gases. That's more than all the transportation in the world combined. Fight climate change with diet change. I'm Emily Deschanel and I'm a vegan.

As Deschanel delivers her thirty-second environmental/animal rights message several screens of written text accompany her verbal message. The first reads, "Emily Deschanel. PETA." The second is an image of the recycle logo (three arrows forming a circle). As she delivers the line, "don't eat meat," the statement "Meat's not green" appears. When she references the UN report we see a green background with different black and white documentary style photographs of factory farms with the single word, "pollution." Following that display is another display with a green background, including a picture of a plate and a portion of raw, red meat encircled with an SUV, cargo ship, train, semi-truck, and a plane. The final image is simply "peta.org."

ANALYSIS

To repeat, we are trying to address the question, Why is there not as much support for the vegetarian/vegan movement as for the organic food movement? The simplest answer may be that it is more difficult to be vegetarian/vegan than to eat organic food. The vegetarian/vegan lifestyle could be construed as "giving up" meat. Public address about "sacrifice" sometimes does not resonate in the US, which may be one reason that President Jimmy Carter faced a difficult rhetorical challenge during the 1979 energy crisis. During his "Crisis of Confidence" speech, President Carter wore a cardigan sweater and asked the American public to cut back on energy use. The appeal was not popular at the time and revealed, perhaps, the challenges inherent in asking for "sacrifice."[19]

To turn to another explanation, a rhetoric of "deficiency" also could be a factor in holding back the vegetarian/vegan movement. For example, a *TIME* magazine article, "Should We All Be Vegetarians?," raised the *fear* of dietary *deficiencies*.[20] The article reported that vegans, especially, might have to contend with calcium deficiency. Calcium deficiency, in turn, is linked to *permanent* conditions, like osteoporosis. This chain of argumentation is not without flaws, but it still has persuasive pull.

Another line of reasoning that might explain the differences between the vegetarian/vegan movement and the organic movement is that the former may be a newer form of social movement, emphasizing identity shift and

cultural change, whereas the latter may be a more traditional social movement, a political and economic movement.[21] In the language of the present
study, the organic movement has politics on its plate, whereas the vegetar-
ian/vegan movement has identity shift on its plate. According to Wendy
Atkins-Sayre, "successful appeals to identity shifts emphasize the familiarity of the new identity—the shared qualities—in order to invite a questioning of the lines of division."[22] Potential adherents to the vegetarian/vegan
movement could "play up" the similarities with non-human animals, that
is, "emphasize consubstantiality."[23] When compared to the organic movement, where purchasing food is a political act, the process of identity shift
requires some additional cognitive and emotional steps.

As we continue to explore the question—Why is there not as much support
for the vegetarian/vegan movement as for the organic food movement?—
Freeman and Johnson and Stewart, Smith, and Denton provide useful perspectives on the stages of social movements that might help frame another
answer. Jo Freeman and Victoria Johnson suggest that social movements
go through five stages: (1) Mobilization, (2) Organization, (3) Consciousness, (4) Strategy and tactics, and (5) Decline.[24] Similarly, Charles Stewart,
Craig Allen Smith, and Robert Denton offer the five stages of (1) Genesis,
(2) Social Unrest, (3) Enthusiastic Mobilization, (4) Maintenance, and (5)
Termination.[25] Using these frameworks to compare the organic food movement with the vegan movement, we conclude that when compared to animal rights, the organic movement may not be a movement at all!

Let us adopt, for a moment, Kenneth Burke's tactic of "perspective by
incongruity."[26] We have been treating the organic food movement as a
strong and more mature social movement and the vegan movement as a
weaker social movement. From this more conventional point of view, the
vegetarian/vegan movement is not as strong in public discourse, because
"As a rule, media coverage of an emerging social movement is either highly
restrained or nonexistent until the movement has been legitimized in the
system."[27] But if the organic food movement is NOT a social movement
then our whole analysis would change. According to Stewart, Smith, and
Denton, "If a social movement maintains an effective organization and its
principles come to match current conventions and practices, it may become
the new order . . . The movement may become the new institution."[28] Pollan
portrays the social history of the organic food movement as running from
granola, to the upper-middle class, and now to the masses.[29] The fact that
organic foods are sold in three-quarters of conventional supermarkets is
testament to the success and, perhaps, the ultimate end of the organic cause
as a social movement.

When a movement has reached its final stage—be it "termination" or
"decline"—"the reformers and revolutionaries of movement days become
the priests of the new order or institution and must perform pastoral functions."[30] Tom Philpott, a featured speaker at the 2008 "Organic Summit,"
humorously refers to this regime change in the book *What White People*

Like, noting that upper-middle-class individuals have replaced church/ mosque/synagogue with farmers' markets and organic food.[31] The growth in farmers' markets suggests there are many such new churches, mosques, and synagogues: According to the USDA in 2010 there were 6,132 farmers' markets in operation in the US, an increase of 16 percent from 2009. Going back to 1994, the first year the USDA began publishing the National Directory of Farmers' Markets, there were 1,755 markets in operation. Our claim that the organic movement has become mainstream and institutionalized is supported by two facts: (a) the number of farmers' markets has more than tripled in only sixteen years and (b) the USDA now is involved in farmers' markets.

We argue that, no longer a social movement, organic has been co-opted as a marketing niche. Many consumers do not have a well-developed consciousness with respect to organic food. Susanne Padel and Carolyn Foster report that consumers vaguely associate organic food with fruits and vegetables.[32] Consumers also loosely connect organic food to health. Gianluigi Guido found that the adjectives used to describe organic food were in two clusters: (a) tasty, good, cheerful, and energetic and (b) genuine, natural, and healthy.[33] Betsy McKay contends that spending the extra money for organic food makes sense only in some circumstances, for example, when one eats a lot of certain types of produce.[34] With respect to the argument that the organic food movement may not anymore be a movement, what is noteworthy about McKay's article is the almost total absence of ethical issues and a moral tone. The article offers common sense advice and business wisdom. The article seems to revolve around consumerism and "value" for the dollar. Whereas one might expect the *Wall Street Journal* to publish this type of account, the article reinforces the concept that the organic food movement is not a social movement, but is one aspect of the purchasing decisions of the consumer who wishes to appear sophisticated.

The move from "movement" to "marketing niche" is reflective of Robert Cathcart's distinction between rhetoric that is managerial versus rhetoric that is confrontational and agitative.[35] The latter is based on vertical versus lateral deviance, according to Bowers, Ochs, Jenson, and Schulz.[36] Rhetorics that are managerial "are designed to keep the existing system viable: they do not question the underlying epistemology and group ethic."[37] Similarly agitation based on vertical deviance "occurs when agitators accept the value system of the establishment but dispute the distribution of benefits or power within that value system."[38] As has long been the case with organic, and evidenced on the current OCA website, "the rhetoric is primarily concerned with adjusting the existing order, not rejecting it. The reformist campaign stays inside the value structures of its existing order and speaks with the same vocabularies of motive as do the conservative elements in the order."[39] The self-defined description of the OCA, "Campaigning for health, justice, sustainability, peace, and democracy," reflects the managerial nature of their rhetoric. The website's persuasive language is "relatively direct and easily understood ideologically."[40] Moreover, in cases of vertical deviance the movement attempts to achieve its goals by making the case to members of the establishment and the agitation "usually ends when the establishment makes the appropriate concessions or adjustments to the demands."[41] In the case of organic we see this relationship between agitation and the establishment in multiple ways: the long established tactic of taking the organic cause directly to the government for labeling and regulation, the appeals to science as authority during the Alar scare, and the use of the mainstream media (*60 Minutes*) to publicize, polarize, and mobilize consumers.

Understanding the organic cause as managerial also suggests it belongs in the classification of innovational movement as well, because these groups act "with the expectation that the changes it demands will not disturb the symbols and constraints of existing values or modify the social hierarchy."[42] The distinction between managerial/innovational and confrontational is relevant not simply because it allows us to correctly classify contemporary organic movement rhetoric, but because of what the classification implies about subsequent strategies.

A critical reading of the website of the Organic Consumers Association reveals that the underlying paradigm is based on a target audience of the "consumer." This and other evidence suggest that the organic food movement is no longer countercultural, but may have been co-opted by an even more dominant paradigm—the Market. In an interview for the book *Global Values 101*, Harvey Cox stated: "I did not see any religious movement or other kind of movement that could challenge the enormous power that the market—the market as God—seems to have acquired in our time and our society."[43] This blunt assertion, one that places a theological spin on Karl Polanyi's position that the market has become the dominant contemporary institution, was accompanied by a poignant cry: "Is there anything in the world, anything at all, that should be excluded from the category of commodity?"[44] With Cox, we also see the awesome power of the market, a market that is not a metaphor for God, but is worshipped as God-like.

Even the Alar scare, which some count as the beginning of the modern organic movement,[45] can be seen in market terms. Or Deschanel's critique, that buying a hybrid isn't enough, points to the use of a market-driven strategy that links purchasing hybrids with saving the environment. The organic battle over "tolerances" in exposure to chemicals, as well as the framing of the debate in terms of risk management, seems to fall within a market-based perspective, rather than a social movement worldview.

When a movement has succeeded in becoming part of the establishment, "the movement-turned institution will face a new generation of reformers and revolutionaries who become dissatisfied with the new order."[46] In the case of organic, current public discourse reveals a concern that, if not running out of gas, the organic movement is being transformed. Some commentators are worried about the direction of that transformation. Michael Pollan offers a warning about Wal-Mart taking the organic movement to the mass level:

> Organic is just a word, after all, and its definition now lies in the hands of the federal government, which means it is subject to all the usual political and economic forces at play in Washington. Inevitably, the drive to produce organic food cheaply will bring pressure to further weaken the regulations, and some of K Street's finest talent will soon be on the case. A few years ago a chicken producer in Georgia named Fieldale Farms persuaded its congressman to slip a helpful provision into an appropriations bill that would allow growers of organic chicken to substitute conventional chicken feed if the price of organic feed exceeded a certain level. That certainly makes life easier for a chicken producer when the price of organic corn is north of $5 a bushel, as it is today, and conventional corn south of $2. But in what sense is a chicken fed on conventional feed still organic? In no sense but the Orwellian one: because the government says it is.[47]

The term "organic," which took more than ten years of social activism to define, now may be only a government and big business label.

Confrontational rhetoric, in contrast to managerial rhetoric, "emanates from outside the system."[48] "Lateral deviance" is the phrase for the actions and rhetoric that occur "when the agitators dispute the value system itself and seek to change or replace it with a competing value system."[49] Francione contends that "we may be said to suffer from a sort of moral schizophrenia"[50] with respect to our thinking about animals. As the young girl in the PETA video says grace, she speaks to the large disparity between what we say about animals and how we treat them. She directly confronts the disjuncture between words and deeds and offers up a confrontational solution, "go veg," from outside the system: PETA.

Giving voice to the turkey's experience in her shocking prayer, she reminds her family of burning the turkey's feathers off while they are still alive, kicking the turkey around like a football, stomping on their little turkey heads and of all the "poop" in the turkey they are about to eat. With this rhetorical move she literally confronts her family and symbolically confronts the entire meat-eating culture:

> The enactment of confrontation gives a movement its identity, its substance and its form. No movement for radical change can be taken seriously without acts of confrontation. The system co-opts all actions which do not question the basic order, and transforms them into system messages. Confrontational rhetoric shouts "Stop!" at the system, saying, "You cannot go on assuming you are the true and correct order; you must see yourself as the evil things you are."[51]

And as the family members cringe, and nonverbally position themselves to reject the food, we see that she has succeeded in telling them to "Stop."

In our fourth artifact, wherein Deschanel presented her message in the form and style iconic of the public service announcement, there was one key difference. Unable to get television air time because PETA was rejected by all major networks, PETA had to "air" its commercials on its website to a very limited audience rather than on television to a more general public. In this way, the message emanates from outside the system, consistent with Cathcart's view of confrontational rhetoric. The substance of Deschanel's message also confronts the portion of the public that would identify as green or environmentally concerned. Specifically telling viewers that you cannot call yourself an "environmentalist" and continue eating meat, she names the contradiction. In this rhetorical challenge to the status quo, she identifies the hypocrisy of the environmental movement and argues that you cannot make social change through consumer purchases alone (i.e., buying a hybrid).

Yet, as a mainstream media celebrity, Deschanel herself can be seen through the lens of a managerial rhetoric. Thus, this text is significant in that it suggests a confrontational message wrapped in a managerial package! The last line in the testimonial, "I'm Emily Deschanel and I'm a vegan," is significant because it summarizes this relationship: I look like your average beautiful celebrity on the outside but I am a radical on the inside.

CONCLUSION

If the organic movement has been so successful that it faces "losing its soul," what are the lessons for the vegetarian/vegan movement? If "organic" has reached the terminal stage of social movements, then whither shall the vegetarian/vegan movement go next? At present, mired in conflicting strategies, the future of the vegetarian/vegan movement is not easy to predict.

If the movement follows the path of the organic movement, then conventional logic suggests that vegans might want to campaign for a clear certification process and for labeling: "Meat free!" We already are accustomed to seeing in motion pictures the disclaimer that "No animals were hurt in the making of this film." The organic movement gained strength by promoting standards and labeling. One could argue that the organic movement actually was a labeling movement that co-opted the communication networks of farmers and the US Department of Agriculture. Vegetarians and vegans inclined to take this route may note that we also have seen successful campaigns against growth hormones in cow's milk that have resulted in the "RBST Free" label, as well as labels proclaiming "gluten-free" and "dairy-free." In the short-term, more vegan activism around labels might strengthen the movement. However, there are other plausible, alternative futures.

Lyle Munro, writing from the perspective of the lived experiences of animal protectionists, notes that "a feature of the politics of animal protection is the tendency towards organizational specialization, which means that organizations often work on single issues . . ."[52] Thus, we often see quite specific calls or campaigns in public discourse, such as to "Save the whales!" The vegan movement might find it challenging to overcome this type of specificity in food and lifestyle advocacy with broader framing.

Erik Marcus indirectly offers the vegan movement yet another alternative. With reference to animal rights, Marcus calls for "an all-new movement . . . one that is specifically designed to weaken and ultimately eliminate animal agriculture."[53] He calls this new movement the "Dismantlement Movement": a third way, beyond welfarism and beyond animal rights. Begging the question if one can start a movement and create a consciousness with organization and not too much spontaneity,[54] can the vegan movement create a brand new movement to fit its particular ideology?

Another voice, Bruce Friedrich (who is an official with PETA), suggests that veganism is about reducing suffering.[55] Veganism is not a dogma. For Friedrich, the key is for vegans to live their values. His set of values includes: opposition to human exploitation, environmentalism, healthy living, and kindness.[56] These values are to be enacted each day, with all the human and non-human animals that one meets.

We can see what "kindness" as a value in everyday life looks like in the lives, for example, of members of the Society of Friends (Quakers). Kindness may be seen in a barn-raising or in the stance of pacifism. Kindness is interpersonal in one sense; kindness is political in another sense. As veganism embodies kindness, Friedrich seems to argue, it will help reduce the suffering of animals and also will attract interest and converts.

Similar to Friedrich's value called "kindness," Joanne Stepaniak proposes a value called "dynamic harmlessness."[57] In fact, Stepaniak offers a code of vegan ethics: (1) Vegans are sensitive to issues of suffering, (2) Vegans value awareness of all life forms, (3) Vegans adjure violence, and (4) Vegans expand the principle of harmlessness.[58] She argues that food is just one aspect of being vegan.[59] Therefore, one can distinguish between vegan living as opposed to the "dietary vegan."

If one broadens veganism beyond dietary veganism, then the social movement is more than a food movement. The broader social movement could be said to center around the values of kindness, compassion, and dynamic harmlessness. As Stepaniak points out, this version of the vegan movement is akin to the philosophy of Mahatma Gandhi. Gandhi, however, saw his philosophy linked to anti-colonialism, independence, and nationalism. One might wonder if veganism will forge similar links, appropriate for the twenty-first century.

Lawrence Finsen and Susan Finsen see ecofeminism as a powerful force for opposing domination of all sorts.[60] They suggest that feminists and civil rights activists may be natural allies for the animal rights movement and, by extension, the vegan movement. Or as Deschanel suggests in "Testimony," there are powerful relationships between environmentalism and animal rights.

In conclusion, we have offered several answers to the question, Why is there not as much support for the vegetarian/vegan movement as for the organic food movement? It would be a mistake for the reader to think that we are advocating one viewpoint. All of the perspectives discussed in this study are found in contemporary public discourse. Some are explicit and some are implicit in the four examples cited in this chapter. In all likelihood, the multiple perspectives, taken together, have considerable explanatory power. In fact, exploring the intersection of these perspectives in public discourse about food, and the tensions among them, may lead not only to a better understanding but also to possible courses of action.

ACKNOWLEDGMENTS

The authors would like to thank Joshua Frye and the anonymous reviewers for their helpful comments on earlier drafts of this chapter.

NOTES

1. Michael Pollan, *The Omnivore's Dilemma: A Natural History of Four Meals* (New York: Penguin, 2006), 143.
2. Thomas Frank, "Why Johnny Can't Dissent," in *Commodify Your Dissent: Salvos from the Baffler*, ed. Thomas Frank and Matt Weiland (New York: W. W. Norton and Company, 1997), 34.
3. Joseph Heckman, "A History of Organic Farming: Transitions from Sir Albert Howard's War in the Soil to the USDA National Organic Program" (*Weston A. Price Foundation* for Wise Traditions, 2007), accessed September 15, 2010, http://www.westonaprice.org/farm-a-ranch/history-of-organic-farming
4. Pollan, *Omnivore's Dilemma*; Craig J. Thompson and Gokcen Coskuner-Balli, "Countervailing Market Responses to Corporate Co-optation and the Ideological Recruitment of Consumption Commodities," *Journal of Consumer Research* 34 (2007): 135–36.
5. Nanette Hansen, "Organic Food Sales See Healthy Growth," *MSNBC*, September 4, 2011, accessed September 15, 2011, http://www.msnbc.com/id/6638471.
6. Melanie Warner, "What Is Organic? Powerful Players Want a Say," *New York Times*, November 1, 2005, Business Section.
7. Catherine Greene and Carolyn Dimitri, "Organic Agriculture Gaining Ground," *USDA Economic Research Service*, September 2002, accessed October 15, 2010, http://usda.gov/publications/aib7771.
8. *Annual Stakeholders Report*, 2008, 10.
9. Michael Pollan, "Naturally," *New York Times*, May 13, 2001, section 6, 30, accessed October 11, 2010, LexisNexis.
10. Philip Shabecoff, "Apple Industry Says It Will End Use of Chemical," *New York Times*, May 16, 1989, A1, accessed October 11, 2010, LexisNexis.

11. "One Bad Apple," *PRWatch*, The Center for Media and Democracy, 2nd quarter 1997, vol. 4, no. 2, accessed September 7, 2011, www.prwatch.org/prwissues/1997Q2/alar.html.
12. This estimate comes from www.museum.tv/archives.
13. David Shaw, "Alar Panic Shows Power of Media to Trigger Fear," *Los Angeles Times*, September 12, 1994, A19, accessed October 11, 2010, http://articles.latimes.com/keyword/alar.
14. Peter Singer, *Animal Liberation: A New Ethics for Our Treatment of Animals* (New York: Avon, 1975), 7.
15. Carrie Packwood Freeman, "Embracing Humananimality: Deconstructing the Human/Animal Dichotomy," in *Arguments about Animal Ethics*, ed. Greg Goodale and J. E. Black (Lanhman, MD: Lexington, 2010), 11.
16. Gary L. Francione, *Rain without Thunder: The Ideology of the Animal Rights Movement* (Philadelphia: Temple University Press, 1996/2005 with corrections), 149–50.
17. Erik Marcus, *Meat Market: Animals, Ethics, and Money* (Boston: Brio Press, 2005), 83.
18. Tara Kelly, "PETA's Porn Website to Promote Vegetarian Message," *Huffington Post*, September 21, 2011, accessed October 4, 2011, http://www.huffingtonpost.com/2011/09/21/peta-plans-porn-website_n_972497.html.
19. "Is He Serious," *New Republic*, December 28, 1979, 179, 2.
20. Richard Corliss et al., "Should We All Be Vegetarians?," *Time Magazine*, July 15, 2002, accessed October 18, 2010, www.time.com/magazine/article.
21. Wendy Atkins-Sayre, "Articulating Identity: People for the Ethical Treatment of Animals and the Animal/Human Divide," *Western Journal of Communication* 74 (2010): 311.
22. Atkins-Sayre, "Articulating Identity," 314.
23. Ibid., 325.
24. Jo Freeman and Victoria Johnson, eds., *Waves of Protest* (Lanham, MD: Littlefield, 1999).
25. Charles J. Stewart, Craig A. Smith, and Robert E. Denton, *Persuasion and Social Movements* (Long Grove, IL: Waveland, 2007).
26. Kenneth Burke, *Attitudes Toward History* (Berkeley, CA: University of California Press, 1984).
27. Susan Dente Ross, "Their Rising Voices: A Study of Civil Rights, Social Movements, and Advertising in 'The New York Times,'" *Journalism and Mass Communication Quarterly* 75 (1998): 518.
28. Stewart, Smith, and Denton, *Persuasion and Social Movements*, 104.
29. Pollan, *Omnivore's Dilemma*.
30. Stewart, Smith, and Denton, *Persuasion and Social Movements*, 104.
31. Tom Philpott, "Not Just for White People Anymore: How the Organic Movement Can Regain Its Relevance," *Grist*, June 27, 2008, accessed September 30, 2010, www.grist.org.
32. Susanne Padel and Carolyn Foster, "Exploring the Gap between Attitudes and Behaviour: Understanding Why Consumers Buy or Do Not Buy Organic Food," *British Food Journal* 107/108 (2005): 606–25.
33. Gianluigi Guido, *Behind Ethical Consumption: Purchasing Motives and Marketing Strategies for Organic Food Products, Non-GMOs, Biofuels* (Bern; New York: Peter Lang, 2009), 61.
34. Betsy McKay, "When Buying Organic Makes Sense and When It Doesn't," *Wall Street Journal*, Eastern Edition, January 16, 2007, 249/12, D1–D2.
35. Robert Cathcart, "Movements, Confrontation as Rhetorical Form," in *Readings on the Rhetoric of Social Protest*, ed. Charles E. Morris III and Stephen H. Browne (State College, PA: Strata, 1978), 95–103.

36. John W. Bowers et al., *The Rhetoric of Agitation and Control*, 5th ed. (Long, Grove, IL: Waveland, 2009).
37. Cathcart, "Movements, Confrontation," 97.
38. Bowers et al., *The Rhetoric of Agitation and Control*, 7.
39. Cathcart, "Movements, Confrontation," 97.
40. Bowers et al., *The Rhetoric of Agitation and Control*, 7.
41. Ibid.
42. Ralph R. Smith and Russell Windes, "The Innovational Movement: A Rhetorical Theory," in *Readings on the Rhetoric of Social Protest*, ed. Charles E. Morris III and Stephen H. Browne (State College, PA: Strata, 1975), 85.
43. Kate Holbrook, *Global Values 101: A Short Course* (Boston: Beacon Press, 2006), 210.
44. Ibid., 216.
45. Pollan, "Naturally," 30.
46. Stewart, Smith, and Denton, *Persuasion and Social Movements*, 104.
47. Pollan, "Naturally," 30.
48. Cathcart, "Movements, Confrontation," 96.
49. Bowers et al., *The Rhetoric of Agitation and Control*, 7.
50. Gary L. Francione, *Introduction to Animal Rights: Your Child or the Dog?* (Philadelphia: Temple University Press, 2000), xxi.
51. Cathcart, "Movements, Confrontation," 100.
52. Lyle Munro, *Confronting Cruelty: Moral Orthodoxy and the Challenge of Animal Rights* (Leiden; Boston: Brill, 2005), 93.
53. Marcus, *Meat Market*, 79.
54. Freeman and Johnson, *Waves of Protest*.
55. Bruce Friedrich, "Effective Advocacy: Stealing from the Corporate Playbook," in *In Defense of Animals: The Second Wave*, ed. Peter Singer (Malden, MA; Oxford: Blackwell Publishing, 2006), 191.
56. Bruce Friedrich, "A Vegan Lifestyle Is Necessary to Stop the Mistreatment of Animals," in *The Rights of Animals*, ed. Debra A. Miller (Detroit: Greenhaven Press, 2009), 121.
57. Joanne Stepaniak, *The Vegan Sourcebook* (Los Angeles: Lowell House, 1998), 2.
58. Ibid., 13.
59. Ibid., 113–14.
60. Lawrence Finsen and Susan Finsen, *The Animal Rights Movement in America: From Compassion to Respect* (New York: Twayne Publishers, 1994), 252.

4 "Food Talk"
Bridging Power in a Globalizing World

John R. Thompson

It is difficult to avoid the proliferation of food discourse around us. It comes in the form of food media in TV and films and numerous food blogs dotting the Internet. Farmer's markets preach the benefits of "eating local" and can be found sprouting up everywhere. Grocery stores sell a narrative with their fish, meat, and vegetables, recognizing that many twenty-first century consumers moralize their food purchases. Everyday headlines recount food riots, food safety breaches in the industrialized system, and someone's favorite blending of ethnic cuisine with local ingredients. Food-based social movements such as Slow Food blend the local with the global to rally everyone around a multicultural potluck of public address.

Food supplies a language for many motives in our current milieu. Mary Eberstadt explored the reversal of social mores between food and sex over the last few decades.[1] James McWilliams deployed food talk as a means of indicting at least some new food movements.[2] The United Nations Food Program simultaneously lobbies on behalf of the hungry in many localities while also driving a homogenizing global food regime through the Codex Alimentarius, a way of categorizing food that removes culture from its description. Punks in Seattle use food to protest a wasteful hierarchical capitalist food system,[3] whereas the Southern Foodways Alliance talks of food on its website as a racial and geographic healer, "a common table where black and white, rich and poor—all who gather—may consider our history and our future in a spirit of reconciliation."[4]

Put simply, food rhetoric is not the province of a single worldview and, indeed, makes for some strange dining companions. Much scholarly ink has been spilled in the category of food studies, but more is afoot here than the flowering of an academic topic. Numerous authors have carved a genre at the border of scholarly and popular literature that creates overnight bestsellers about food.[5] Cultural and media critics and their more popularized incarnations have used these food discourses to assay many aspects of the social world. Like many, I am a fan of their work.

Yet, it is difficult to explain the existence of any sub-genre of this discourse without a self-reflective turn back to the explosion of discourse (e.g., food safety is big news because we are concerned about where our food comes from as evidenced by eat local movements and the like). So, this chapter's highest (and possibly unattainable) goal is to begin teasing out an explanation for why food talk has become so dominant in so many genres in such a short time— without relying on a circular explanation. To understand food talk, then, I hope to step at least somewhat outside it.

Food talk. You likely read right past the term in the previous paragraph. It so captures this discursive milieu *of, about, and articulated through* food that its uniqueness is easily overlooked. This chapter takes that phrase seriously. Food talk is rising as a first language of political and cultural claims-making and is crossing many boundaries and topics. In that light, food talk is similar to the emergence of rights talk in the twentieth century. Rights talk became a *first language* for political claims-making, a set of rhetorical elements with an inventory of meanings[6] by which individuals positioned themselves—and others—in a world organized by a nation-state system. Food talk bears similarities to rights talk. My goal here is not to claim that the entire inventory of meanings embodied in food talk is completely developed, only that changing conditions—writ largely as *globalization*—are driving us to grope once again for a language of identification and agency.

By reading food talk against rights talk, I argue that a rhetorical homology links twenty-first-century food talk with twentieth-century rights talk. That homology involves a discursive building block of *fundamental identity*. By adding the modifier "fundamental" to Kenneth Burke's notion of all rhetoric relating to identification,[7] I mean to indicate a primitive discursive structure that necessarily emerges at times of change in the social and political organization of the world. *Fundamental identity* serves to locate the individual in a moment of change, providing resources for navigating that change and relating to others in that moment.

To illustrate fundamental identity at work in our current milieu, I will briefly explore one grammatical unit of this food talk, the popular phrase "eat local." In that analysis, I will argue that the rhetorical key to understanding "eat local" and the discourses built upon it lies in the "eat" rather than the "local" as is often assumed. "Eat local," I argue, is an act-based grammar that builds on this fundamental identity structure, laying the foundation for a generative bottom-up politics of a globalized era. Put another way, the eater is hunting for agency in a globalized world.

A globalized world, however, is a big place with many forces and definitions of globalization with which to contend. So, I begin with a brief outline of my approach to globalization.

GLOBALIZATION, DISCURSIVE HISTORY, AND RHETORICAL HOMOLOGIES

This section's goals are to briefly sketch an approach to globalization rooted in the work of Kenneth Burke and then to position Barry Brummett's concept of the rhetorical homology—itself derived from Burke—as a tool to link the emergence of twentieth-century rights talk with twenty-first-century food talk.[8] Before making that link, I want to acknowledge that the word *globalization* covers a great deal of territory and the first task is to wrestle it onto a rhetorical playing field.

It is difficult to reduce globalization to a single force—be it economic, cultural, political, or colored by new immigration, new communications technologies, or other phenomena. Globalization entails all these things, much like a many-headed beast possesses a plethora of brains and snapping jaws extending from a single body. Scholars tend to study the pieces by deploying the language of our various disciplines, languages that highlight one set of snapping jaws over others (i.e., economists speak of globalization in economic terms, anthropologists in cultural terms, etc.).

I mean to sidestep the snapping jaws here and make a stab at the body of the beast. *Globalization* describes a set of changing conditions that transcend the nation-state as the fundamental organizing unit of the world. According to Anthony Giddens, "Globalization has something to do with the thesis that we now all live in one world."[9] Risks, problems, culture, markets, and virtually everything else have escaped the control of the nation-state and democratic processes. Attending that *notion* is the real, perceived, and increasing inadequacy of the ways we have talked about a world that was safely sub-divided into nation-states, political units that could mediate our positions, relationships, responsibilities, and rights as we strut the planet. This inadequacy shows up in a variety of forms. For instance, critic Nancy Fraser has observed the need for a new "grammar" of justice enabling the discussion of issues that are global in scope "as transnational social movements contest the national frame within which justice conflicts have historically been situated."[10] Fraser wrestles with a language of justice forged within a national frame that does not scale to our new conditions.

Fraser's call is echoed elsewhere on other topics, as critics and average rhetors struggle to represent the world—and their place within it—under these changing conditions. They use a language superseded by globalizing conditions or stretched beyond its discursive limits. For instance, the language of citizenship—once effectively material in consequence in a world organized as nation-states—is often no longer adequate for securing a place in the world. Some have attempted to stretch the ideograph of <citizenship> beyond the nation-state through such grammatical units as *global citizenship* or *cosmopolitan citizenship*.[11] Yet, by relying on a nation-state grammar, these theorists must simultaneously postulate the creation of global institutions and governing layers to secure citizenship—institutions and layers that largely do not exist.

Elsewhere in America, immigration concerns have spawned the term "anchor baby" to re-fashion the political identity of children born to undocumented immigrants in the US. Whereas this particular rhetoric is wrapped in a form of nationalism, it is driven by the crumbling of borders in a globalizing, multicultural world. Even those calling for a new definition of citizenship in the US Constitution acknowledge that the location of birth is no longer an adequate marker of identity, as seen in this statement uttered by US Representative Duncan Hunter (California) at a Tea Party rally in Southern California: "And we're not being mean. We're just saying it takes more than walking across the border to become an American citizen. It's what's in our souls."[12] A similar sentiment can be found in the Bush administration's reclassification of Jose Padilla, born in Brooklyn, from the category of "citizen" to that of "enemy combatant" without constitutional rights. Where he was born, according to arguments in court papers, had no bearing on who he was. The globalizing moment trumped the well-trod discourse of citizenship found in the arguments Padilla mounted for his rights.[13]

These disjunctures occur in a rhetorical chasm, a gulf between a way of talking about the world that no longer matches underlying conditions, and a discourse that has yet to fully form to replace it. This phenomenon has been studied before in Kenneth Burke's Depression Era writings in *Permanence and Change* and *Attitudes Toward History*.[14] Burke was working to understand a world in which a "superstructure of certainties"[15] and that superstructure's attending language had toppled and no longer fit the conditions of the world.

Burke elaborated this view of individual and social disorientations under changing conditions into a discursive theory of history. Burke argued that history is divided into discursive eras where a "collective poem" or way of talking about the world arises from shared conditions and reinforces those conditions. This shared language structures people into the world. However, those conditions shift over time, forcing people to stretch their shared meanings until these meanings reach their "Malthusian limits" and fall apart because they no longer match conditions. Various shards of that collective poem vie to re-organize the world under these new conditions.[16]

Drawing on Burke, rhetorician Barry Brummett articulated a critical tool that can be used to track these shards across disjunctures. A *rhetorical homology* is a single discursive structure that generates texts across genres and time, providing "templates with which we might order our life experiences."[17]

> These discursive homologies cut across history and locations but must always be reindividuated, to use Burke's term, in texts and experiences at particular junctures of time and place. The way in which discursive structure orders text and experience is always both rhetorical and formal, always providing motives in the exigencies of the immediate moment and connecting the moment formally to other texts and experiences across time and space.[18]

The notion of the rhetorical homology helps to uncover the existence of a rhetorical building block that provides the starting point for different discursive genres at different times and places and under different conditions. It is a linkage between discourses in much the same way that a given Lego piece could be used to construct a robot in one construction kit or a Harry Potter diorama in another. However different the ultimate constructions, they are held together by certain underlying commonalities and the rules attending those commonalities. In Brummett's terms, the building blocks might be used differently depending on just what life experiences require ordering.

To bring this full circle, arguing the existence of a rhetorical homology linking disparate discourses across two centuries—one dominated by nation-states and the second giving way to increasingly globalized politics, economics, and transnational cultures—is to track one of the shards of the disintegrating discourse as it connects with new conditions. To have impact, that shard must be elaborated into a discourse ordering the relevant life experiences lived under new conditions.

For the purposes of the current argument, *fundamental identity* is a discursive structure elaborated into rights talk in one era and food talk in the next. As Burke argued that identification is the fundamental aim of rhetoric—even beyond persuasion—it follows that fundamental identity would be a building block of discursive eras groping toward consolidating a collective poem through which to organize the social world.

FUNDAMENTAL IDENTITY IN TWO ERAS

I recognize that in some fashion I am comparing the public rhetoric of the civil rights movement with that of food bloggers writing about last night's dinner. Nevertheless, to argue the existence of a rhetorical homology is not to claim that each utterance is equivalent on all points or to collapse different genres of texts into a single category. Indeed, rhetorical homology has been used to link texts that possess significant differences or are located on radically disparate nodes of the Left/Right political spectrum.[19]

Reading rights talk and food talk against each other results in a rhetorical homology that might be phrased like so: Nation-state citizens adopted the language of what Michael Schudson called the "rights-bearing citizen" to orient themselves in the shifting sands of the twentieth century.[20] As globalizing forces in the twenty-first century supersede the rights-guaranteeing nation-state, individuals are reasserting a vernacular rhetoric of fundamental identity—but under significantly altered conditions. With no clear entity, such as a nation-state, charged with guaranteeing a position in such a supranational system, the fundamental identity being asserted is arguably the most fundamental possible: We are all eaters. The everyday act of eating (along with the many practices of cooking, shopping, gardening, etc. that it entails) provides a set of symbolic elements from which this discursive structure can usefully emerge.

The most direct description of rights talk as a discourse of fundamental identity comes from Schudson's tracing of the meaning of American citizenship through the decades. Schudson cast the late-twentieth-century milieu in which he wrote as the time of the "rights-bearing citizen," a definition and discourse of what it meant to be an American citizen.[21] Yet, this definition of fundamental identity was not invented out of whole cloth, as Schudson himself noted. It was a re-individuation of fundamental American identity that followed from the "informed citizen" of the progressive era. One of the benefits of this elaboration of fundamental identity was that it not only defined an individual citizen, but also provided an elaborated discourse by which one could identify "the other" (i.e., the Western development of *human rights* as a way of differentiating democracy from totalitarian regimes). Thus, the civil rights movement possessed an accepted vernacular through which America was able to atone for some sins as African-Americans and others fought for equal treatment under the law.

This shift of rights talk from a "technical language" to a vernacular rhetoric allowed fundamental identity to be articulated broadly, drawn on by disparate individuals and peoples across populations and power dynamics. As Gerald Hauser argued, such a well-spring of common rhetorical resources to discuss common problems pulls more people into a public sphere that might otherwise be dominated by institutions.[22] Rights talk not only provided a language for claims-making by many sides, but also, in so doing, proliferated fundamental identity across the many twists and turns of twentieth-century history.

Richard Primus argued that the American language of rights grew out of the need to redefine Americans as one era gave way to another.[23] The Bill of Rights, thus, was drafted as a way to define American government as something fundamentally different from the then-recent experience of British subjecthood. This theme animates rights talk through the ages as what Primus called "a process of concrete negation of past evils is a leading dynamic of change in the content of rights."[24] Likewise, a discourse of "human rights" was launched following World War II as a way of defining Western nations in opposition to totalitarianism. It was also a way for Western nations to atone for various sins, including the internment of Japanese-Americans, Jim Crowe laws, and the treatment of Jews that led up to Hitler's Final Solution. By constructing any human being as a rights-bearing entity, human rights discourse re-individuated the fundamental identity structure to a world recovering from massive war and brutal fascism while adjusting to a Cold War and the threat of nuclear annihilation. It provided the rhetorical underpinnings of the American civil rights movement and elaborated the fundamental identity structure into a global discourse.

However, Burke's "collective poem" can be stretched only so far until it reaches its Malthusian limits. Conditions ultimately change beyond the scope of the discourses that organize the world. Globalizing forces have de-centered the nation-state's role in creating identity and agency. What was once so certain is now so fluid. We live in a world with more moving parts than we have had for some time, what Arjun Appadurai described as "a general rupture in the tenor of intersocietal relations,"[25] Jurgen Habermas called a "time of transitions,"[26] and Michael Hardt and Antonio Negri described as a transition to an *empire* of capital.[27] However described, I contend that as part of this reformulation of the world, fundamental identity as a discursive building block is finding a new expression, and it is emerging in the proliferation of food discourses.

Identity and food have been bound together in numerous eras. For instance, Mary Douglas argued that a Hebrew view of racial and cultural purity intersected the daily practice of preparing food and eating, ultimately producing kosher rules. To reach to my notion of fundamental identity, change is important.[28] Appadurai wrote about Indian cookbooks that circulate only within India in an effort to promote the many regional cuisines of that diverse nation into the convergence of an Indian national identity as India takes a greater role in the world.[29] Richard Wilk observed the Central American nation of Belize (formerly British Honduras) struggling to recover an indigenous cuisine to throw off the taint of generations of British occupation and reassert a fundamental identity.[30]

This notion that food intersects with identity can be found in popular media as well, and it takes on the character of a globalizing world. Elizabeth Rosenthal wrote in *The New York Times* of the erosion of the so-called Mediterranean Diet in the very Mediterranean Basin that spawned this healthy and luxurious combination of vegetables, legumes, meats, fish, and red wine.[31] A new generation of youth, according to Rosenthal, is eating fast-food hamburgers in an attempt to assert a globalized identity separate from their parents and ancestors. Elsewhere, the *Times* also reported on new immigrants to New York City and the many ways they adapt their daily food regimens to strike a hybrid identity, straddling the city they live in and the culture they come from.

> Most families had been forced by necessity to come up with short versions of their cuisine. Many had settled on bastardizations of American classics. A popular dish, for example, is spaghetti and meatballs, but Koreans served it with kimchi on the side, while some Kenyans cut hot red peppers into theirs. Just as intriguing are the national staples that have been subtly adapted to American grocers. A Korean family offered a steaming rice bowl with sliced nori (the seaweed paper used in sushi), bologna and a raw egg. Ji Yoon Yoo, who lives in Jersey City and often works late selling real estate, makes an Americanized version of pa jun, the Korean scallion pancake, several nights a week.[32]

Hybridity, according to Marwan Kraidy, is the "cultural logic of globalization."[33] That hybridity is highly salient (read "fundamental") to the new immigrant's sense of identity in the moment of transnational change and can be written into daily practices through food.

This same notion of transnational change, food, and the creation of fundamental identity animates a broad genre of food blogs. In this genre, cooks and eaters from one culture find themselves living in another place.[34] They blog, in part, to establish this transnational identity that is fundamental, at least at that moment in time, to who they are. Blogs are one form that has taken shape and soared in popularity as food talk has shifted from the realms of food celebrities to a vernacular rhetoric. Pollan himself has noted that one function of this food media is to teach people a grammar they might use in everyday life: "[W]e learn how to taste and how to talk about food."[35]

This same vernacular, then, provides the conceit of new shows on the recently established Cooking Channel. For instance, David Rocco, an Italian-American, returns to Florence to rediscover the original cuisine that seasoned the hybrid cuisine of his youth. In another show, Luke Nguyen returns to his family's native Viet Nam to celebrate that culture's unsung cuisine. Both of these shows elaborate this fundamental identity structure into a globalized world of transnational movements. These cooks return to a fundamental identity through these shows, in essence inviting anyone of similar heritage along for the ride. However, the shows rely on the globalization of cultural foods and the language that attends them for their connection to an audience. Put another way, if I were not already familiar with or at least curious about eating like a Vietnamese peasant, I lack the grammatical resources to engage the show.

Like human rights discourse, food talk also provides resources for constructing "the other" in a globalizing moment. Coverage of food riots around the world often relies on food talk for its animation. Just like human rights cast all people as equal in fundamental ways as a right-bearing entity, food talk puts all people on the same plane as *eaters*. The rhetorical process is similar to the way that human rights discourse appropriated rights talk to construct both democratic citizens and those living under other regimes as equals. Elsewhere, large agri-businesses appropriate food talk for their own versions of creating fundamental identity in this moment of change. By claiming that they are working to feed an exploding global population, they argue that their fundamental identity at this globalizing moment is that of a compassionate innovator with the best interests of eaters everywhere in its heart. The claim stands in stark contrast to those who demonize Monsanto and others as profiteers and pirates, driving the globalization of the food system. Yet, food talk supplies the grammar of both constructions.

To sum up, the excavation of this discursive structure enables one to trace fundamental identity as it energized rights talk in the twentieth century and now is splintering as globalizing conditions erode the collective poem of a world organized through a nation-state system and its attending discourses (e.g., citizenship) and structures. Fundamental identity must therefore be re-individuated to a new era and it can be found in food discourse.

EAT LOCAL, ACT GLOBAL

I turn now to a brief application of this insight to test its critical purchase. My goal is to provide a unique critique of some aspect of food talk. I choose the popular phrase "eat local" because of its seeming simplicity, connotations to globalizing forces, and its widespread use. These words can be found in many places, from Whole Foods Markets grocery stores, to farmers' markets and sustainable food centers around the world, to the Slow Food movement, to various incarnations of food television. This is a widely distributed phrase by any reckoning.

My first move here is to disabuse the reader of leaping to the obvious—but misleading—conclusion that "eat local" is what Burke described as a scenic grammar, a text rooted in a place, a setting or environment that calls other things into existence.[36] It is an understandable and certainly tempting conclusion that "eat local" is aimed at differentiating a given place from a larger globalizing world that de-centers people and places. Such an analysis privileges the word "local" in the phrase and summons the local-global binary to salience. Rather, I argue here that the word "eat" presents greater insight into the rhetorical nature of the phrase, casting it as an act-based grammar, a hunt for a generative politics in a time of globally driven change.[37]

What is local in this locution? The answer is a bit muddled. At my nearest Whole Foods here in Austin, the produce marked "local" has a qualifier that defines local as grown in Texas. Whereas that certainly makes it more local than, say, California-grown produce, this produce could have traveled as much as a day in a truck to reach me. Produce from certain other states and northern Mexico is no less local as the crow flies. Local, then, begins to abstract itself from a certain place or scene. In that sense, the rhetorical power of "eat local" lies more in its paradoxical wide distribution as a means of establishing identity. Said differently, "eat local" functions as a rhetorical resource for claims-making at a moment of globalizing change.

This somewhat intangible, globally tinged status of "local" is inherent in the rhetoric of the Eat Local Movement. The website *Eat Local Challenge*, an advocate of this philosophy, promotes a hierarchy of food choices that includes "fair trade" labeled foods.[38] Such goods are globally sourced and certified by certain organizations as being products grown, harvested, and produced with environmentally sound activities and fair labor practices. In that sense, global goods can qualify as at least a form of "local" consumption. Likewise, the Slow Food movement has taken up the causes of preserving regional foodstuffs and cultural practices. Yet, Slow Food's local focus is also attended by the global. It is a global movement, using the global Internet medium. This seeming contradiction is an example of what

Kraidy preferred to call "critical transculturalism," where social practices actively link localities and social contexts, and create a rhetorical resource to resist globalization's cultural hegemony.[39] Put another way, there is a considerable element of the "global" in "local" food discourse.

I point out these inconsistencies simply to problematize the face-value analysis of "eat local" and to suggest that "local" might not be the most important part of the "eat local" imperative. If we shift our lens to "eat," something new begins to emerge. The verb connotes action to be taken by the *eater*. This overlooking of the act is consistent with the analysis of what Burke called "act-based grammar."

> But if the scene of action is there already, and if the nature of the agent is also given, along with the instrumental conditions and the purposes of action, then there could be novelty only if there were likewise a locus of motivation within the act itself, a newness not already present in elements classifiable under any of the other four headings [of Burke's Pentad].[40]

The phrase "eat local" has an implied subject—the eater, or for my purposes the fundamental identity of the moment. It also gives a location of that subject—local. In Burke's estimation, with those things spelled out, the *act* is the most interesting source of critique and when we critique the grammar of "act," we must think in terms of a "paradigm of action," not just a single act.[41] So, "eat" in this construction is about more than just eating. Eating to maintain bodily functions would fall into what Burke termed "motion," an autonomic movement without motivation. Action is inspired by motivation.

Here, I shift from the precise text "eat local" to what Roderick Hart called the critic's "imaginative leap from text to idea."[42] The act-based grammar of "eat local" provides a call for a paradigm of action under globalizing conditions, a hunt for agency in a moment of change. This search for agency is consistent with the nation-state's decreasing ability to protect its citizens from globalizing forces. To the degree that rights provided some level of tangible agency in the nation-state-organized world it is an agency that is eroding.

"Eat local," then, is not a replacement for agency. It is a *call* for agency expressed in an act-based grammar readily available to the eater. "Locavore," therefore, is an identity based on empowerment and action.

CONCLUSION

That the world has changed because of globalization is obvious. What is less obvious is that we have yet to describe those changes to ourselves in a way that replicates the nation-state's sense of identity and agency. Many institutions spew out white papers and jargon and virtually no political speech is complete without a few mentions of the term *globalization*. Yet, the everyday language—the vernacular, the first language that takes on material status in our lives—has yet to emerge. Until it does, we will grope to connect fundamental identity to a stable discourse.

When the world appears to change under our feet, it makes sense that we might first want to know who we are under these new conditions. Fundamental identity, as a discursive structure, can likely be found in many elaborated discourses, cutting across time, location, and subject matter. Globalization offers ample opportunities for the *search for* and *assertion of* fundamental identity.

Now, my argument suggests that we are being reduced from "Americans" or "Indians" to "eaters." That might sound like a leap to some and maybe inelegant to others. So be it. I would remind us that globalization has created a time in which we cannot agree on what it means to be an American. There are those who think "anchor baby" is a more useful term than "citizen" to describe some children born within these borders. Likewise, you can be the *citizen* of a nation one minute and an *enemy combatant* the next. Nations such as Germany and France are having their own parallel discussions. Identity and agency have become fluid at best.

It is worth wondering what happens from here. Globalization is a process, not an event. The nation-state is slipping from its singular role as organizer of the world, yet it seems an exaggeration to suggest it will not continue as a primary player in the world. Will food discourses and the attendant media forms continue to be so popular? Or will our sense of who we are solidify as conditions gain some stability? Will some other first language emerge to carry the structure of fundamental identity?

It will all depend on our attitudes toward history. Whatever does happen, rhetorical homology will provide a tool for critiquing it.

NOTES

1. Mary Eberstadt, "Is Food the New Sex?," *Policy Review* 115 (April/May 2009), accessed September 14, 2011, http://www.hoover.org/publications/policy-review/article/5542.
2. James McWilliams, *Just Food: Where Locavores Get It Wrong and How We Can Truly Eat Responsibly* (New York: Little, Brown and Company, 2009).
3. Dylan Clark, "The Raw and the Rotten: Punk Cuisine," in *Food and Culture: A Reader, Second Edition*, ed. Carole Counihan and Penny Van Esterik (New York: Routledge, 1997), 411.
4. "SFA Vision Statement," *Southern Foodways Alliance*, www.southernfoodways.com.
5. The list is growing but for a representative sample see: Barbara Kingsolver, *Animal, Vegetable, Miracle: A Year of Food Life* (New York: Harper Collins, 2007); Marion Nestle, *Food Politics* (Berkeley: University of California Press, 2002); Michael Pollan, *The Omnivore's Dilemma: A Natural History of Four Meals* (New York: Penguin Press, 2006); Eric Schlosser, *Fast Food Nation* (New York: Harper, 2002).

6. Roderick Hart et al., *Political Keywords: Using Language That Uses Us* (New York: Oxford University Press, 2005).

7. Kenneth Burke, *A Rhetoric of Motives* (Berkeley: University of California Press, 1969), 26.

8. Barry Brummett, "Rhetorical Homologies in Walter Benjamin, The Ring and Capital," *Rhetoric Society Quarterly* 36 (2008): 449.

9. Anthony Giddens, *Runaway World: How Globalization Is Reshaping Our Lives* (New York: Routledge, 2003), 7.

10. Nancy Fraser, *Scales of Justice: Reimagining Political Space in a Globalizing World* (New York: Columbia University Press, 2009), 1.

11. For global citizenship, see David Held, *Global Covenant: The Social Democratic Alternative to the Washington Consensus* (Cambridge: Polity Press, 2004); for cosmopolitan citizenship, see Robert Went, "Economic Globalization Plus Cosmopolitanism?," *Review of International Political Economy* 11 (May 2004): 337.

12. Marc Lacey, "Birthright Citizenship Looms as Next Immigration Battle," *The New York Times*, January 4, 2011, accessed January 5, 2011, http://www.nytimes.com/2011/01/05/us/poliutics/05babies.html.

13. I do not intend to re-hash the tortured history of Jose Padilla, an American citizen classified as an "enemy combatant" and stripped of his citizenship rights. For a history of his case see the *New York Times* at http://topics.nytimes.com/top/reference/timestopics/people/p/jose_padilla/index.html.

14. See Kenneth Burke, *Permanence and Change: An Anatomy of Purpose*, 3rd ed. (Berkeley: University of California Press, 1954); Kenneth Burke, *Attitudes Toward History* (New York: The New Republic, 1937).

15. Burke, *Permanence*, 173.

16. Burke, *Attitudes*, 111.

17. Brummett, "Homologies," 454.

18. Brummett, "Homologies," 454.

19. See Jason Black, "Extending the Rights of Personhood, Voice, Life Sensate to Others: A Homology of Right to Life and Animal Rights Rhetoric," *Communication Quarterly* 51 (Summer 2003): 312; Kathryn Olson, "Detecting a Common Interpretive Framework for Impersonal Violence: The Homology in Participants' Rhetoric on Sport Hunting, 'Hate Crimes,' and Stranger Rape," *Southern Communication Journal* 67 (2002): 215.

20. Michael Schudson, *The Good Citizen: A History of American Civic Life* (Cambridge: Harvard University Press, 1998).

21. Ibid, 9.

22. Gerald Hauser, *Vernacular Voices: The Rhetorics of Publics and Public Spheres* (Columbia: University of South Carolina Press, 1999), 78.

23. Richard Primus, *The American Language of Rights* (Cambridge: Cambridge University Press, 1999).

24. Ibid, 27.

25. Arjun Appadurai, *Modernity at Large: Cultural Dimensions of Globalization* (Minneapolis: University of Minnesota Press, 1996), 2.

26. Jurgen Habermas, *Time of Transitions* (Cambridge: Polity Press, 2006).

27. Michael Hardt and Antonio Negri, *Empire* (Cambridge: Harvard University Press, 2000).

28. Mary Douglas, "Deciphering a Meal," in *Food and Culture: A Reader*, 2nd ed., ed. Carole Counihan and Penny Van Esterik (New York: Routledge, 1997), 44.

29. Arjun Appadurai, "How to Make a National Cuisine: Cookbooks in Contemporary India," in ibid., 289.

30. Richard Wilk, "'Real Belizean Food': Building Local Identity in the Transnational Caribbean," in ibid., 308.

31. Elizabeth Rosenthal, "Fast Food Hits Mediterranean; A Diet Succumbs," *The New York Times*, September 23, 2008, accessed September 15, 2011, http://www.nytimes.com/2008/09/24/world/europe/24diet.html.
32. Leslie Kaufman, "For Dinner (and Fast), the Taste of Home," *The New York Times*, February 11, 2009, accessed February 11, 2009, http://www.nytimes.com/2009/02/11/dining/11immi.html.
33. Marwan Kraidy, *Hybridity, or the Cultural Logic of Globalization* (Philadelphia: Temple University Press, 2005).
34. The list is far too long to include here. But, as a representative sample: French Kitchen in America (http://frenchkitcheninamerica.blogspot.com), David Liebovitz's quite popular food blog (http://davidliebovitz.com), The Fat Expat (http://thefatexpat.blogspot.com).
35. Michael Pollan, "Out of the Kitchen, Onto the Couch," *The New York Times*, August 2, 2009, accessed August 2, 2009, http://www.nytimes.com/2009/08/02/magazine/02cooking-t.html.
36. Burke, *Grammar*, xvi.
37. Burke, *Grammar*, 64–67.
38. See www.eatlocalchallenge.com.
39. Kraidy, *Hybridity*, 151.
40. Burke, *Grammar*, 65.
41. Ibid., 66.
42. Roderick Hart, *Modern Rhetorical Criticism*, 2nd ed. (Boston: Allyn & Bacon, 1997), 34.

5 Food, Health, and Well-Being
Positioning Functional Foods

Alison Henderson and Vanessa Johnson

DISCOURSES OF "HEALTHY" FOOD

In the Western world, where "healthy" food is largely constructed within a medical paradigm, healthy usually means the well-being of humans, and healthy food is frequently narrowly defined in terms of the essential material nutrients for human health. Recent advances in food science technology, coupled with increased consumer interest in healthy foods and beverages, have enabled food-producing organizations to create and market food products that claim physiological benefits beyond the need for basic nutrition. These *functional foods* have sparked considerable public debate despite growing in popularity and availability. As the boundaries between foods and medicines are simultaneously becoming blurred and being reconstructed, the resulting complexity of medical and market information draws on multiple alternative discourses, and creates challenges that are played out rhetorically. For example, within a medical paradigm, food producers use new biotechnologies to manufacture foods that combine food elements in novel ways to "fix" health problems, such as osteoporosis. Yet, *Anlene*, a milk product designed to help combat osteoporosis, was initially promoted without a clear health warning that the product should not be consumed by those taking blood thinning drugs for heart conditions.[1] Intriguingly, competing discourses about the health value of "natural" foods inform the positioning of products like New Zealand manuka honey; yet, such "natural" products are increasingly sold in the form of "health supplements" (such as royal jelly), and as an ingredient in manufactured foods (like muesli bars), as well as in a raw or unprocessed form.

Mats Alvesson and Dan Kärreman suggest that the term *discourse* can be considered on multiple levels, including both "discourse"—the text, talk, and behavior of individuals within everyday interactions at a micro level—and "Discourse"—the prevalent systems of thought, and the vehicle by which socially constructed meanings can be understood at a macro level.[2] In this chapter, we discuss the interaction of "discourse" and "Discourse" in relation to the development of functional foods. For example, "discourse" might refer to the language and terminology used specifically by food technologists at a food-producing organization, whereas "Discourse" might refer to the body of thinking underpinning such terminology, such as bio-medicine.

The term "functional food" originated in Japan in the early 1980s, although the linking of food and optimal health is not new. In 400 BC Hippocrates espoused the tenet, "let food be thy medicine and medicine be thy food," [3] and many cultures share long-held, deep-rooted beliefs in food's health-giving properties.[4] Yet, it was Japan's academic researchers, government, and food industry that began to identify and promote the health benefits of specific foods and food elements. Although the first recorded functional food product sold in Japan was a fiber-enriched soft drink, "Fibre Mini,"[5] most functional food studies have focused on solid foods, such as Benecol Margarine, Golden Rice, and Cardia Salt.[6] Yet, functional beverages—for example, probiotic yoghurt-based drinks and milk/orange juice enriched with calcium, omega 3, or fiber—are becoming increasingly popular.[7]

Varying reasons have been proffered for the rapid development and popular appeal of functional foods. For food producers these include advances in science enabling new product development,[8] an expanding global marketplace,[9] a concerned and interested media,[10] higher overall disposable consumer incomes,[11] and a highly competitive food market where new product development is critical.[12] From a public policy perspective, health issues that might be addressed by consuming functional foods include high medical costs due to an aging population, increased chronic illness, and greater public awareness of health and diet.[13] From a consumer perspective, Jennifer Gray et al. argue that consumers are ready for a positive, proactive approach to food consumption as opposed to the negative "reduce and avoid" dietary approach of prior decades.[14]

However, stakeholders in the fields of medicine and nutrition, science, policy, and business have yet to agree on a single definition of functional foods.[15] To some degree all foods are functional in that they provide some form of nutritional benefit(s),[16] and many terms are used interchangeably— for example, health foods, phytochemicals, nutritional foods, super foods, pharmafoods, and designer foods, adding to the confusion for consumers, health and education professionals, retailers, and legislators.[17] Maurice Doyon and JoAnne Labrecque offer the following as a working definition:

> A functional food is, or appears similar to, a conventional food. It is part of a standard diet and is consumed on a regular basis, in normal quantities. It has proven health benefits that reduce the risk of specific chronic diseases or beneficially affect target functions beyond its basic nutritional qualities.[18]

Functional foods, however, require different understandings from consumers, educators, and retailers, and require different legislation. As the boundaries between food and medicine become blurred, existing legislation differentiating food and medicine is no longer easily applied.[19]

Since their introduction, the development of functional foods has created debate and controversy.[20] Tensions exist around the definition, ethos, and health-benefit claims of functional foods.[21] The lack of international consensus and lag in effective regulation have led to conflicting and sometimes exaggerated health claims, causing confusion, mistrust, and anger from consumers and interest groups toward food producers and regulators.[22] Such confusion, mistrust, and anger are pronounced when consumers fail to see the benefits of eating functional foods.[23] As Dilip Ghosh says, "regulation is important in food innovation because it governs the means by which health benefits can be translated into messages for consumers."[24] Many consumers see functional foods as a potentially cost-effective, preventative approach to healthcare.[25] Yet, other consumers are more skeptical than ever before about trying new products claiming to provide "extra" health benefits, uncertain if products are being marketed simply to increase food producers' profits.

The degree of trust in regulations thus becomes important. On the one hand, public policy seeks to take a regulatory approach to manage food safety and food consumption patterns; on the other hand, individuals are asked to take responsibility for their own healthy food choices, health, and well-being. The choice of what counts as healthy food is then ostensibly left to consumers, in a context where food producers, medical professionals, governments, regulatory authorities, and other interest groups debate the parameters and complex issues of food and health consumption.

In this chapter, we illustrate the organizational assumptions and hidden relations of power evident in the normalized practices of functional food production. We refer to an empirical study of beverages developed specifically to enhance sports performance and active lifestyles. Sportspeople participating in social or competitive individual and team sports, and those performing at an elite level, continually look for ways to out-perform, out-train, and out-recover their opponents, and improve on their personal benchmarks. Furthermore, coaches, physical trainers, and medical professionals agree that correct nutrition is critical to optimal performance, especially as the exertion levels of competitive sportspeople often mean a well-balanced diet of nutrients at the recommended daily intake is simply not enough.[26] Many claims are made about the benefits of functional foods and beverages in terms of energy, performance, concentration, stamina, increased muscle mass, or recovery. However, in the sports food market some products have clearly shown little efficacy,[27] whereas others make exaggerated claims about active ingredients, which are usually present in amounts far below those shown to be effective, sometimes without full evaluation of the potential benefits and risks associated with their use.[28]

Our examination of organizational communication with internal and external stakeholders demonstrates how food producing organizations use rhetorical strategies to manage these tensions as they juggle multiple identities and engage with the broadest range of stakeholders possible.

RHETORIC, IDENTITY, AND PERSUASION

Rhetoric involves "the uses of symbolic and non-symbolic resources for persuasion in instances where more than one outcome is possible and the outcome can be affected through persuasive means."[29] The rhetorical construction of texts expresses the meanings food producers attribute to "functional foods" as they make sense of and attempt to influence their operating environment. The language and symbols used by food producers are linked to organizational values and strategies, to values prevalent in society, and to current discourses related to what counts as "healthy" food. Rhetoric, then, is the use of language (symbols) to unite people or induce cooperation; it is purposive, has motive, and involves symbolic action.[30] A rhetorical act is a strategy for identification or persuasion; it provides an orientation to a situation and help in adjusting to it.[31] In issues management communication, as Timothy Kuhn suggested, a rhetorical perspective allows an examination of the process of influence—the struggle over meanings.[32] Organizations often use competing rhetorical strategies that emphasize particular values and marginalize their opponents' values—for example, in relation to competing food products.

George Cheney and Daniel Lair argued that organizations are constituted by rhetoric in the sense that rhetoric plays a part in persuasion and identification at both micro and macro levels in the process of organizing, as well as in the management of issues.[33] Identity is thus a crucial intangible asset. Rather than being conceived as a static construct, organizational identity is actively (re)created, (re)framed, and (re)negotiated as situations demand.[34] For example, a food-producing organization may need to reposition its identity if a competitor introduces a new product in the same product category. When McDonald's introduced fruit and vegetables into its Happy Meals, other fast-food producers were also challenged to reframe their identity in relation to healthy foods.

It is increasingly recognized that the boundaries between internal and external organizational communication have become blurred, such that identity and image need to be considered from the multiple perspectives of all organizational stakeholders. Cheney described the nature of organizational rhetoric as the management of multiple identities, and suggested that "similarity and difference mutually implicate one another, exist in ongoing dialectical tension, and provide the formative context for what we call our 'identity.'"[35] For individuals and organizations such socially constituted aspects of identity may thus sometimes be conflicting.

According to Rajesh Sethi and Larry Compeau, organizations with multiple identities will be better prepared to "respond to a wider range of environment and stakeholders because they can draw upon a wider range of self-referential frames."[36] However, having multiple identities can also hinder an organization by pulling it in different directions, creating identity "overload."[37] As Stefan Sveningsson and Mats Alvesson argue, identity is central to meaning production, decision-making, action-taking (external communication), and social relations (interaction).[38]

Given the aggressive nature of the food industry, organizational identity and reputation are crucial for producers of functional foods. The operating environment for functional foods provides unstable ground, especially as some functional foods are at the cutting edge of food science technology. Organizations must, therefore, accurately represent health claims in relation to new products that push technological and legislative boundaries. A positive reputation creates competitive advantage by opening up new market opportunities; reduces barriers to competition; and enables a firm to attract top recruits, business partners, and investors.[39] An organization with a sympathetic reputation may also attract new customers, create brand loyalty, and generate word-of-mouth endorsement, which may lift sales or create an assumption of higher quality allowing for premium price charges.[40] Firms with a favorable reputation can exert influence in government circles, acquire support from financial analysts and opinion leaders,[41] and generate positive media stories.

The rhetoric of organizational decision-making then is critical to identity and reputation. How an organization rationalizes the multiple public positions of its stakeholders is linked to how it manages its multiple identities and images.[42] Additionally, organizations often rationalize their strategic positioning retrospectively to make sense of uncertainties created by managing multiple public positions and identities.[43] Such choices may have lasting consequences for organizational reputation, especially in relation to controversial sociopolitical issues such as those surrounding functional foods. We need to examine the taken-for-granted assumptions inherent in organizational positioning, and the processes used to manage that positioning, as organizations navigate complex, changing, and often contested operating environments, so that dominant paradigms—such as bio-medical paradigms in relation to healthy foods—can be challenged and re-examined. This was particularly evident, for example, in the widespread debate about genetically modified foods at the time of the Royal Commission on Genetic Modification in New Zealand.[44]

CLAIMING MATERIALITY: HEALTH BENEFITS FOR SPORTS PERFORMANCE

In this section, we describe the findings from a case study of a food- and beverage-producing organization in Aotearoa, New Zealand. We illustrate how food and beverage producers negotiate various discourses related to what counts as "healthy" food, as they develop new functional food products. We examine the rhetorical construction of meanings and positions

evident in interviews and formal organizational documents and discuss the
discursive, strategic premises for that positioning—that is, how values are
represented and expressed as the organization attempts to influence both
internal and external stakeholders.

The Case Study Organization

The case study organization was originally a New Zealand company
(referred to here as EnZedCo) established in the 1960s to manufacture and
distribute fruit juice under the oversight of the New Zealand Apple and
Pear Board. Today, the organization is privately owned by overseas interests and comprises a small central office and manufacturing site, and a relatively large distribution team with more than nine hundred staff across New
Zealand and Australia. EnZedCo manufactures and distributes more than
twenty non-alcoholic beverages—energy drinks, fruit juices, fruit drinks,
pure waters, sports waters, soft drinks, and milk drinks—and leads the
New Zealand market in both energy and juice drinks. Our study focuses
on the research and development (R&D) and marketing (Marketing) teams
involved in new product development. It illustrates the tensions negotiated
by many food producers as they consider competing discourses about what
counts as healthy food and make strategic decisions about the development,
production, and marketing of healthy food products. Our study examines
EnZedCo's assumptions about food and health issues, the specific assumptions made about sportspeople and sports performance, and the consequent
tensions that emerged in relation to functional foods for health and sports
performance.

We conducted semi-structured interviews with marketing and research
and development staff who were key decision-makers. We asked questions
related to the images and labels given to beverages and food; the research
and development of the organization's functional products; consumers;
product marketing; and communications. We also examined a small range
of formal organizational documents, including EnZedCo's website, television advertisements, and promotional pamphlets. We looked at the rhetorical constructions evident in the interview texts and documents, and used a
thematic analysis to identify patterns within the data.[45]

The range of products referred to in our case study includes two sports
drinks: a hypotonic product for elite sportspeople, and an isotonic sports
drink for lifestyle sportspeople, as well as energy drinks and juice drinks.
All of these could be described as functional foods, delivering particular
health benefits.

Rhetorical Constructions of "Healthy" Food

Marketing and R&D staff differed in their responses to the question: "What
does the term 'healthy' mean?" in relation to food and beverages. Two
related themes emerged; the R&D team talked about specific physiological

outcomes, like hydration and energy, which in the following example are measured in terms of calories:

> Nutrition and Claims Manager: A water-based product, which to me would be the healthiest in terms of low calories.

In contrast, Marketing staff were more cautious about referring to "healthy" specifically:

> Marketing Manager/Hydration: We don't kinda go out and go this is a "healthy" drink.

Marketers commented that consumers like the idea of being healthy, but explicit use of this term can be viewed as too exercise-oriented, "hard core," and guilt-inducing. Instead the Marketing team used words with all-encompassing connotations:

> Brand Manager/Sports Beverages: A balanced diet, looking after your body . . . good choices, taste and enjoyment, well-being, goodness, holistic.

In one advertisement, a sports beverage is even referred to as, "that's healthier and *still tastes great*" (emphasis added), and the tag line on the label of a pure water bottle states, "Have your cake and drink me"—you can "enjoy life" (eat the cake) and still "live healthily" (by drinking the pure water). Two distinct organizational perspectives are thus clearly evident in product descriptions. On the one hand, the organization seeks identification with "healthy living"—taking care of oneself, and making sensible nutritional choices—and, on the other hand, with "enjoying life"—consuming beverages for taste and pleasure.

Both R&D and Marketing staff commented that products might deliver *different* health benefits to *different* consumers; for example, hypotonic drinks are not designed to be consumed in large quantities except following extended exercise:

> Product Development Manager: The classic one would be our [hypotonic sports drink] . . . you don't want to be drinking *six bottles* of it a day health-wise, but as part of sport that's what we designed it for. [Emphasis added]

Marketing staff also suggested that consumers choose what is healthy relative to who they are, their lifestyle, and what they are doing at the moment of consumption:

> Brand Manager/Sports Beverages: All our beverages, none of them are bad. So I'd say all of them are used within a balanced and healthy diet, you can manage yourself.

The responsibility for defining "health," and which products will be of most benefit, is thus assumed to lie with the consumer.

There was general consensus between R&D and Marketing staff that functional products give consumers a physiological effect:

> Marketing Manager/Energy: So there's functional ingredients which deliver *efficacy* for the consumer. So there's a *benefit*, there's a clear *benefit* beyond just perception and taste and hydration. [Emphasis added]

But three of the four staff in the Marketing team used the word "promise" in relation to functionality:

> Marketing Manager/Hydration: [It provides] more than just the basic requirements . . . something that *promises* an ingredient or a benefit over and above that. [Emphasis added]

The word "promise" suggests an assurance of functionality; yet, health claims cannot be made for products that have not undergone clinical trials, so such "promises" to consumers are in some cases open to interpretation. They *imply* functionality in order to appeal to a range of target markets. The hypotonic sports drink was scientifically formulated and clinically tested, but the newer isotonic sports drink was not clinically tested. The intended target audience for the hypotonic drink was consumers who are highly competitive sportspeople, who do intense exercise, are concerned about nutrition, and are achievement-oriented:

> Brand Manager/Juice: It's got a very, very . . . specific function around faster rehydration . . . and a *good choice for athletes* . . . when you are doing extreme exercise. [Emphasis added]

However, consumers perceived that the hypotonic product was *exclusively* for top echelon sportspeople with extreme nutritional requirements, such as elite athletes like Olympic medalist/world champion triathlete Bevan Docherty, who was featured in several product advertisements:

> Brand Manager/Juice: The challenge is . . . with [the hypotonic sports drink] is that it can become too elite in terms of, "oh it's not for me, it's only for elite athletes" . . . as hard core I guess as the likes of the Bevan Dochertys . . . so in terms of marketing it is, it's actually quite challenging.

In order to extend the target market, the isotonic sports beverage was developed to appeal to consumers wanting to be physically active and successful, and to enjoy a variety of active lifestyles:

Brand Manager/Juice: We associate it [the isotonic product] with active healthy people, for people into sports and not sports specifically . . . you don't have to be a sportsperson to be drinking it, but sort of relates more to that sporty type of person, that's . . . on the go and active and . . . just out enjoying life.

From participants' comments, it became apparent that consumers are looking for more and more functionality out of their drinks. In other words, the demand for functional foods is assumed to be driven by the consumer. Yet, several comments indicated that consumer motivation was more about trying new, trendy products that look good, taste good, and sound good for you rather than being concerned about actual functional benefits:

Nutrition and Claims Manager: Visual cues . . . have a huge influence on consumer purchase and the mainstream consumer of sports drinks is not a sports person, and the visual cues that they are looking for are colour and that opacity . . . It looks intense and *brightly coloured* . . . gives them an impression of *potency* . . . they are couch potatoes or the weekend warriors. [Emphasis added]

Such comments describe the importance of image and lifestyle in identification with a product. In fact, participants also talked of educating consumers:

Brand Manager/Sports Beverages: It was almost like an education job, you had to do with consumers, to tell them about what guarana was and educate them as to the benefits . . . a benefit that consumers can identify with.

It seems that EnZedCo believes consumers see functionality as "trendy," providing products that might lessen feelings of guilt and create identification in terms of lifestyle. Perhaps genuine functional benefits will be lost on these consumers, and developing innovative, functional beverages with genuine health benefits may not be as worthwhile as creating beverages that address consumer concerns about image.

Research and Development: Making Health Claims

Both R&D staff and Marketing staff agreed that there are two levels with regard to what can be legally claimed. "Soft" claims referred to general functional benefits, whereas "hard" claims referred to scientific/evidence-based claims:

Marketing Manager/Hydration: Vitamin B . . . it has a function over and above just hydration or being a nice taste . . . it's a pretty soft, soft function.

Vitamin B is viewed as "soft" because you cannot claim a *measurable* physiological effect. A number of factors constrain the development of products with "hard" benefit claims, including technological complexity, cost,
time, the depth of research required, the need for scientifically supported
evidence, and the rigors of regulations. Only one beverage (the hypotonic
sports drink) within the sports beverages range has functional benefits that
can be claimed as "hard":

> Nutrition and Claims Manager: The nutrition and health-related
> claims standard . . . requires you to have enough evidence to support
> your claims and that is why we had to do another clinical trial which is
> more in depth and gave a lot more concrete evidence.

However, thus far, EnZedCo's sole product with "hard" benefits has not
had superior sales over its major competitor product. It has a market limited to competitive sportspeople, consistent with the earlier premise that
mainstream consumers identify with lifestyle imagery rather than specific
health benefits.

When asked about constraints on health claims, participants were quick
to highlight legislative constraints:

> Brand Manager/Sports Beverages: Absolutely there are constraints . . .
> from governing bodies . . . certain things you can and can't say on
> packaging.

Food Standards Australia New Zealand (FSANZ) currently allows both
nutrition claims and health claims. Nutrition claims tell consumers about a
nutritional property—for example, how much calcium is in a food. Health
claims are currently regulated by a transitional Standard 1.1A.2, and the
only health claim that can be made about a serious disease is the benefit of
maternal folate consumption for women.[46] A new health claims standard
is currently under development, and will mean that claims must not be
misleading and must be scientifically substantiated. This new standard will
regulate *three* types of claims: nutrition content claims, general-level health
claims, and high-level health claims. Development of this new standard is
due for completion by late 2011.

Interestingly, the research and development of an innovative product frequently push the boundaries of current legislation, and this presents unique
challenges:

> Nutrition and Claims Manager: Companies who have been innovative
> can actually launch a new product . . . where the food legislation or the
> foods standard hasn't actually caught up, so we are always ahead of the
> legislation and sometimes that puts us in a sort of a grey or precarious
> area where . . . the legislation hasn't come up to speed with our invention.

Participants were clearly concerned about the effectiveness of legislation in monitoring competitors' products and the resulting consumer cynicism about functional foods and beverages:

> Brand Manager/Sports Beverages: In relation to functional products [there] is a real cynicism from the New Zealand public . . . I think we as a New Zealand population have been exposed to products that have been deemed to be functional in terms of giving us good stuff . . . and then you find out that they're potentially not as good as you thought.

In contrast, participants were adamant that EnZedCo's functional products are genuinely effective:

> Nutrition and Claims Manager: I can put my hand on my heart and say that the [hypotonic sports drink] . . . [it's] a product which works and it can support its claims.

Participants said that they aimed to comply with regulations, set a good example for the rest of the industry to follow, and provide consumers with genuinely beneficial products.

Challenges and Tensions in Relation to the Development of Functional Foods

The different perspectives of Marketing and R&D staff in EnZedCo were acknowledged to result in some tensions. Marketing staff saw these tensions as positive, if at times frustrating:

> Brand Manager/Juice: Sometimes there's a bit of tension between the marketing team . . . and the technical side . . . but I think it's a good tension . . . you know we've gotta from a marketing perspective try and come up with the best and most compelling way to say it and the technical in terms of how can you say that in the right way.

But R&D staff implied that they must monitor the claims made by Marketing staff closely and that this was somewhat resented:

> Nutrition and Claims Manager: You actually have to be very careful on what you say on the pack because marketers will inevitably try and push you to try to make more overt claims.

Further tensions were expressed between remaining competitive and maintaining product credibility and scientific validity. The Nutrition and Claims Manager's comments illustrate this:

Nutrition and Claims Manager: It's been a challenge . . . we have tried to stay unique and true to its origins so that's been one of the biggest challenges . . . how to grow the brand, but still retain that credibility and those strong [hypotonic sports drink] credentials that loyal [hypotonic sports drink] followers were purchasing this product for.

In trying to manage multiple brand identities for both "serious" sportspeople and "lifestyle" sportspeople, EnZedCo is concerned it will lose credibility among health professionals and elite sportspeople, with the possible demise of a genuinely beneficial product. In sum, if the organization over-extends itself trying to appeal to too many different consumers it may eventually find it struggles to appeal to any of them.

Interestingly, both Marketing and R&D staff agreed that there were additional tensions related to the desire to "do good" and have a positive health impact, and at the same time make a profit:

Brand Manager/Juice: It's not just to make money, I mean it is at the end of the day, but we are certainly driven by a bigger purpose than just making money at all costs . . . trying to build brands and develop products that are *good* for people. [Emphasis added]

EnZedCo is committed to innovation, which is referred to as "trailblazing" and described on the organization's website as follows:

We're innovators, not imitators. At [EnZedCo] we challenge the status quo. People look to us because we think differently. It's what makes us [EnZedCo]. We are bold . . . We aren't scared to try new things. That's why we lead and others follow.

It is clearly important to the organization that it is identified by relevant external stakeholders as innovative, industry-leading, and technologically capable, but that this also leads to profit opportunities:

Marketing Manager/Energy: It's all around where the white space is . . . finding unmet territories which provide incremental business opportunities and in marketing terms that is a really hard nut to crack. A brand like [Energy Drink Brand] is a once in a lifetime thing.

Such comments suggest the organization is innovating to both "trailblaze" and "cash in" on business opportunities.

Tailoring Communication to the Targeted and Mainstream Consumer

EnZedCo seeks to build the credibility of its functional sports drinks through athlete sponsorship and endorsement by health professionals.

In order to balance communication with different target markets so that both competitive sportspeople and lifestyle sportspeople can identify with EnZedCo products, advertisements *switch* between an elite athlete and a "regular person" to promote sports beverages:

> Brand Manager/Juice: It's quite interesting actually if you see the [sports drink] comms over time, sometimes it will be Bevan [Docherty], then it will go back to more of an approachable inclusive sort of an ad and then, oh we need to dial up credibility so we'll go back to sort of athletes.

The rhetorical construction of two different appeals is clearly evident in advertisements. One television advertisement aimed at sportspeople and promoting the hypotonic sports drink features the following comment from Bevan Docherty:

> You know when you're pushing yourself to the limit you need to be smart about what you're actually putting in. Hydration is fuel to me so you know I've got to pump the right sort of fuel in just to keep the engine going. [Hypotonic sports drink], it's got everything I need.

A second advertisement promoting the isotonic lifestyle sports drink is aimed toward the mainstream consumer and features a "regular person":

> I may never play first division. I may never be selected for Man U. I may never hold aloft the World Cup. But there are some moments when it sure as hell feels like I could. This is me, Matt Trainer, in my zone.

Interestingly, in these television advertisements, functional benefits of the isotonic sports drink are never mentioned specifically, and on billboards, package labels, and the sports drink website, general information is given precedence rather than scientific detail about each of the drinks; such messaging clearly targets the "lifestyle" consumer rather than the serious athlete. On package labels more detailed information about functionality is placed in a less prominent position. However, the Nutrition and Claims Manager was concerned about this shift in information priority:

> Nutrition and Claims Manager: I couldn't even find some of the clinical stuff [on the hypotonic sports drink] or the support material [on the website] . . . it is there, but it's been stripped right back, so my concern is that the actual credibility and science behind it could be lost.

Those who want more detailed information—a much smaller target market—seem to be required to do extra work to find it.

By developing two products with such different functional appeal—that is, trying to be "all things to all people"—EnZedCo may lose credibility with elite sportspeople, coaches, and professional interest groups. Further-more, in trying to appeal to such a breadth of stakeholder groups, the orga-nization must be extremely wary of pushing regulatory boundaries, as the generation of "exaggerated" health claims and marketing messages could lead to a severe erosion of trust and reputation.

ORGANIZATIONAL TENSIONS AND RELATIONS OF POWER

Our case study has explored the assumptions a food producer makes about functional foods for health and sports performance, and how these assumptions impact decision-making, research and development prac-tices, and external communication. EnZedCo rhetorically constructed *functional foods* as having genuine physiological and health advantages for "serious" sportspeople and other professional external stakeholder groups, but as embodying trendiness, novelty, and a lifestyle image for the mainstream consumer—"having your cake and eating it too." The need to appeal to multiple stakeholder groups led to the creation of separate products for differing target markets, steering the organization away from the single branded identity it originally intended. The findings show that the organization experienced a series of dilemmas: how to be "all things to all people," sustain a competitive advantage, make a profit, and promote good nutrition. The small scale of the study referred to in this chapter pre-vents wider generalization of the findings, but suggests an opportunity for further research. It would be valuable to explore differences and/or simi-larities in assumptions, decision-making, and actions across a variety of food-producing organizations that produce functional foods outside the area of sports performance.

This research illustrates how food and beverage producers negotiate var-ious discourses related to what counts as "healthy" food, as they develop new functional food products. As food producers try to appeal to multiple and sometimes divergent stakeholder groups, they manage multiple identi-ties and draw on a variety of discourse premises to rhetorically construct their positions in relation to what counts as "healthy" foods.

On the one hand, the functional foods industry is driven by medical sci-ence and nutrition discourses, and this expert knowledge sets the ground for the physiological benefits that can be claimed, using scientific evidence. However, at the same time, in Western society, power is vested in the con-sumer, whose preferences determine which products are likely to survive in a competitive marketplace. The responsibility for "healthy" decisions is then deemed to lie with the consumer.

Additionally, at a time when new food technologies represent the "cut-ting edge" of biotechnology development, the regulatory power of gov-ernments lags behind the research and development of new products;

production of novel food technologies actually leads the generation of regulation. As debate about the exact definition of functional foods and nutraceuticals continues, it is not yet clear whether functional foods fall within the realms of medicine or the food industry. At present, the failure of regulatory bodies to define the parameters of nutrition and health claims for these innovative products creates further tensions and challenges for medical professionals, the food industry, consumers, and other interest groups (like sports professionals). The question of the *discursive control* of such health claims for the products of new food technologies is thus one that warrants further attention.

ACKNOWLEDGMENTS

This chapter has been developed from research conducted as part of a three-year research study (2010–12) generously supported by a Fast Start Marsden grant, administered by the Royal Society of New Zealand.

NOTES

1. "Anlene Brand of Milk Products Will Carry Warnings about Blood-Clotting Risks," *Medindia*, http://www.medindia.net/news/view_news_main.asp?x=13047.
2. Mats Alvesson and Dan Kärreman, "Varieties of Discourse: On the Study of Organizations through Discourse Analysis," *Human Relations* 53 (2000): 1125–49.
3. Clare M. Hasler, "The Changing Face of Functional Foods," *Journal of the American College of Nutrition* 19 (2000): S6.
4. Israel Goldberg, "Functional Foods: The New Wave of Foods for the Next Millennium," *Nutrition in Clinical Care* 3 (2000): 257–58.
5. Kerry Chamberlain, "Food and Health: Expanding the Agenda for Health Psychology," *Journal of Health Psychology* 9 (2004): 467–81; Linda Tapsell, "Functional Foods: An Australian Perspective," *Nutrition and Dietetics* 65 (2008): 523–26.
6. Chamberlain, "Food and Health," 467–81; Martijn Katan and Nicole de Roos, "Promises and Problems of Functional Foods," *Critical Review of Food Science Nutrition* 44 (2004): 369–77; Mari Niva, "Can We Predict Who Adopts Health-Promoting Foods? Users of Functional Foods in Finland," *Scandinavian Journal of Food and Nutrition* 50 (2006): 13–24.
7. Jane Kolodinsky et al., "Sex and Cultural Differences in the Acceptance of Functional Foods: A Comparison of American, Canadian, and French College Students," *Journal of American College Health* 57 (2008): 143–49; Niva, "Can We Predict," 13–24; Abby Thompson and Paul Moughan, "Innovation in the Foods Industry: Functional Foods," *Innovation: Management, Policy and Practice* 10 (2008): 61–73.
8. Saikat Basu, James Thomas, and Surya Acharya, "Prospects for Growth in Global Nutraceutical and Functional Food Markets: A Canadian Perspective," *Australian Journal of Basic and Applied Sciences* 1 (2007): 637–49;

Tsuneo Hirahara, "Key Factors for the Success of Functional Foods," *Bio-Factors* 22 (2004): 289–93.

9. Niva, "Can We Predict," 13–24.

10. Ioannis S. Arvanitoyannis and Maria van Houwelingen-Koukaliaroglou, "Functional Foods: A Survey of Health Claims, Pros and Cons, and Current Legislation," *Critical Reviews in Food Science and Nutrition* 45 (2005): 385–404.

11. "Market Profile of Functional Foods in Japan," New Zealand Trade and Enterprise (2009), accessed September 25, 2011, http://www.nzte.govt.nz/explore-export-markets/market-research-by-industry/Food-and-beverage/Documents/functional-foods-market-in-Japan.pdf

12. American Dietetic Association, "Position of the American Dietetic Association: Functional Foods," *Journal of the American Dietetic Association* 109 (2009): 735–46.

13. Basu, Thomas, and Acharya, "Prospects for Growth," 637–49; Maurice Doyon and JoAnne Labrecque, "Functional Foods: A Conceptual Definition," *British Food Journal* 110 (2008): 1133–49; Hirahara, "Key Factors for the Success of Functional Foods," 289–93.

14. Jennifer Gray, Gillian Armstrong, and Heather Farley, "Opportunities and Constraints in the Functional Food Market," *Nutrition and Food Science* 33 (2003): 213–18.

15. Gyorgy Scrinis, "Functional Foods or Functionally Marketed Foods? A Critique of, and Alternatives to, the Category of 'Functional Foods,'" *Public Health Nutrition* 11 (2008): 541–45.

16. Doyon and Labrecque, "Functional Foods," 1133–49; Lotte Holm, "Food Health Policies and Ethics: Lay Perspectives on Functional Foods," *Journal of Agricultural and Environmental Ethics* 16 (2003): 531–44; Katan and de Roos, "Promises and Problems," 369–77; Robert Russell, "Functional Food Fables," *Nutrition in Clinical Care* 3 (2000): 259–60; Doris Schroeder, "Public Health, Ethics and Functional Foods," *Journal of Agricultural and Environmental Ethics* 20 (2007): 247–59; Tapsell, "Functional Foods," 523–26.

17. Chamberlain, "Food and Health," 467–81; Janne Lehenkari, "On the Borderline of Food and Drug: Constructing Credibility and Markets for a Functional Food Product," *Science and Culture* 12 (2003): 499–525; Marcel B. Roberfroid, "Global View on Functional Foods: European Perspectives," *British Journal of Nutrition* 88 (2002): S133–38.

18. Doyon and Labrecque, "Functional Foods," 1144.

19. Walter H. Glinsmann, "Functional Foods in North America," *Nutrition Reviews* 54 (1996): S33–37.

20. Katan and de Roos, "Promises and Problems," 369–77; Scrinis, "Functional Foods orFunctionally Marketed Foods?," 541–45.

21. Schroeder, "Public Health, Ethics and Functional Foods," 247–59; Peter Williams and Dilip Ghosh, "Health Claims and Functional Foods," *Nutrition and Dietetics* 65 (2008): 589–93.

22. Dilip Ghosh, "Functional Food and Health Claims: Regulations in Australia and New Zealand," *The Australian Journal of Dairy Technology* 64 (2009): 152–54; Martin Hahn, "Functional Foods: What Are They? How Are They Regulated? What Claims Can Be Made?" *American Journal of Law and Medicine* 31 (2005): 305–40; Peter Jones, "Clinical Nutrition: 7. Functional Foods—More Than Just Nutrition," *Canadian Medical Association Journal* 166 (2002): 1555–63; Rebecca W. Naylor, Courtney Droms, and Kelly Haws, "Eating with a Purpose: Consumer Response to Functional Food Health Claims in Conflicting Versus Complementary

Information Environments," *Journal of Public Policy and Marketing* 28 (2009): 221–33; Robert Russell, "Functional Food Fables," *Nutrition in Clinical Care* 3 (2000): 259–60.

23. Kendall Powell, "Functional Foods from Biotech—An Unappetizing Prospect?," *Nature Biotechnology* 25 (2007): 525–31.

24. Ghosh, "Functional Food and Health Claims," 152.

25. American Dietetic Association, "Position of the American Dietetic Association: Functional Foods," 735–46.

26. Wataru Aoi, Yuji Naito, and Toshikazu Yoshikawa, "Exercise and Functional Foods," *Nutrition Journal* 5 (2006): 15–22.

27. Ibid.; Louise Deldicque and Marc Francaux, "Functional Food for Exercise Performance: Fact or Foe?," *Current Opinion in Clinical Nutrition and Metabolic Care* 11 (2008): 774–81.

28. Deldicque and Francaux, "Functional Food for Exercise Performance," 774–81; Ron J. Maughan, "The Sports Drink as a Functional Food: Formulations for Successful Performance," *Proceedings of the Nutrition Society* 57 (1998): 15–23.

29. George Cheney and Daniel J. Lair, "Theorizing Organizational Rhetoric: Classical, Interpretive, and Critical Aspects," in *Theory Development in Organizational Communication*, ed. Dennis K. Mumby and Stephen K. May (London: Sage, 2005), 9.

30. Sharon Livesey, "Global Warming Wars: Rhetoric and Discourse Analytic Approaches to Exxon Mobil's Corporate Public Discourse," *Journal of Business Communication* 39 (2002): 117–48; Karyn Rybacki and Donald Rybacki, *Communication Criticism: Approaches and Genres* (Belmont, CA: Wadsworth, 1991).

31. Kenneth Burke, *A Rhetoric of Motives* (Berkley: University of California Press, 1969); Sonja K. Foss, *Rhetorical Criticism: Exploration and Practice*, 3rd ed. (Long Grove, IL: Waveland Press, 2004); Sonja K. Foss, Karen Foss, and Robert Trapp, *Contemporary Perspectives on Rhetoric*, 2nd ed. (Prospect Heights, IL: Waveland Press, 1991).

32. Timothy Kuhn, "The Discourse of Issues Management: A Genre of Organizational Communication," *Communication Quarterly* 45 (1997): 188–210.

33. Cheney and Lair, "Theorizing Organizational Rhetoric."

34. Stuart Albert and David A. Whetten, "Organizational Identity," in *Organizational Identity: A Reader*, ed. Mary J. Hatch and Majken Schultz (New York: Oxford University Press, 2004), 89–118; Bey-Ling Sha, "Exploring the Connection between Organizational Identity and Public Relations Behaviours: How Symmetry Trumps Conservation in Engendering Organizational Identification," *Journal of Public Relations Research* 21 (2009): 295–317; Stefan Sveningsson and Mats Alvesson, "Managing Managerial Identities: Organizational Fragmentation, Discourse and Identity Struggle," *Human Relations* 56 (2003): 1163–93.

35. George Cheney, *Rhetoric in an Organizational Society: Managing Multiple Identities* (Columbia: University of South Carolina Press, 1991), 13.

36. Rajesh Sethi and Larry Compeau, "Social Construction, Social Identity, and Market Orientation of the Firm," in *Conference Proceedings 13* (Chicago, IL: American Marketing Association, 2002), 183.

37. Ibid., 183–84.

38. Sveningsson and Alvesson, "Managing Managerial Identities," 1163–93.

39. Nigel O'Connor, "UK Corporate Reputation Management: The Role of Public Relations Planning, Research and Evaluation in a New Framework of Company Reporting," *Journal of Communication Management* 6 (2001): 53–63; Maktoba Omar, Robert Williams Jr., and David Lingelbach, "Global

Brand Market-Entry Strategy to Manage Corporate Reputation," *Journal of Product and Brand Management* 18 (2009): 177–87; W. Timothy Coombs and Sherry J. Holladay, "Unpacking the Halo Effect: Reputation and Crisis Management," *Journal of Communication Management* 10 (2006): 123–37.

40. Coombs and Holladay, "Unpacking the Halo Effect," 123–37; Dirk Gibson, Jerra Gonzales, and Jaclynn Castanon, "The Importance of Reputation and the Role of Public Relations," *Public Relations Quarterly* 51 (2006): 15–18; Omar, Williams, and Lingelbach, "Global Brand," 177–87; O'Connor, "UK Corporate Reputation Management," 53–63.

41. Prema Nakra, "Corporate Reputation Management: 'CRM' with a Strategic Twist?," *Public Relations Quarterly* 45 (2000): 35–42; Coombs and Holladay, "Unpacking the Halo Effect," 123–37; Elif Karaosmanoglu and T. C. Melewar, "Corporate Communications, Identity and Image: A Research Agenda," *Brand Management* 14 (2006): 196–206.

42. Alison M. Henderson, C. Kay Weaver, and George Cheney, "Talking 'Facts': Identity and Rationality in Industry Perspective on Genetic Modification," *Discourse Studies* 91 (2007): 9–41.

43. Karl E. Weick, Kathleen Sutcliffe, and David Obstfeld, "Organising and the Process of Sensemaking," *Organization Science* 16 (2005): 409–21.

44. Tee Rogers-Hayden and R. Hindmarsh, "Modernity Contextualises New Zealand's Royal Commission on Genetic Modification: A Discourse Analysis," *Journal of New Zealand Studies* 1 (2002): 41–62.

45. Virginia Braun and Victoria Clarke, "Using Thematic Analysis in Psychology," *Qualitative Research in Psychology* 3 (2006): 77–101.

46. "Australia New Zealand Food Standards Code," *Food Standards Authority Australia New Zealand (FSANZ)*, 2011, accessed September 25, 2011, http://www.foodstandards.gov.au/foodstandards/foodstandardscode.cfm.

6 Parsing Poverty

Farm Subsidies and American Farmland Trust

Maxwell Schnurer

This chapter attempts to unpack the political representations that defend American agriculture subsidies. If you typed "farm subsidy" or "agricultural support" in Fall 2010 into the search engine *Google*, the first result for your search would be farmland.org, whose preview message is: "Agricultural subsidies—get the facts from our experts."[1] The link leads viewers to American Farmland Trust—the leading *proponents* of big agricultural subsidies. If you look carefully you can see the "sponsored link" message. Following the American Farmland Trust link provides the opportunity to unpack a case of propaganda in its invitational stage.[2] We get a chance to look at how American Farmland Trust avoids the global criticisms of farm subsidies while re-presenting subsidies as transformed via its Average Crop Revenue Election (ACRE) program.

METHODOLOGY: PROPAGANDA ANALYSIS

This chapter centers on the production of popular knowledge by controlling the access to information about farm subsidies. The goal is to better understand how the widely criticized farm subsidies are defended and presented to those who casually search for information. Randal Marlin's work on propaganda has been influential in considering how propaganda is created and sustained.[3] Using a careful rhetorical analysis of the pages that cascade from the sponsored American Farmland Trust link, we can get a stronger understanding of how agricultural subsidies are recuperated and marketed to the American citizenry.

The critical process in this chapter is to make visible the operation of power and to increase the awareness of savvy media consumers. Although this author cannot pay for a sponsored link, the hope is that the title of this article will come up in future searches and provide some opportunity for rejoinder.[4]

THE PROBLEM: US FARM SUBSIDIES

Among the people of the globe who are starving, many point to Western food subsidies as the cause. Large American agricultural businesses benefit from government financial support, which creates artificially low prices for crops like corn, wheat, rice, cotton, dried milk, soybeans, and other easily exportable crops. Those crops then undercut those who try to grow food in their home communities. The result is that farms and food traditions wither in the face of cheap food and fiber imported from the US.

Representatives of non-governmental farming organizations from fifty developing nations met in India during Fall 2009 to coordinate their opposition to subsidies in the upcoming World Trade Organization (WTO) meeting. Forming the Food and Agriculture Organization (FAO), the group identified the harm from these trade policies as mass global starvation, arguing that "over one billion people are now going hungry, with about 150 million more people experiencing hunger as a result of the current food crisis."[5]

In a letter detailing its complaints, the FAO blames agricultural subsidies for the devastation brought to food sustainability. "The subsidized products flow into developing countries' markets, representing unfair competition to local farmers, destroying livelihoods and increasing hunger. The NGOs point out that even where export subsidy limits exist, the US and the EU regularly violate them and dump their agricultural products on developing countries' markets, ruining farming communities."[6] The complaints of advocates from developing nations, in the streets and in trade rounds, have centered on the impact of American agricultural subsidies.

But it isn't just international critics who recognize the harms of farm subsidies. Bob Waldrop, the president of the Oklahoma Food Cooperative, also a farmer, describes the relationship. "I think the overproduction here in the United States of certain commodity crops has had the effect of driving a lot of farmers out of business in other countries. We subsidize corn and wheat, so a lot of it gets produced and small farmers in other countries can't compete with that."[7] Throughout the global south, American farm subsidies are identified as the cause of millions of people's starvation, impoverishment, and death.[8]

There have been a number of attempts to put limits on the US subsidies, but in every instance the US government has bucked global opinion. In August 2009 Brazil was awarded $294.7 million in sanctions against the US in a World Trade Organization judgment. Brazil charged that the cotton from the US had been illegally subsidized. The World Trade Organization agreed, and charged the US to cut cotton subsidies by 82 percent. The US refused and did nothing.[9]

Despite the dramatic global commentary, farm subsidies are enveloped in a controlling discourse within North American media. Particularly, financial support for farmers has earned favorable political status contextualized as a way to prevent the *loss of the family farm*. These justifications usually come with a certain amount of nostalgia about American farming tradition, arguably obscuring farming in other nations. The rise in power of farming states and their political representatives, tied to the moral panic about declining numbers of farmers, sanitizes any critical public dialogue and virtually silences any discussion of the impact of US agricultural supports on citizens of developing nations.[10]

This chapter examines the use of defensive discursive strategies used to re-articulate farm subsidies laid out in the 2009–10 website of the rancher/ farmer advocacy group American Farmland Trust. The goal of this study is to explore how the American Farmland Trust rhetorically defends against the global critics of agricultural subsidies.

Following a long tradition of ideological criticism, we propose to examine contemporary public discourse in the US associated with "the family farm" and "farm subsidies." The specific focus of this study is the rhetoric of the American Farmland Trust and its website (www.farmland.org). To articulate the ideological position of the American Farmland Trust, we will have to position American Farmland Trust as lobbyists rather than as a community social movement group. Through an examination of the American Farmland Trust's website we will examine the rhetorical methods and strategies that defend farm subsidies in the US.

CO-OPTION AND AVOIDANCE: AMERICAN FARMLAND TRUST

American Farmland Trust was formed in 1980 and grew along with the Reagan-era Farm Bill. Its mission "is to help farmers and ranchers protect their land, produce a healthier environment and build successful communities." As the leading advocate for farmers and ranchers, its support and power are central to the continued existence of American agricultural subsidies. John Winthrop Jr., board chair of American Farmland Trust, explains: "Our work on the 2008 Farm Bill in the past year has helped to give agriculture and conservation a larger role in shaping federal farm policy than ever before."[11]

How important is American Farmland Trust in the defense of farm subsidies? Stephanie Mercier, chief economist of the US Senate Agriculture Committee, explained that the American Farmland Trust was instrumental in creating the Farm Bill legislation *itself*, contributing some of what she refers to as "innovative policy approaches."[12]

Those "innovative" ideas brought the combined power of the American Farmland Trust and the National Corn Growers Association together, to push for the new system of farm subsidies, which they called Average Crop Revenue Election or ACRE.[13] Mercier argues that it was the corn lobby and American Farmland Trust that created and guided the ACRE program into the Farm Bill.[14]

Starting with its sponsored *Google* links, American Farmland Trust successfully influences the access to information and thus circumvents the ability of a reasonable person to understand its actual position on farm subsidies. Using jargon and misdirection, the American Farmland Trust websites related to farm subsidies suggest that the group is a reform-oriented, pro-family farming organization. It is entirely possible that someone opposed to farm subsidies might inadvertently give his or her support to American Farmland Trust.

The sponsored link allows the advocacy group to encourage Internet searchers to find the American Farmland Trust's "spin" on the subject first in their search results. Searching for "Farm subsidy," "food subsidy," or even "Farm Bill" will also bring up the American Farmland Trust's digital advocacy to the top of your results page. The link is supposed to take the reader to the organization's position on farm subsidies but, once clicked, American Farmland Trust mentions the phrase only once. Instead, the sponsored link simply leads to a page inviting two ways to support American Farmland Trust.

On the left side of the American Farmland Trust page viewers are invited to sign up for a free bumper sticker reading: *No farms, no food*, and on the right side, viewers are invited to sign a petition intended to "urge your lawmakers to protect our farms and food." Nowhere is the advocacy or goals regarding farm subsidies visible for the viewer. Instead it is implied that American Farmland Trust is on the side of small-scale farmers.

The web page is visually disingenuous—the banner ad shows a ripe tomato and the images on the page are of a traditional tiny farm represented by an antique tractor. The side banner offers more encouragement to the first-time visitor, leading the viewer to believe that they are viewing a small farm–friendly group. The side banner offers such options as: "dine out for farms," "America's favorite farmer's markets," and "seven ways to save farmland." Even the tiny black and white logo of American Farmland Trust is the shadow image of a classic North American farm complete with a silhouetted silo. All of these cues are intended to suggest that the American Farmland Trust website is part of the American agricultural movement—far from the lobbying group pushing for the needs of large-scale farm corporations and ranchers.

If you move further into the website, you can find some policy discussion about the Farm Bill. Under the banner headline "What's next for the 2008 Farm Bill," American Farmland Trust outlines a discussion of almost every concern of American consumers *except* farm subsidies.

> The passage of the 2008 Farm Bill launches a new era for American farm and food policy. While we did not secure every gain we sought, the legislation makes many improvements by including:
>
> • Support for local foods
> • Significant new funding for conservation and farmland protection
> • Change in how agriculture subsidies are calculated
>
> Rising global food demand, spiking food and fuel prices and the ever-present threat of development are pressuring America's farmers and

ranchers. That's why American Farmland Trust worked so hard for the farm bill's conservation and local foods measures—tools that farmers need now more than ever. **Now AFT is taking these gains to the next level to protect more farm and ranch land, expand local food production, and help farmers and ranchers combat climate change and protect our drinking water.** [Bold in original][15]

Tactically the passage invites readers to understand American Farmland Trust as an outsider group, which is strange considering that it is the central advocate *for* the farm bill and spent millions to lobby and control the message.[16]

Even more interesting is how the passage emphasizes the environmental gains and local food benefits from the bloated farm bill. The conjunction of 'food' and 'farm' suggests to readers that AFT is an advocacy group for farmers' markets and local food initiatives. More powerfully, American Farmland Trust also implies that there are imminent threats to farmers and ranchers (food demand, food and fuel prices, and threats of development)—fear appeals that distract from the discussion about price supports for farmers.

The main reason for price supports (farm subsidies) is to create a steady financial income for farmers so they won't quit farming. But rather than explaining the justifications for subsidies, the passage suggests that the intentions of the Farm Bill are protecting land and water and fighting global warming—all arguably things harmed by large-scale subsidized ranching and farming.

It is worth looking carefully at the two boxes inviting the web page viewer to participate on behalf of American Farmland Trust. One is an offer for a free *No farms, no food* bumper sticker. The other is an invitation to sign a petition to be sent to Congress to let them know "you support a new direction in farm and food policy."

These representations are particularly crafty. The *No farms, no food* bumper sticker is a clever ultimatum that is literally true, but also represents an antagonistic rhetorical positioning. It ensures that anyone who disagrees with those who sport the bumper sticker will be tarred with the label of being against farming (and perhaps threatened with starvation).

No farms, no food doesn't say anything about the size of the farms, or the degree to which they actually provide food for communities (as opposed to corn for ethanol). Instead the phrase insulates criticism of *any* farms, and lumps together the causes of small-scale, organic farming with those of the largest agricultural corporations.

The invitation to sign the petition is supported with some of the most abstract, open-ended promises and vague, almost universally positive goals. With nothing specific, signees indicate that they are supporters of American Farmland Trust and invite their names to be used as weight in American Farmland Trust's advocacy.

The legislative home for what we are calling farm subsidies is in the 2008 Food Conservation and Energy Act (FCEA, often called the "Farm Bill"). The FCEA is an extension of the 1996 Farm Bill, which formalized export subsidies (monies directly paid to crop producers who exported to other nations), and the Marketing Loan Program (which lends to farmers until their crops come in). These are the primary engines that create cheap export crops and lead to flooding of markets and cascading global poverty.

Financial support for farmers whose crops are failing hinges on the backdrop of the emotionally distraught 1980s telethons that publicized the plight of the American farmer. Willie Nelson and his Farm Aid concerts helped to crystallize the crisis of the American farm and provide the political weight to fund farms, whose consolidation under exceptionally large agricultural businesses centralized profits. Industrialization meant that the larger farming conglomerates got exponentially larger on federally supported cheap grain and smaller farms became increasingly niche producers.

The dual, competing imperative of funding farmers (to both help small farmers, and to produce more food) helped to insulate the farm subsidy programs from political criticism and created a series of loopholes that enabled large producers to gather enormous amounts of subsidy money and—especially in the case of corn—build an infrastructure to ensure massive production at record-breaking low prices. "Because nearly 70 percent of the subsidies go to the top 10 percent of agricultural producers, the recent prosperity is not seen or felt among many small-to-medium-size growers who keep the struggling counties of the Great Plains alive."[17]

We finally get an outline of American Farmland Trust's position on subsidies on its page "An overview of subsidy payments." On this page, American Farmland Trust further distances itself from the old ideas of subsidies by outlining the *benefits* of subsidies (stable food supply, food security in case of extreme weather, and keeping down farmer debt), but also describes the *criticisms* of farm subsidies (failure to help small farms, overproduction, and crowding out subsistence farming). They position themselves as insider-reformers whose proposed ACRE program solves the criticisms of farm subsidies.[18]

Perhaps in response to the tainted name of subsidies, the language of the American Farmland Trust websites relies on the distinctions between traditional farm subsidies and its new ACRE (Average Crop Revenue Election) program. American Farmland Trust suggests that the new ACRE program will offer better protection, is supported by agricultural groups, is optional, removes market distortions, and will save money.

Is ACRE a real change? The fact that the ACRE program doesn't address the threat of cheap American food to the global food supply suggests that the reforms presented have nothing to do with the international critique of American subsidies. Instead, these 'reforms' are in fact mostly tied to the symbolic changes associated with the name.

ACRE was "a concept developed by the National Corn Growers Association and American Farmland Trust," said Mercier, the chief economist of the US Senate Agriculture Committee. "It was included originally in Chairman (Tom Harkin's) mark in the Senate Agriculture Committee, where it was modified. Further modifications were made in conference committee." ACRE's adoption is sort of an "anomaly" in the political process, said Mercier. It was supported by only a handful of groups and senators. Under those circumstances, "such programs don't normally get into a farm bill."[19]

Touted as representing reform, ACRE is insurance for price dropping in crops, precisely the problem that American export food dumping has been accelerating all these years. Because the government guarantees to pay farmers when price dips, American farmers are insulated from market trends that might otherwise encourage them to plant fewer or different crops. Let's note how Ralph Grossi describes ACRE in an American Farmland Trust press release:

> The ACRE program is an important element of reform that is not well understood. It represents a fundamental reform in how U.S. commodity programs operate—**reducing market distortions, cutting direct payments, reducing loan deficiency payment rates, and freeing up funding for other priorities.** This is an historic change. ACRE allows producers to choose a market oriented, risk management tool that adjusts with market prices and pays farmers only when they need it—when they suffer a real loss in revenue.
>
> Existing policies are based on politically set target prices and loan rates that distort the market. We know many farmers want this choice and we expect **more than 50-million acres to be enrolled in the program.** It is a small step for farmers but a giant leap forward for U.S. farm policy now—and sets the stage for future improvements. [Bolding in original][20]

On the American Farmland Trust website, the discussion about subsidies is almost entirely shifted to a discussion of ACRE. The value of ACRE as a rhetorical location to redefine farm subsidies can't be overstated. This new name allows American Farmland Trust to re-articulate the conversation about subsidies to be about the new program, thus sidestepping most of the prominent critiques while insulating itself in a cloud of excess verbiage suggesting that ACRE is a less costly form of crop insurance. American Farmland Trust outlines the distinction between farm subsidies and ACRE and in that maneuver re-positions ACRE as helping needy farmers, something few readers can oppose.

> Farms and ranches are inherently prone to variations in prices and yields. Government programs help protect our food supply, but the

farm subsidies in the 2002 Farm Bill only protected price, not loss in crop yield, and were unwieldy, inefficient and supportive of only a few producers.

Developed and championed by AFT and the National Corn Growers Association, the new Average Crop Revenue Election (ACRE) program restores the concept that a farm safety net should provide help only when producers are in need after suffering from a loss beyond their control.[21]

The only place American Farmland Trust deals with the global crisis of farmers against subsidies is a tepid acknowledgment that the new ACRE program might help get the US out of WTO scraps.

> *Reduction in Marketing Loan Program rates by 30 percent.* This reduction begins to address one of our most troublesome international trade concerns, which has triggered WTO trade disputes. It doesn't solve all of the United States' international trade problems, but it is a step in the right direction.[22]

But will the changes of ACRE mean an end to World Trade Organization troubles for the US? Not likely. Noting the likely increase in payments to farmers enrolled in the ACRE program, the European Commission's agriculture directorate-general has published a report arguing that despite the attempt to frame ACRE as distinct from subsidies, the commissioner will argue that they are trade-disrupting. "ACRE is likely to be classified as product-specific 'amber box' support. The 'amber box' classification groups measures with trade-distorting impacts that consequently have to be capped."[23]

ACRE gets a particularly scathing description in a *Washington Post* editorial, where the *Post* claims that the provision would mean $18 billion more in agricultural subsidies and a deep incentive for large-crop farmers to overproduce.

> Starting in 2009, farmers can choose to trade in some of their traditional subsidies in return for a government promise to make up 90 percent of the difference between what they actually made from farming and their usual income. In principle, this provides farmers a federal safety net only in those years when prices or yields fall drastically— that is, when they really need one. Congress added the optional ACRE program to the bill as a sop to reformers who, sensibly, wanted to replace the current subsidy system with a simpler insurance-style program. Such a wholesale change would, indeed, have been a real reform. But since the farm bill continued direct payments and other old-style subsidies, no one expected huge numbers of farmers to volunteer for the new ACRE deal.[24]

Then farmers got a look at the bill's formula for determining benefits under ACRE. It pegs the subsidies to current, record-high prices
for grain, meaning farmers would get paid if prices fall back to their
historical and, for farmers, perfectly profitable norms. A program that
started out as a streamlined insurance policy against extraordinary
hardship has mutated into a possible guarantee of extraordinary prosperity. Small wonder that, as *The Post*'s Dan Morgan reports, a farming blog is urging farmers to sign up for ACRE, which it describes as
"lucrative beyond expectations."[25]

As noted by the *Washington Post*, food prices were at an all-time high
in 2008. Central to this elevated price has been the impact of subsidized
corn to make ethanol and corn syrup (and quite a bit more—consider the
arguments presented by Michael Pollan on the political economy of corn
in *The Omnivore's Dilemma*).[26] One likely outcome of the new ACRE
program will be the substantial increase in cheap grains—precisely the
complaint of poor farmers in developing nations and of progressive American farming movements.

The Food and Agricultural Research Institute at the University of
Missouri-Columbia reported in 2008 that ACRE provides a substantial
increase in monies paid for subsidies, primarily for large grain producers.

> The ACRE program could have significant effects on producer income
> and taxpayer costs. On a crop year basis, the program increases net
> farm program payments by an average of more than $1 billion per year
> and the potential expenditures are much larger. Given program rules
> and estimated payments, the ACRE program appears much more likely
> to appeal to producers of feed grains, wheat and soybeans than to pro-
> ducers of cotton, rice and peanuts.[27]

One of its crucial findings is that, in fact, ACRE's payments will likely
increase production of crops. The program doesn't address the primary
criticism of developing world farmers—overproduction and export of agricultural goods that are painfully cheap. The ACRE program would protect farmers who planted large plots from shifting prices. This creates an
even greater incentive to produce and, with excessive returns, probably to
export. The University of Missouri-Columbia report continues:

> Because ACRE payments are tied to planted acreage, they are expected
> to affect crop production decisions. Production increases for crops
> where expected ACRE payments are larger, and the total area devoted
> to production of 12 major crops increases slightly.[28]

ACRE will not reduce the production of cheap food-stuffs in the US.
First, the program is optional, so for crops whose price remains high,
farmers can retain conventional subsidies. Second, the construction of

the program seems to be built to favor large businesses that farm many acres. There is a requirement that participants assume a twenty percent reduction in direct payment rates and a 30 percent reduction in marketing loan guarantee and loan deficiency payments in order to enroll. This suggests that participants would need a bankroll to survive.[29]

The gap of coverage means that the only businesses who can afford to use ACRE are massive planters of subsidized crops.

Essential to the linguistic shift away from farm subsidies is the development of ACRE as an alternative—rhetorically and politically—to subsidies. Most centrally, this allows American Farmland Trust to position itself as opposed to farm subsidies, while still essentially lobbying for them.

IMPLICATIONS OF AMERICAN FARMLAND TRUST RHETORIC

How are farm subsidies sold to the American public when they are a bane to so many millions of the world's poor? The strategies and tactics presented in these few web pages are valuable blueprints to understand how discourse on food provides opportunity for corporate interests to redefine what the public knows. In this case, using five tactics of propaganda American Farmland Trust is able to gain credibility and influence over the issue of farm subsidies.

First, the creators of the website displaced the critiques about the harms of US farm subsidies through *avoidance*. Despite being led to a page promising political experts analyzing agricultural subsidies, viewers are led to a page where the two main choices are simply to support American Farmland Trust. There is no acknowledgment or even outline of the complaints about American farm policy by the rest of the world. Instead the American Farmland Trust describes them as "international trade concerns." It barely uses the terms farm subsidies, instead transmogrifying financial supports for farmers into acronyms like ACRE, which present little structural difference, but offer expansive discursive opportunity to shift away from a previously laden term.

Second, American Farmland Trust uses the power of *naming* to influence readers who encounter the ACRE program. The use of the new acronym ACRE to describe the slightly reformed crop-support policy allows the group to distance itself from the terminology of subsidies. This tactic is called naming, and is a relatively common tool of propagandists.

A government may choose to title legislation that drastically cuts back on funding for education, as "An act for the improvement of Education," treating as a truth what is at best only debatably so. A great deal of effort and expense is often required to counteract impressions so formed. Name-calling in general is a powerful force for influencing opinion because names are easily remembered.[30]

In this case, American Farmland Trust named the new program ACRE, which not only is memorable but also has metonymic connection to farming. The acronym uses the antiquated scale of measurement, in this case for the purposes of implying a connection to farms measured in "acres," despite the fact that farms measured in miles or hectares are more likely to take advantage of the program.

Third, American Farmland Trust *controls the access to information* about farm subsidies. By paying for its politics to be found at the top of *Google* searches, it increases the likelihood that viewers will search out and be connected to its political goals. This maneuver is done by obscuring its policy positions and implying political support for family farms through leading search terms. American Farmland Trust pays *Google* to guide searchers to its policy position, which allows it to obscure criticism and dissent.

Fourth, the group uses *farming imagery* that suggests small, rural family farming not only for the purposes of nostalgia, but also to gather contextual credibility. In this case the bumper sticker campaign of *No farms, no food* suggests an entwined relationship between food consumers and producers—obviating any difference that might be drawn between large and small or organic and conventional farming. The implied common cause between food reformers and large corporate agriculture is a crafty hijack of activist energy. This lumping together borrows the credibility of farm reformers and displaces the ideas of change to continue the current farm policies.

Despite advocating for the needs of large farmers, the pages of the American Farmland Trust website use farming images and connections to farmers' markets to connect its cause to small farms. While avoiding any discussion of organic or scale of food production, the American Farmland Trust website visually and rhetorically connects itself as part of the "civic agriculture movement."[31] The general presentation of the American Farmland Trust website stresses local communities and food from small farms and uses particular images to develop perceptual credibility through association.

Fifth, the American Farmland Trust website *takes advantage of the moral panic* of informed consumers who want local/organic food because of the fears elicited about big agri-business. It positions the responsibility for farm policy in the hands of consumers, who actually have very little power over the financial incentives that bankrupt small family farms and centralize growing power in the hands of a few corporations.

This rhetorical inversion relies on a certain amount of knowledge among consumers. They use the anxiety generated by those conscious about healthy local food and then align their cause as parallel, despite being oppositional.

Tactically, American Farmland Trust identifies the criticisms of the farm bill and then argues that the adoption of new ACRE program will solve all the problems with farm subsidies.

This inversion of capacity for change is a wonderful tactic to induce guilt in those whose farmers' markets end in October and have to shop in corporate supermarkets or buy imported produce. Consider the myriad threads of engaged activists who've influenced the public knowledge of farms: Willie Nelson and Farm Aid, vegetarian advocates, farmers' market organizers, community supported agriculture (CSAs), permaculture movements, health food stores, *Mother Earth News*, Schlosser's *Fast Food Nation*, and Michael Pollan among other authors. Considered in whole, these activists have changed the way we understand food in the last twenty years. They also include a political awareness about farm subsidies and their impact.

CONCLUSION

If the purpose of these agricultural movements is to *raise* awareness, then the purpose of the American Farmland Trust website is to *harness* and *reinvest* that awareness into the lobbying for the status quo, that is, to support a system of continued farm subsidies.

How are farm subsidies defended in the US? How are the cries of the farmers of the globe diffused, responded to, and re-articulated to *support* farm subsidies—the very policies they critique? Poor farmers, in the US and abroad, cannot afford the kind of systematic information campaign that American Farmland Trust can. Businesses with a profound interest in how terms like *farm subsidies* are understood by the public can use propaganda to influence the very fabric of what we know.

In the example used in this chapter, we get a chance to view the development and implementation of intellectual trickery. The present analysis makes more evident how public policy discussions can be guided, obscured, and sanitized. With the visibility of these persuasive tools, readers can auto-critique similar examples of propaganda.

NOTES

1. *American Farmland Trust*, accessed October 12, 2010, www.farmland.org.
2. Propaganda is distinguished from persuasion. This is propaganda because it impedes the ability of readers to understand who is persuading them or, in this case, of what they are being persuaded. Propaganda obscures the creator or the medium of the message in an attempt to gain credibility without sharing the actual biases (political location) of the message creator.
3. Randal Marlin, *Propaganda and the Ethics of Persuasion* (Peterborough, Ontario: Broadview Press, 2002), 95–96.
4. Marlin makes this potential for engagement with propaganda clear in his text. "Propaganda analysis that exposes types of ambiguity and the ways

in which attention is captured and directed by the propagandist performs a useful service by alerting us to possible manipulation by others" (95).

5. "World Trade Body's Policies Caused Global Food Crisis," *Africa News*, September 23, 2009, LexisNexis Academic.
6. Ibid.
7. Jim Stafford, "Feed Me—Does US Policy Fight Global Hunger?," *McClatchy Tribune Business News*, May 18, 2008, LexisNexis Academic.
8. To make the case stronger, some scholars have considered what the impact of a reduction of US farm subsidies would be. In a 2009 report on Kenya sponsored in part by the Carnegie Endowment for International Peace, the United Nations Economic Commission for Africa (UNECA), the United Nations Development Programme, and the Kenyan Institute for Research and Policy Analysis, lead author Eduardo Zepeda estimated what the impact of an end to US and European agricultural subsidies would do to Kenya, noting: " . . . the gains for Kenya would primarily come from the elimination of subsidies to exports of agricultural goods in the EU and the United States that would make their products more competitive; to a lower extent, gains would also come from reductions in domestic support for agriculture in the developed world . . ."
9. "US Hit with 300m WTO Sanction in Cotton Fight," *New Zealand Herald*, September 1, 2009, LexisNexis Academic.
10. A good example of this kind of writing is found in the book *Farm Aid: A Song for America*. Thoughtful progressive Jim Hightower outlines the stakes and also reinforces the norms identified earlier. "But there's also been a shove-back in the countryside, where farmers have been refusing to go quietly, as bankers, speculators, chemical peddlers, genetic manipulators, global commodity traders, monopolistic processors, and retailers—as well as the politicians of both parties they own—combine to shove the family farm out of existence, leaving our food supply in the grasping hands of a few globalized, industrialized, agribusiness profiteers" (135).
11. "About American Farmland Trust," *American Farmland Trust*, www.farmland.org/about/message/default.asp.
12. David Bennett, "Senate Ag Committee Economist Offers Farm Bill Post Mortem," *Southeast Farm Press*, April 8, 2009, 17, LexisNexis Academic.
13. Mercier also noted that the complaints from other nations represented in the World Trade Organization had little impact on the discussion of the US Congress. "Consequently though, the international (scene) had little or no influence on members of Congress when it came to putting together the (new) farm bill" (Bennett, "Senate Ag Committee").
14. It's worth noting the relationship between corporate agriculture money and large universities. Presumably, faculty at Iowa State helped to build the credible intellectual weight for the ACRE program. This argument is supported by the academic claims of the program while it was in development (at that point called the Revenue Counter-Cyclical Program) by the National Corn Growers Association. " . . . the National Corn Growers' Public Policy Action Team spent two years developing the Revenue Counter-Cyclical Program, drawing on state corn grower associations and Iowa State and other universities for analysis of the program's features." Laws, Forrest, "Corn Growers: RCCP would close hole in safety net," *Southwest Farm Press*, April 19, 2007: 10, accessed March 12, 2012, www.southwestfarmpress.com/corn-growers-rccp-would-close-hole-safety-net-0
15. "What's Next for the 2008 Farm bill," *American Farmland Trust*, http://www.farmland.org/actioncenter/no-farms-no-food/farm-bill.asp.
16. American Farmland Trust, "Annual Report 2008," p. 20, http://www.farmland.org/about/annualreport/documents/AFT_ar2008.pdf.

17. Timothy Egan, "Even with Subsidies, Farmers Are Worried; Letter from America," *The International Herald Tribune*, December 27, 2004, Lexis-Nexis Academic.
18. "Overview of the Farm Bill: History of Subsidy Payments," *American Farmland Trust*, http://www.farmland.org/programs/farm-bill/history/usfarmsubsidies.asp.
19. Egan, "Even with Subsidies."
20. David Bennett, "ACRE Program Reviews Less Than Positive," *Southeast Farm Press*, April 1, 2009, 22, LexisNexis Academic.
21. American Farmland Trust, "ACRE Is Reform," http://www.farmland.org/programs/campaign/documents/AFT-FarmPolicyCampaign-ACREisReform_051208.pdf.
22. "Farm Subsidies," *American Farmland Trust*, http://www.farmland.org/programs/farm-bill/analysis/farmsubsidies.asp.
23. Luc Vernet, "EU/US: Commission Says New US Farm Bill Trade-Distorting," *Europolitics*, February 5, 2009, LexisNexis Academic.
24. Please note that the development of this program was specifically intended to allow the US to report subsidies to the WTO. "The program was designed to allow the United States to report BRP [base revenue protection] payments to the World Trade Organization as 'Green Box' support" (Laws, Ibid., 10).
25. *Washington Post*, "Pasture of Plenty: You Thought You Knew How Bad the Farm Bill Was," May 22, 2008, A25, LexisNexis Academic.
26. Michael Pollan, *The Omnivore's Dilemma* (New York: Penguin Press, 2006).
27. Food and Agricultural Research Institute at the University of Missouri-Columbia, "The Food, Conservation and Energy Act of 2008," http://www.fapri.missouri.edu/outreach/publications/2008/FAPRI_MU_Report_08_08.PDF.
28. Ibid., 12.
29. Ron Smith, "ACRE Decisions Depend on Crop Base, Yield History," *Southwest Farm Press*, May 21, 2009, LexisNexis Academic.
30. Marlin, *Propaganda and the Ethics of Persuasion*, 100–101.
31. Joan Dye Gussow, "Here Comes the Future," in *Farm Aid: A Song for America*, ed. Holly George-Warren (Emmaus, PA: Rodale Books, 2005), 194.

7 Pardon Your Turkey and Eat Him Too

Antagonism over Meat Eating in the Discourse of the Presidential Pardoning of the Thanksgiving Turkey

Carrie Packwood Freeman and Oana Leventi-Perez

To celebrate the Thanksgiving holiday for at least the last twenty years, the president of the United States has hosted a press conference during which he uses his executive powers to pardon the life of a turkey gifted to him from the National Turkey Federation, an agri-business industry group. Considering the reality that the president (and millions of Americans) will indeed eat a turkey as the traditional centerpiece of their Thanksgiving meal, this utopian spectacle of a life-saving public pardon for one bird reveals an antagonism—a discursive rupture disclosing an opening between the hegemonic advertising rhetoric of the meat industry and the counter-hegemonic vegan rhetoric of animal rights. We wondered what this hypocritical ritual—this animal sacrifice in reverse—implies regarding American attitudes and anxieties about killing non-human animals for food.

"Carnism" is the term psychologist Melanie Joy coined to describe the hegemonic, taken-for-granted ideology that implicitly justifies American culture's choice to eat animals.[1] The two main institutions that legitimize carnism are the government and the media. The government legitimizes the system through legalizing the mass slaughter and consumption of non-human animals and limiting their legal status to that of property, and the media "maintain the invisibility of the system and reinforce the justifications for eating meat."[2] Justification relies on institutions and the public supporting three myths: "eating meat is normal, natural, and necessary."[3]

In examining the legitimizing discourse of these two institutions, we discuss the results of our critical discourse analysis of White House press transcripts of the turkey pardoning ceremony as well as its news media coverage, starting with President George Bush Sr. in 1989 to President Obama in 2010. As the highest elected leader, how does the US president treat the pardoning, turkeys, and the practice of eating animals? And as the watchdog of government and agenda-setters of public policy, how do the news media cover this pardon? Is it largely a whimsical human interest story, or do they view it as a hard news opportunity to investigate factory farming or the ethics of eating animals? How seriously do they take this pardoning ceremony, and how is the turkey and his/her interests represented? What does the media discourse reveal about America's identity as a meat-eating public?

This chapter contributes to an understanding of the rhetoric of food and its connection to power structures by first situating the national turkey pardoning ceremony in context of a review of literature on: presidential pardons, animal sacrifice, meat's role in celebratory eating, modern animal agri-business practices and laws, meat industry rhetoric versus vegan rhetoric, and news media coverage of farmed animals.

As authors and vegetarians (eaters of tofu-turkey), our discourse analysis is informed by an animal rights perspective that acknowledges that non-human animals are fellow sentient individuals who deserve to be valued inherently rather than instrumentally as tools/property.[4] Peter Singer described discrimination against sentient non-humans as an unjust, "speciesist" bias that fails to recognize their natural interest in enjoying life and avoiding suffering.[5] Animal rights philosophy advocates that humans eat a plant-based (vegan) diet that avoids the domestication, enslavement, exploitation, or killing of animals.[6] If sentient animals deserve rights, then the legal, institutionalized annual mass slaughter of billions of beings for unnecessary human food is nothing short of criminal—a subject certainly worthy of scholarly scrutiny.

LITERATURE REVIEW

History of the Presidential Pardon

In the US, executive clemency is rooted in the pardoning power of the British monarchs.[7] Given that pardons were considered a personal gift from the monarch, "an act of grace," and were not subject to scrutiny, this power was often used for monetary and political gain.[8] The US Constitution gives the president the power to "grant reprieves and pardons for offenses against the United States."[9] The pardon can take several forms: (1) A full pardon allows the offenders to walk away as if they had never been convicted; (2) A partial pardon relieves the offender of some of the consequences of his/her act; (3) Amnesties, which are usually granted to groups of people, imply that the offense will be forgotten; (4) Reprieves postpone the execution of the sentence; and (5) Commutations substitute a lesser for a harsher sentence.[10] One major criticism of the contemporary federal clemency system is that not enough pardons are granted to deserving offenders.[11] Jeffrey Crouch argues that, in recent history, presidents have avoided risk by granting pardons only in cases that pose no political threats, and mostly to "well-vetted offenders who have waited years for a decision, committed nonviolent offenses, or both."[12]

The origin of the presidential pardoning of turkeys is disputed, as some believe President Truman was the first to pardon a turkey in 1947.[13] It was not until 1989 that President George H. W. Bush first pardoned the turkeys received for Thanksgiving, initiating an annual tradition.[14] Since then, a turkey and an alternate, chosen in case the first bird is unable to "perform," have been pardoned each year. The alternates are sometimes called "Vice Turkeys."[15] Until 2005, the pardoned turkeys were sent to a working farm in Frying Pan Park in Herndon, Virginia, "where many died within months."[16] After that, they were sent to one of the Disney resorts. In 2010, as Disneyland started looking for new attractions, Washington's Mount Vernon Estate in Virginia became the turkey's new destination.[17]

Factory Farming and Turkeys

For the 97 percent of Americans who eat animals,[18] animal products comprise over a quarter of the average American's caloric intake.[19] To satisfy this high demand, the USDA estimates agri-business kills over nine billion land animals annually, the majority of which are birds.[20] Specifically, 250 million turkeys are slaughtered annually, with approximately a fifth of these eaten on Thanksgiving day.[21] The scale of the slaughter necessitates that modern animal farming employ industrial methods, warehousing animals in "factory farms," also called "confined animal feeding operations" (CAFOs).[22]

A turkey CAFO will house hundreds or thousands of birds, averaging just three square feet of space per individual.[23] Their beaks and toes are painfully clipped off without anesthesia, a cheap manipulation meant to reduce the lethalness of aggression caused by the frustratingly dense, unnatural conditions for these social animals. Because they are bred to have abnormally large chests to meet consumer demand for breast meat, turkeys frequently suffer lameness and heart attacks due to obesity. In fact, they can no longer mate naturally, and the artificial insemination process is a rough and stressful sexual violation.[24] When deemed optimally profitable, the turkeys are crammed into trucks and transported to the slaughterhouse. The stressful and fast-paced slaughtering process involves them being shackled upside down by their feet, with their heads run through an electric stunning bath before a worker slits their throats. Conscious or not, they are run through the scalding bath and dismembered on a production line.[25]

No federal laws exist to protect animals while on the farm (only in transport), and the Humane Slaughter Act doesn't cover birds. State anti-cruelty laws often exempt standard agricultural practices, so cruelty prosecutions are rare.[26] However, animal protection groups have started passing statewide reforms via the referendum process, which subverts agri-business lobbyists, to provide animals more space in accordance with public opinion.[27]

Consumers often wonder if organic or free-range is much better.[28] Federal organic standards do not dictate much regarding humane treatment, as it is more about increasing consumer health benefits. But standards do prevent birds from being genetically modified and allow them access to the outdoors, even though they can still be warehoused. This is similar to "free-range" categories that don't guarantee that each bird makes it outdoors and don't specify length of time outdoors nor the quality of that experience.[29]

Animal Sacrifice and Celebratory Meat-Eating

The food symbolism associated with highly ritualized special events reveals a lot about the society in which it is constructed.[30] Historically, the symbolic value of meat consumption was derived from the scarcity of this resource, reserved for the wealthy. In prehistoric society, meat distribution was traditionally associated with "royal" status, thus setting one of the preconditions for social inequality.[31] Animal sacrifice was a phenomenon of early domesticity, but through widespread domestication, animals gradually lost their spiritual symbolic dimensions and were viewed more instrumentally. Richard Bulliet notes that sacrificial ceremony's decline was ironically marked by an increase in animal slaughter, concluding that "the decline in blood sacrifice does not equate to a rise in the humane treatment of animals."[32]

Historian Kimberly Patton claims the sacrificial animal is considered special from the rest of the flock—a more perfect specimen with a relationship to God.[33] Michael Pollan proposes that the religious rituals related to animal sacrifice reflect humanity' s historic discomfort and shame over the killing of animals for food, even when necessary for survival: "Many cultures have offered sacrificial animals to the gods, perhaps as a way to convince themselves it was the gods' appetite that demanded the slaughter, and not their own."[34] Humane Society President Wayne Pacelle notes that animal sacrifice represented a "highly personal moral tension" over killing the innocent; the ritualistic ceremony is meant to show remorseful respect and offer atonement, "washing away the taint of violence."[35] Bronislaw Malinowski's ethnographies found that, to ease the guilt, many cultures prefer to believe that animals (whether hunted or sacrificially killed) offer themselves voluntarily.[36]

Today, meat eating is rooted in the dominant economic and philosophical systems of capitalism and anthropocentrism. In a world that celebrates consumerism as a given right, and where material and economic growth is deemed essential for human progress, non-human animals are mere resources for human use. In her culinary analysis of American culture, Barbara Willard concludes "The primary theme is the glory of meat in a capitalist environment: Meat, it's a good investment for the body, the family, the economy, and the land."[37]

Pro-Meat and Anti-Meat Rhetoric

"Beef. It's what's for dinner," was the popular slogan for the American beef industry's advertising campaign in the early 1990s. The campaign's slogan implies that animals exist to be eaten, and mutes carnivorous imagery with the traditional representation of the family dinner.[38] And fast-food advertising often promotes meat-eating as central to hedonistic heterosexual male bonding in defiance of femininity and social or ecological responsibility.[39] This way, both producers and consumers distance themselves from the reality of animal consumption. Mass terms like "meat," "hamburger," and "leather" used instead of "dead animal," "cow," or "skin" encourage consumers to forget that they are eating or using a dead animal.[40] According to ecofeminist Carol Adams, this muting is typical for the colloquial speakers' pleasurable talk of meat. Whether used literally or figuratively, meat is an omnipresent, positively evocative symbol in American culture.

The symbolic values that meat takes can be situated within a broader political-cultural context, and can mirror the entire American belief system.[41] To study the social meanings the American marketplace assigns to meat, Bettina Heinz and Ronald Lee[42] applied a Burkean cluster analysis to fifty meat-based texts, which revealed six associational clusters: Product (where the discourse of meat consumption dissociates the product of consumption from the living animal), Food (where meat is established as natural human food, associated with entertainment), Meal (here meat is the one food that makes a meal and is seen as a necessity), Tradition (messages in popular culture establish meat consumption's traditional place in US life, giving it pious and patriotic connotations), Masculinity (meat-eating is a masculine activity), and, finally, Health (here meat consumption is placed in the context of healthier eating). Overall, this analysis concluded that contemporary culture structures perceptions so that the raising and killing of animals for food becomes a taken-for-granted, natural part of life. Cultural taboos demand the invisibility of meat production and, by obscuring the violence, meat products are made more palatable.

Contrarily, in the much less pervasive pro-vegan rhetoric, American animal activists focused on framing problems with meat as: cruelty and suffering; commodification of animals; harm to humans and the environment; and needless killing. Activists primarily blamed factory farming and sometimes advocated for less cruel farming practices, but the most common solution was for consumers to go vegan or reduce animal product consumption.[43]

Journalistic Coverage of Farmed Animals

The commercial influence of a pervasive and legalized meat industry is strong, which may account for why speciesism and the ideology of carnism are cultural values that Freeman found national news tends to impose on audiences, naturalizing and legitimizing the exploitation of farmed animals.[44] This discriminatory perspective is so naturalized that journalists and the public often don't acknowledge it as a bias. To prevent dissonance, Joy notes people defensively distort reality by internalizing carnism through three cognitive processes: They objectify animals, de-individualize animals to prevent identification and connection, and dichotomize animals into separate categories, such as edible/inedible.[45] These cognitive processes are similar to the three framing processes Freeman found the US national media typically use when constructing farmed animals: Journalists deny animals' individual identities, commodify beings into bodies, and fail to acknowledge animals' emotions and ethical aspects of their predicaments.[46] Additionally, Joy claims media often legitimize carnism through: omitting strong exposés that challenge agri-business, prohibiting animal rights perspectives, and diminishing the scope of farmed animal cruelty by portraying it as isolated scandals rather than systemic problems.[47]

METHODOLOGY

As communication scholars, we take a Foucauldian social constructivist stance in noting the fundamental power of communication, namely discourse, to make meaning and construct truth on a topic rather than communication merely reflecting an existing and fixed reality.[48] In this study we view the government and the media as powerful players actively constructing, participating in, and maintaining a discursive regime of truth defining the meaning of turkeys, Thanksgiving, and carnism within an American cultural context. To examine this, we conducted a critical discourse analysis based on Teun Van Dijk's model, described more as a perspective than a method: "critical discourse studies scholars are typically interested in the way discourse (re)produces social *domination*, that is, the *power abuse* of one group over others."[49] Here we examined discursive themes, both implicit and explicit, that reveal how meaning is made and ideology is functioning. We deconstructed the implicit hypocrisy of publicly celebrating a pardon of one, named turkey while privately killing millions of other nameless turkeys, as it serves as an antagonism. Ernesto Laclau and Chantal Mouffe define antagonism as a limit to a discourse, which reveals inconsistencies undercutting the legitimacy of the discourse's accepted "truth."[50]

Our sample contained transcripts of presidential Thanksgiving press conferences from 1989 to 2010 (except for a lack of access to years 1995–96). And the news media sample for the same two decades consisted of sixty-six stories on the pardoning from major national news organizations: *The Washington Post* (37), *The New York Times* (16), and NPR (13), including hard news, features, and editorials/op-eds (excluding letters to the editor).

We asked the following research questions:

- How seriously is the pardoning ceremony taken and what view of turkeys does that imply? To what extent does the government or journalism consider the turkey's perspective versus an anthropocentric perspective?
- What does the discourse reveal about the function or purpose of the president pardoning a turkey's life on Thanksgiving?
- How do the government and journalism construct America's identity as a meat-eating public? To what extent do they challenge carnism versus support carnism?

FINDINGS

Press Conference Presidential Discourse

White House press conferences generally discussed a turkey's life not in terms of a right to life but in terms of presidents mercifully choosing to spare him from his destined purpose of ending up on the dinner table (what Obama in 2009 called a "terrible and delicious fate"), for a future where he can now enjoy a "life of leisure."[51] Most presidents mentioned "life," focusing on the bird "living out" his years, days, or life at a park. Whereas presidents throughout the 1990s focused on the turkey living *years*, as of 2000 presidents always said *days*, perhaps as a way to imply, rather than openly acknowledge what some journalists and activists reported, that a modern turkey's unnatural body cannot live years.[52] Use of the word "retirement" by all presidents implied the turkey's *job* is to be food, and, having been relieved of this work, he is free to enjoy his "golden years."[53] Clinton emotively described the birds' future as "happy" whereas G. W. Bush often focused on it as safe and comfortable.

The only acknowledged threat to the pardoned turkeys' safety was the presidents' dogs (Ranger, Barney, and Bo). This common prediction, while playful, implies non-human animals are less self-disciplined than humans when it comes to predation. Being implicitly rational and in control, men choose to "spare" the birds, an act presidents sometimes characterized with humane terms such as "compassion" or "mercy." However, in his first ceremony, Obama played into masculine meat-eating stereotypes when he joked that the only thing that saved Courage the turkey was his wife and daughter's intervention because "I was planning to eat this sucker."

No president ever mentions vegetarianism or implies he or others should not eat turkeys, as the ceremony glorifies the agri-business industry and honors the National Turkey Federation executives. In 2009 Obama mentioned he would "take two of their less fortunate brethren [turkeys]" to feed the homeless and said he didn't blame other presidents for eating their turkeys because "that's a good-looking bird." It's assumed that presidents will be eating a non-pardoned turkey, yet the only president who openly admitted this was Clinton in 1999, saying "before I feast on one of the 45 million turkeys . . ."[54] Whereas many presidents lauded this same national statistic of annual turkey consumption, in 1992 a National Turkey Federation executive instead quantified turkeys by total body *weight*, not lives lost, boasting farmers "produce five billion pounds of ready-to-cook turkey meat annually." These millions of birds may be "produced," "served," or "consumed," but were never said to be "killed," "dead," or "slaughtered." Pardoned birds would be spared simply from ending up on the "dinner table," not explicitly from slaughterhouses or the knife. In fact, turkey deaths were sometimes euphemized as a voluntary "sacrifice" on their part[54] or an "irreplaceable contribution" to our Thanksgiving.[55]

Often their deaths were made light of, as almost every presidential ceremony joked about the pardoning. For example, in three ceremonies G. W. Bush used the same "neck-and-neck" pun (presumably referring to the ringing or eating of a bird's neck) to describe the tight race to name the birds in the online contest. In 2007, he said Vice President Cheney wanted to name the turkeys Lunch and Dinner, and in 2003 and 2005, he joked about them not wanting to go to "Frying Pan Park." His puns were timely for the election year in 2004, naming a fictional political group "Barnyard Animals for Truth" and a fake documentary "Fahrenheit 375 Degrees at 10 Minutes per Pound." Presidents liked to play off the dual meaning of the word "turkey," by referencing its derogatory connotation as a description for inept or foolish men—namely politicians. For example, Clinton said 1997 marks the fiftieth year "we give one more turkey in Washington a second chance" and that, in 1999, the agricultural state of Minnesota was no match for DC when it comes to producing turkeys. These self-deprecating insults toward politicians reveal humans' derogatory beliefs about turkeys' mental capabilities (as well as elected officials').

Obama was the only president to mock the pardoning ceremony as beneath the dignity of the president, implicitly belittling the birds' lives. In 2010 he said sarcastically that it was "one of the most important duties that I carry out . . . as the leader of the most powerful nation on Earth. Today I have the awesome responsibility of granting a presidential pardon to a pair of turkeys," and, the previous year, he joked, "There are certain days that remind me of why I ran for this office—and then, there are moments like this—where I pardon a turkey and send it [sic] to Disneyland." He was reluctant to pardon them that year and said he had to do it before he changed his mind, even noting how the 45-pound (pardoned) birds could "feed a lot of folks."

This illuminates another theme—anthropocentrism—where all presidents prioritized human interests. Saving the birds' lives was silly and sweet, but military troops protecting *human* lives was serious and a source of pride to be grateful for each Thanksgiving. No jokes were made when discussing military personnel, needy families, or patriotic Americans at every ceremony. Many presidents talked about being grateful for our free-dom and sense of justice. In 2002, G. W. Bush said, "We remember those in other lands who suffer under oppression, who long for freedom. And we pray that they might one day live in a world at peace and in a free society." There is no mention of the ironic fact that millions of American turkeys (and billions of other farmed animals) languish in America's factory farms and suffer under a legal oppression, not having freedom over their own bodies or lives. When presidents frequently laud the American public for its generosity, good heart, and compassion, they are clearly thinking about the way Americans are supposed to treat fellow *humans*, as it would not be a fair or applicable commentary on how Americans treat non-human beings.

Turkeys themselves are not officially or seriously given a voice or an advocate at the Thanksgiving ceremony. Although the president welcomes and thanks National Turkey Federation executives and turkey farmers who present him with the turkey gifts, he doesn't officially invite any animal protection organizations nor publicly accept gifts of produce or plant-based meats. The ceremony is an agri-business marketing opportunity during which presidents proudly recognize the top turkey-producing states and individual farmers who raised the presidential birds. The gobbling of the turkeys during the ceremony tends to produce laughter and jokes. During the uproar, the president mocks the idea that the turkeys understand what is happening and have anything to say. Almost every ceremony transcript reveals a joke about the turkeys being nervous guests because they don't yet know they are getting a life-saving pardon. Presumably, this is funny so long as it is ridiculous to think a turkey has awareness, rationality, and any ability to purposefully communicate.

In a few cases presidents do acknowledge the subject status of the birds, such as when G. W. Bush directed his welcome at Biscuit himself in 2004. And in 2002 he said he was looking forward to having a conversation with Katie (first female bird pardoned). Yet he got her gender wrong prior to this, and like many presidents, often used the objectifying pronoun "it" to describe birds of any gender. George Bush Sr. tended to correctly say "he." Although presidents often described the birds in objectifying terms regarding looks/size, occasionally they were described by personal-ity, such as G. W. Bush saying Stars was "friendly" in 2003. But the most unique and least objectifying comment in support of turkeys was made by Clinton in 1999:

> One of the most interesting things I've discovered in the seven years we've done this is that turkeys really do have personalities, very differ-ent ones. And most all of them have been quite welcoming to the presi-dent and to the children who want to pet them. On occasion, they're as independent as the rest of Americans. So, Harry, you got your pardon.

Journalism Discourse

Out of the sixty-six news stories examined, we categorized fifty-five as feature stories, seven as hard news, and four as editorials. The vast majority of the feature stories (forty-two) assumed a solely anthropocentric stance, often morphing into human interest stories about Thanksgiving traditions or the pardoning record of presidents. By rendering the birds as edible products, most news stories failed to expose the harsh realities of factory farming and failed to challenge the mainstream ideology of carnism by legitimizing less cruel modes of consumption, such as vegetarianism. Among the feature stories, thirteen contained some less anthropocentric commentary that acknowledged the subject status of the birds, exposed their objectification, or attempted to give them a voice by offering animal rights activist perspectives.

Most of the news stories revolved around humans and their values, anthropocentrism being a dominant theme reflected in both feature stories and editorials. Furthermore, whereas most features discussed the Thanksgiving holiday, its historical importance and associated traditions, consumption of turkey meat was presented as a natural, undisputable part of the celebration. By reinforcing the assumption that turkeys belong on the dinner table, journalists negated the subject status of the bird and perpetuated their conceptualization as products, thus legitimizing the need for factory farming. Following the naturalization of carnism, associations between turkeys and food were trivialized—deprived of any dramatic connotations. For example, in a *Washington Post* feature story, Manuel Roig-Franzia[56] equated turkeys with "pounds of potentially mouth-watering deliciousness," *Washington Post*'s Joe Heim[57] described the birds as "deliciously departed," and NPR's Michelle Norris[58] called the president's introduction at the pardoning ceremony "an important culinary announcement."

Pictures featuring the turkey surrounded by smiling, proud industry representatives rendered obvious the association of the bird with a trophy: The National Turkey Federation offers its largest, best-looking product to the chief of state as proof of its ability to successfully manipulate the breed, a practice some journalists call the future of the industry. The fact that this celebrated exchange takes place at a time when millions of turkeys are inhumanely slaughtered remains largely unacknowledged; instead, caught in the marketing vibe, several feature stories celebrate the National Turkey Federation and Butterball, cite their representatives, and praise their ability to feed the hungry nation, all while recognizing the fact that birds are raised for meat (not longevity) as a given.

In several instances, the turkey pardoning ceremony served as a pretext for human interest stories. The presidential pardoning of *humans*, for example, is discussed in five feature stories and three editorials in which the turkey pardoning is used as an opportunity to critique the president's misuse of his pardoning powers by sparing poultry instead of deserving humans. For example, in a *Washington Post* editorial, Molly Gill expressed hopes that clemency scores will favor humans in the future,[59] and in a *New York Times* editorial, George Lardner[60] briefly mentioned the turkey pardoning before launching a critique of Obama's pardoning record, as does NPR host Mary Louise Kelly.[61] The ethical concerns voiced in these human interest stories do not extend to non-human animals. The life-sparing ceremony for turkeys is considered a mere diversion from the more important, controversial matters, which always involve human subjects.

Additional examples abound of turkey pardoning stories morphing into human interest stories. Wil Haygood[62] used the pardoning of Katie, the first female turkey, as an opportunity to list famous women's achievements in history, whereas Leslie Walker chose to focus on the video tours offered by the White House, which happened to include a webcast of Bush's "playful" encounter with Katie.[63] Whether the stories entertain by telling us how Martha Stewart celebrates Thanksgiving or inform by explaining how the holiday is observed abroad, most fail to give turkeys a voice and acknowledge them as sentient beings with rights and emotions.

A few of the journalists attempted to revert to a less anthropocentric perspective and use the "bird world" as a point of reference, but the validity of this perspective was usually discredited by humorous remarks.[64] For example, in a *Washington Post* feature story, Neely Tucker explained that "in the short, happy life of your farm-raised turkey, the end is a terrible thing to contemplate" and the fact that they are eaten is sad (for them).[65] Journalists poked fun at the turkeys for disregarding human conventions by gobbling back at the president and by having "accidents." At the same time, stories made fun of how the presidential turkeys are treated to upscale human experiences. As birds soil hotel rooms and tables, officials feel the need to excuse this uncivilized, taboo behavior. For example, as the turkeys carelessly proceeded to relieve themselves in the private airport cabin of "Turkey One," the captain reassured us that "Everybody poops."[66]

Several articles described the unfolding of the ceremony, including the preparations and aftermath. Most descriptions focused on appearances: If the birds looked good and acted docile, the event was considered a success. Turkey breeding and the selection of the pardonable turkeys were also discussed, with little or no mention of the horrible lives most birds endure in CAFOs. Furthermore, some journalists followed the birds after the ceremony and reported on how they were transported in a police-escorted motorcade and traveled to their destination with representatives of the National Turkey Federation in a first-class airplane cabin. But few noted the turkeys' stress at being kept in kennels, shuffled through busy airports, barked at by dogs, ironically stored in hotel kitchens, and sometimes even drugged.

Whereas some journalists consider the pardoning ceremony to be royal treatment and others see it as a display of excess, a handful of articles sympathetically described the turkeys as unwilling, terrified participants. The bird's extreme weight, trimmed beak, large size, white color, and lameness were most often used to illustrate his/her unnatural appearance and behavior.

In a *Washington Post* story, Tucker described "real" turkeys in opposition to commercially bred turkeys in order to expose the negative consequences of the human manipulation of the birds' bodies.[67] Tucker explained that, unlike wild turkeys, commercial birds are rendered unable to fly and reproduce on their own, and their lifespan is dramatically shortened.

Few articles acknowledge that the pardoning ceremony serves as a diversion from the realities of factory farming. In this respect, emphasis falls on the pardon as staged performance, with the president and the turkey acting out predetermined, manicured roles. While the president uses this opportunity to show a lighter, playful side to the public, make turkey jokes, and tie in references to patriotism and current political events, the turkey is washed, fluffed, and perfumed (and even drugged on occasion), so as to look pleasing and remain placid while being shuffled around on stage like a prop. Theatrical references abound: The "star"[68] turkey "performs"[69] and has a White House "gig,"[70] the alternate turkey is the "understudy,"[71] and the public witnesses a "bit of holiday theater."[72]

Some stories critiqued this performance, noting the lack of substance in this sugar-coated display of holiday benevolence. A few stories gave critical details, such as the fact that pardoned turkeys are often production birds used for breeding who would not have been slaughtered anyway, most of them die shortly after the ceremony because of in-bred physical ailments, and the president also receives other (frozen) turkeys, which he consumes. Some stories also provided statistics on the millions of turkeys consumed in the US. These insights defined the pardoning as an isolated incident, the purpose and validity of which remain questionable—one that does not reflect/affect the fate of all the other commercially bred turkeys.

The protests staged by animal rights groups during the ceremony provided a context for inclusion of stories about animal abuse in several instances, where words like "slaughter" and "decapitation" balance the benign and happy rhetoric featured in the ceremony.[73] Feature stories sometimes focused in closely to profile a single activist, such as Karen Davis of United Poultry Concerns, a vegan activist, and children's author Lisa Suhai, who advocated for a pig pardon. Although these stories were useful in outlining the differences between the lives of rescued turkeys and those abused by industry, they tended to emphasize the hardships associated with adopting turkeys and serve as a deterrent, emphasizing that "it is not like adopting a kitten or a puppy."[74] Furthermore, as an alternative that could challenge the hegemonic conceptualization of humans as meat-eaters, vegetarianism is rarely mentioned in the news discourse on "Turkey Day." It is mentioned mostly in the stories featuring animal rights activists.

CONCLUSION

What does the discourse reveal about the function or purpose of the president pardoning a turkey's life on Thanksgiving? Given that someone can be officially pardoned only if he or she committed a federal crime, the reasoning behind a ceremony pardoning an innocent turkey deserves examination. The "crime" that warrants a death sentence for millions of birds must be their status as non-humans—exploitable and "delicious." But how would being non-human represent a crime against the US? Perhaps the legalized enslavement and slaughter of millions of individuals belie the myth that America provides "liberty and justice for all." But this guilt-inducing antagonism that calls American integrity into question is hardly treasonous. So the White House doesn't apply a criminal frame to the pardoning and instead employs a retirement frame. Presidents are granting the birds a reprieve from their "job" of serving humans, so they can retire to a life of leisure. This does admit that birds want to live and experience happiness, but the meaningfulness of their lives is belittled by the retirement frame. It connotes an emptiness and lack of utility, as if the birds have nothing to do or to be outside serving humans.

The fact that the presidents avoid violent rhetoric when talking about turkeys on Thanksgiving, and even in some cases euphemistically insinuate the birds willingly make the "ultimate sacrifice" to be a celebratory meal, implies some guilt and discomfort with the unseen massacre. The pardon then fits within an animal sacrifice framework of atonement and a need to cleanse one's guilt. Yet we are calling it an "animal sacrifice in reverse," as the president openly saves two turkeys while legally sanctioning the closed-door killing of millions of others. This demonstrates Bulliet's[75] point that domesticated societies might avoid animal sacrifice, but they kill less ceremoniously in greater quantities.

It is actually the National Turkey Federation that is offering the sacrifice, as its members are the ones who really need forgiveness. They offer up their best specimens as a gift, not for the gods, but for the ruler—the head of the state that grants their business permission to function, largely unregulated. Yet his pardon can be seen as a *rejection* of their sacrificial gift, at least in a largely symbolic sense. The president's pardon embodies the ruling species' discomfort with accepting its self-appointed dominance over other animals—a poignant yet hollow attempt to construct humanity's rule as benevolent and earn its title as the "humane" species.

How seriously is the pardoning ceremony taken and what view of turkeys does that imply? The White House understands the hypocritical and nonsensical nature of the pardon, as evidenced by the way the ceremony is trivialized and mocked through levity. It is a staged performance, with the turkey as the comic star with the silly stage name.[76] This theatrical frame symbolizes its inauthenticity as well as its entertainment purpose. Although they try to disguise the innate commercialism of this PR event by highlighting agriculture's economic impact, ultimately it serves as an advertising opportunity for the turkey industry and the American brand. Therefore it must be made pleasant and entertaining—a mood befitting the consumptive spirit of the holiday. Thanksgiving is about gratitude, and criticism has no place at the table. So the turkey industry is as safe here as the pardoned bird. Journalists often mirror the playful tone, using whimsical pun-filled headlines; as they poke fun at the president, the turkey, and officials, they stimulate their audiences' appetite for festivity as well as food.

To what extent does the government or journalism consider the turkey's perspective versus an anthropocentric perspective? The discourse reinforces the human/animal dichotomy, such that putting turkeys in a human context is a humorous anthropomorphism. The birds flout human conventions by interrupting the president and defecating openly. Emphasizing the birds' lack of humanity enables the discourse to privilege the lives, needs, desires, and luxuries of humans as paramount over the interests of non-humans. The discourse implicitly acknowledges the birds' sentience and *desire* to live, but not their *right* to live. The pardon demonstrates humanity's power to be merciful to animals when it chooses. But it is a hollow and hypocritical gesture, as the government, and the news media for the most part, fails to acknowledge or criticize the everyday cruelties humans impose on millions of non-humans.

How do the government and journalism construct America's identity as a meat-eating public? To what extent does the discourse challenge carnism? As Joy notes, when media maintain the invisibility of animal suffering, it perpetuates the view of American carnism as "normal, natural, and necessary."[77] Meat was indeed portrayed as normal and natural (with some journalistic critique of unnatural modern farming), but its status as necessary was a gray area. Needy families were in need of a donated holiday turkey to satisfy their hunger, yet the presence of animal rights activists in some stories reminded the public that humans don't *need* animal-based foods. But holiday feasting isn't about merely meeting needs; it is about celebrating abundance and indulgence, as symbolized by meat at the table.

The discourse also fits Heinz and Lee's[78] social meanings of meat as a traditional, healthy main meal, presided over by men. The one exception may be meat as product, as the live turkey's public presence shatters the comfortable distance Americans tend to put between the animal and his or her flesh. This connection with an individual, named bird probably explains the necessity for the pardon, as both the president and the public don't want to meet their meat.

Other examples of a discursive challenge to carnism include when President Clinton[79] acknowledged that the birds each have different personalities. He even counted them *as* Americans, saying they are just as independent. And a few journalists did criticize the hypocrisy of the event, noting the president eats a turkey anyway and the pardoned turkeys don't live long. Animal rights activists generally served as the only prod for journalism to construct a more critical frame and foreground factory farming and, in some cases, its antidote, vegetarianism.

Yet, despite these exceptions, the discourse generally conveyed that the president pardoning a Thanksgiving turkey is as traditional, joyful, and natural as Americans eating one. This maintains the hegemony of a carnistic culture, thereby avoiding spoiling America's appetite or its humane identity.

NOTES

1. Melanie Joy, *Why We Love Dogs, Eat Pigs, and Wear Cows: An Introduction to Carnism* (San Francisco: Conari Press, 2010), 29–30.
2. Ibid., 103.
3. Ibid., 96.
4. Gary Francione, *Rain without Thunder: The Ideology of the Animal Rights Movement* (Philadelphia: Temple University Press, 1996), 4; Tom Regan, *The Case for Animal Rights* (Berkeley, CA: University of California Press, 1983), 235–43.
5. Peter Singer, *Animal Liberation* (London: Random House, 1990), 6.
6. Regan, *Case for Animal Rights*, 331–51; Francione, *Rain without Thunder*, 109–202.
7. Jonathan Menitove, "The Problematic Presidential Pardon: A Proposal for Reforming Federal Clemency," *Harvard Law & Policy Review* 3, no. 2 (2009): 449.
8. Ibid., 449.
9. Ibid., 447, Article II, Section 2, Clause I of Constitution.
10. Kathleen Dean Moore, *Pardons: Justice, Mercy, and the Public Interest* (New York: Oxford University Press, 1989), 5.
11. Menitove, *Problematic Presidential Pardon*, 453; and Jeffrey Crouch, *The Presidential Pardon Power* (Lawrence, KS: University Press of Kansas, 2009), 147.
12. Crouch, *Presidential Pardon Power*, 2.
13. "Truman Trivia," *Truman Library and Museum*, www.trumanlibrary.org. But library staff can find no records of Truman pardoning a turkey.
14. Joe Heim, "At White House, President Obama's Pardons Prevent Turkeys' Shellacking," *Washington Post*, November 24, 2010, www.washingtonpost.com.
15. Manuel Roig-Franzia, "Thankfully, Bush Never Had an Ax to Grind," *Washington Post*, November 27, 2008, www.washingtonpost.com.
16. Elizabeth Bumiller, "Two Turkeys Pardoned, with First-Class Tickets," *Washington Post*, November 23, 2005, www.washingtonpost.com.
17. Jessica Gresko, "Thanksgiving Turkey with Presidential Pardon Will Head to George's Place Instead of Mickey's This Year," Associated Press, November 20, 2010, *The Yule Blog*, accessed March 10, 2012, http://blogs.sj-r.com/yuleblog/index.php/category/turkey
18. Peter Singer and Jim Mason, *The Ethics of What We Eat: Why Our Food Choices Matter* (Emmaus, PA: Rodale, Inc., 2006), 4.
19. Gidon Eshel and Pamela Martin, "Diet, Energy and Global Warming," *Earth Interactions* 10 (2006): 4–5.
20. "Farm Animal Statistics: Slaughter Totals," *HSUS*, per USDA, last updated 2011, http://www.humanesociety.org/news/resources/research/stats_slaughter_totals.html. Additionally, Singer and Mason, 112, estimate Americans kill seventeen billion sea creatures annually.

118   *Carrie Packwood Freeman and Oana Leventi-Perez*

21. "Turkey Facts & Trivia," *National Turkey Federation*, www.eatturkey.com. Americans eat forty-six million turkeys at Thanksgiving and twenty-two million at Christmas.
22. Daniel Imhoff, introduction to *CAFO Reader: The Tragedy of Industrial Animal Factories*, ed. Imhoff (Watershed Media, 2010), xiii–xviii; and Singer and Mason, *Ethics of What We Eat*, part I.
23. "Factory Poultry Production," *Farm Sanctuary*, http://www.farmsanctuary.org/issues/factoryfarming/poultry/.
24. Singer and Mason, *Ethics of What We Eat*, 28.
25. "Factory Poultry Production," *Farm Sanctuary*.
26. Paige Tomaselli and Meredith Niles, "Changing the Law," in *CAFO Reader*, ed. Daniel Imhoff (Watershed Media, 2010), 317–19.
27. Ibid., 319.
28. "Agency Reports," *USDA*, www.usda.gov. 88 percent of Americans eat turkey on Thanksgiving, but only 1 percent of these turkeys are organically raised.
29. Singer and Mason, *Ethics of What We Eat*, Ch. 8 and 14.
30. Janay Nugent and Megan Clark, "A Loaded Plate: Food Symbolism and the Early Modern Scottish Household," *Journal of Scottish Historical Studies* 30, no. 1 (2010): 48.
31. Richard Bulliet, *Hunters, Herders, and Hamburgers* (New York: Columbia University Press, 2005): 123.
32. Ibid., 133.
33. Kimberly Patton, "Animal Sacrifice: Metaphysics of the Sublimated Victim," in *A Communion of Subjects: Animals in Religion, Science, and Ethics*, ed. Paul Waldau and Kimberly Patton (New York: Columbia University Press, 2006), 391–405.
34. Michael Pollan, *The Omnivore's Dilemma: A Natural History of Four Meals* (New York: Penguin Press, 2006), 331.
35. Wayne Pacelle, *The Bond: Our Kinship with Animals, Our Call to Defend Them* (New York: Harper Collins, 2011), 40.
36. Ibid., 41–42.
37. Barbara Willard, "The American Story of Meat: Discursive Influences on Cultural Eating Practice," *Journal of Popular Culture* 36, no. 1 (2001): 116.
38. Bettina Heinz and Ronald Lee, "Getting Down to the Meat: The Symbolic Construction of Meat Consumption," *Communication Studies* 49, no. 1 (Spring 1998): 86.
39. Carrie Packwood Freeman and Debra Merskin, "Having It His Way: The Construction of Masculinity in Fast Food TV Advertising," in *Food for Thought: Essays on Eating and Culture*, ed. Lawrence Rubin (Jefferson, NC: McFarland & Company, 2008), 277.
40. Carol Adams, *Neither Man nor Beast: Feminism and the Defense of Animals* (New York: Continuum, 1994): 27–28.
41. Ibid., 32.
42. Heinz and Lee, "Getting Down to the Meat."
43. Carrie Packwood Freeman, "Framing Animal Rights in the Go Veg Campaigns of U.S. Animal Rights Organizations," *Society & Animals* 18, no. 2 (2010): 163.
44. Carrie Packwood Freeman, "This Little Piggy Went to Press: The American News Media's Construction of Animals in Agriculture," *The Communication Review* 12, no. 1 (2009): 98.
45. Joy, *Why We Love Dogs*, 117.
46. Freeman, "This Little Piggy Went to Press," 13.
47. Joy, *Why We Love Dogs*, 103.

48. Stuart Hall, *Representation: Cultural Representations and Signifying Practices* (London: Sage, 1997), Ch. 1; Michel Foucault, *Power/Knowledge* (Harvester: Brighton, 1980), 131.

49. Teun Van Dijk, "Critical Discourse Studies: A Sociocognitive Approach," in *Methods of Critical Discourse Analysis*, ed. Ruth Wodack and Michael Meyer (Washington, DC: Sage, 2009), 63.

50. Ernesto Laclau and Chantal Mouffe, *Hegemony and Socialist Strategy: Towards a Radical Democratic Politics* (London: Verso, 1985), 126–27.

51. Bush ceremony, 2005. See "President Pardons "Marshmallow and Yam" in Annual Turkey Ceremony," *The White House, President George W. Bush*, November 22, 2005, accessed March 9, 2012 , http://www.georgewbush-whitehouse.archives.gov/news/releases/2005/11/20051122–1.html.   "Turkeys' Big Day at the White House," National Public Radio (NPR), November 22, 2005, accessed March 9, 2012, http://www.npr.org/templates/story/story.php?storyId=5024034

52. This may be in response to David Montgomery's critical exposé of the lack of living, pardoned birds: "Not Quite a Slice of Poultry Paradise; Pardoned Turkeys Live a Lonely Life," *Washington Post*, November 24, 2000.

53. Clinton ceremony, 1997. See "Speech by President at National Turkey Pardoning Ceremony," November 26, 1997, accessed March 9, 2012, http://archives.clintonpresidentialcenter.org/?u=112697-speech-by-president-at-national-pardoning-ceremony.htm

54. Clinton ceremonies, 1994, 1999. See, for example, Tamara Jones, "Talking Turkey; Giving Bill The Bird (I), *Washington Post*, November 24, 1994, B1.

55. Bush ceremony, 1992. See, for example, "Thanksgiving Turkey Pardon," November 24, 1992. *C-Span Video Library*, accessed March 9, 2012, http://www.c-spanvideo.org/program/Thank. See also, Lloyd Grace, "Bush's Poultry Duties; The President Pardons Tom Turkey," *Washington Post*, November 25, 1992, A1

56. Roig-Franzia, "Thankfully, Bush . . ."

57. Heim, "At White House, President Obama's . . ."

58. Robert Siegel and Michelle Norris, "Turkey's Big Day at the White House," *All Things Considered*, NPR, November 22, 2005, http://www.npr.org/programs/all-things-considered

59. Molly Gill, "Turkeys 2, Humans 0," *Washington Post*, November 27, 2009.

60. George Lardner, "No Country for Second Chances," *New York Times*, November 23, 2010.

61. Mary Louise Kelly, "Obama Pardons Turkeys, But No Humans," *All Things Considered*, NPR, November 24, 2010, http://www.npr.org/programs/all-things-considered

62. Wil Haygood, "At the White House, A Different Drumstick; Katie Joins a Fabled List of Female Firsts," *Washington Post*, November 27, 2002.

63. Leslie Walker, "A Web Vista of the Oval Office," *Washington Post*, December 1, 2002.

64. Heim, "At White House, President Obama . . ."

65. Neely Tucker, "A Pardon with All the Trimmings; Two Turkeys Toasted, Not Roasted," *Washington Post*, November 18, 2004.

66. Dana Milbank, "Pardon Me!" *Washington Post*, November 21, 2007.

67. Tucker, "Pardon with All Trimmings."

68. Kim Severson, "In Some Households, Every Day Is Turkey Day," *New York Times*, November 22, 2007.

69. Linton Weeks, "Wattle They Think of Next?," *Washington Post*, November 23, 1995 and Heim, "At White House, President Obama . . ."

70. Mary Jane Solomon, "At Thanksgiving, Poultry in Motion," *Washington Post*, November 21, 1997.
71. Montgomery, "Not Quite a Slice of Poultry Paradise."
72. Margaret Colgate Love, "Pardon People, Too, Mr. President," *Washington Post*, November 12, 2010.
73. Gail Collins, "A Tale of Two Turkeys," *New York Times*, November 25, 2009.
74. Severson, "In Some Households."
75. Bulliet, *Hunters, Herders & Hamburgers*, 133.
76. Themes for names usually related to food (Pumpkin & Pecan, Apple & Cider, Biscuits & Gravy), patriotism (May & Flower, Liberty & Freedom, Stars & Stripes), or humor (Flyer & Fryer).
77. Joy, *Why We Love Dogs*, 96.
78. Heinz and Lee, "Getting Down to the Meat," 86.
79. Incidentally, Clinton went vegan in 2010.

8 Resignified Urban Landscapes
From Abject to Agricultural

Natasha Seegert

ROOTED AND UNROOTED BODIES

The Material Landscape: Bodies in Contact

Diesel exhaust, the coo of mourning doves, multi-hued pansies, the tang of steer manure, and the piercing clang of Trax invade the corner of what was once a vacant city lot. The urban and the agricultural meld. The People's Freeway Community of Salt Lake City sits adjacent to I-15 and spans several neighborhoods that provide easy access to other interstates and expressways.[1] Freeways are synonymous with ephemeral, fast-paced movement. And individuals, locked inside their exoskeletons of steel and glass, conjure anything but the idea of community. Indeed, as one drives west on 900 S., the freeway signs urge one's body forward, encourage speed as one approaches the on-ramp, and do not invite an engagement with the neighborhood, which only seems to get in the way when the stoplight impedes constant motion. The freeway signs subtly imply: You are not here; you are supposed to be "there." If the stoplight turns red and forces your car to pause at the corner of 900 S. and 200 W., your arrested flight may cause you to pause in the present moment, where you might notice large, wooden boxes overflowing with flowers and vegetables during the summer, which in the spring come to life with snow peas, chard, herbs, and pansies of every hue. It is a space teeming with roots that nourish bodies and communities, but it is a space with a transitory future. This space is the People's Portable Garden (Figure 8.1). This garden is more than simply a progressive model of urban planning. It also challenges basic theoretical assumptions about what space can mean *and* how it is resignified. In addition, it challenges the distribution of the sensible, of what is heard and of what is seen.

Gardens typically signify a rootedness to place, both literally and figuratively. Putting seeds in the ground signals a tie to a specific piece of earth, an act grounded in hope with a focus on a future connection. The People's Portable Garden confuses these connections. As the name implies, these gardens are portable. Like the transitory vehicles that rush by, the beds too are nomadic and will someday change locations when the city finds the

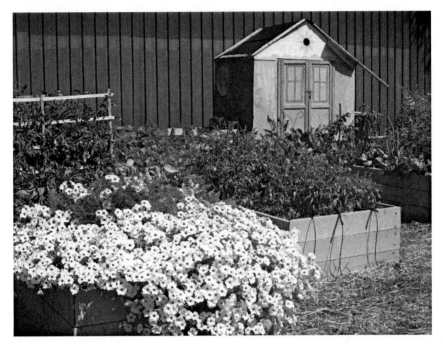

Figure 8.1 Vegetables and flowers overflow garden boxes in the 2009 growing season. Photo provided by Wasatch Community Gardens. Reproduced with permission.

need to develop the formerly vacant plot where the garden beds currently sit. The portable nature of these gardens reflects the urban landscape, but with a twist. The city is always changing: spaces are transformed through development of "empty" lots; old buildings are demolished and new structures spring to life. The unfixed urban environment is not necessarily associated with rooted, organic life. Certainly there are the stray dandelions or trees of heaven that are impudent and strong enough to force their way through cracks in asphalt, but normally the urban jungle is constructed of concrete and steel that resist such fugitive plants. Such locations of industrial modernity are where the community garden can shock the sensibilities of what an urban space is, or can be. The greenery jolts our vision and reminds us that the organic can, and does, intermingle with the concrete. A garden reminds us that the city need not simply be pavement, but can also invite the agricultural—albeit on a small scale—into its rigid formation. In essence, the city is marked by the organic world and the organic world is simultaneously marked by the urban.

The People's Portable Garden enacts this hybridity by disrupting the urban landscape with its green agriculture. Such hybridity is also marked by the unexpected contact of disparate bodies. The urban-agricultural

emerges in encounters among human bodies, non-human bodies, and physical bodies. Just as unseen bodies become seen, what was pushed away and
abjected from our perception emerges in a space that permits the *possibility*
of resignified and transformed political bodies. At this corner lot the invisible becomes visible and we begin to question what exactly a city means.
What is permissible in the urban realm? How do other fugitive plants—in
this case vegetables—break the asphalt and challenge the definitions of a
city? What potential opportunities exist that expand sensations and meanings? How does a community garden exert political force?

Bodies in the Institutional Wasteland: Challenging Systems of Being

The community members who rent these thirty-six plots for twenty-five
dollars a growing season have known from the beginning that their garden
beds will someday move and something else will take root in that corner
lot. Ironically, it is the presence of a billboard, whose steel pole roots itself
into the garden soil, which anchors and makes possible the presence of the
garden at all (Figure 8.2). In many ways, the billboard makes visible how
our physical spaces, and the possibilities of imagination to transform those
spaces, are tied to our economic system. When the billboard lease expires,
the city plans to sell the land for redevelopment, possibly for an apartment
building, a parking lot, or whatever the latest needs are in 2012. Until that
happens, the corner lot of 900 S. and 200 W. is marked and transformed
with the presence of garden beds, and the material presence of the garden
transforms the nature of the People's Freeway Community. Material bodies, both human and non-human, transform urban space.

As one looks at the empty site of what would become the People's Portable Garden, one can see a space of possibilities where meanings of what is
permitted are unraveled (Figure 8.3). In this space of possibility, creativity,
imagination, and politics germinate and sprout. The empty lot can be more
than a parking lot. A parking lot is not actually seen and registered whereas
an urban garden is far more likely to be seen, to be noted, and to shock our
sensibility of what an urban space is. This ability to be seen required unexpected negotiations as well as institutional standing. This city-owned plot
managed by the Redevelopment Agency (RDA) of Salt Lake City was initially proposed as a possible parking lot for the neighborhood. Two University of Utah students who heard that the RDA was offering a $50,000 grant
for this city block saw the potential for something different. These students,
Lauren and Marianne, approached the city with some other ideas. However, their bodies—young, twenty-something, female college students—fell
outside of the realm of what Jacques Rancière refers to as the "sensible."[2]
The distribution of the sensible is an embodied experience addressing what
is apprehended through the senses—what is seen and heard, and, I would
add, what is smelled and felt.[3] Rancière holds that there are some bodies

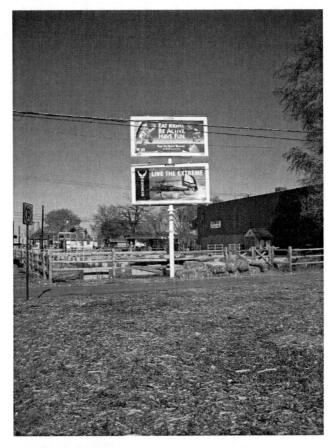

Figure 8.2   A billboard plants its steel roots into garden soil.
Photo taken by Natasha Seegert.

left outside of politics, bodies that are marginalized and unseen.[4] The voices of these young college students were not heard due to their lack of institutional standing. As a result, Lauren and Marianne approached the non-profit organization Wasatch Community Gardens and proposed that it serve as an umbrella organization for the garden. With this institutional backing, they were then granted standing by the RDA to approach the community and discuss other possibilities, possibilities that did not include the tarry wonders of asphalt.

These two students, Lauren and Marianne, stressed the importance of letting the neighborhood take on the project so that their own visions could unfold. This approach meant that hidden talents, such as carpentry skills, leadership roles, as well as planning and design skills, had the space to emerge. It also created opportunities for subverting traditional gender

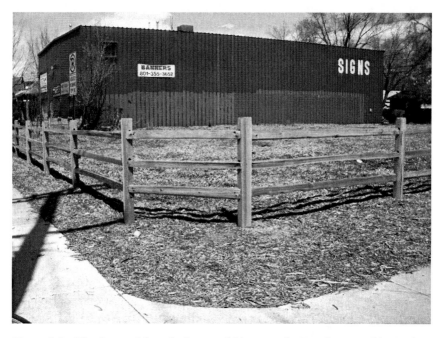

Figure 8.3 The "empty" lot of what would become the People's Portable Garden. Photo provided by Wasatch Community Gardens. Reproduced with permission.

roles, specifically those associated with masculine, mechanical labor. The creation of the thirty-six boxes, each measuring sixteen feet long, four feet deep, and twenty-two inches wide, was so time-intensive that it required all community members, regardless of past experience or gender, to take part in the physically demanding tasks of sawing wood, cutting metal, and drilling holes. Beth Hinderliter et al. assert that such subversions are part of the role of art:

> The task of art today is not to make the invisible visible through the recontextualization of given information, but to reconfigure the visible and its spectacular economies in a way that reconfigures society's current division into parties and disrupts the distribution of social roles.[5]

It was not simply the garden that disrupted the space of the city block. The act of creating the garden also challenged traditional notions of "how things are done." These activities subverted notions of time itself. Because the project was taken on by students who do not hold a 9–5 schedule like the RDA does, the planning meetings and the construction of the boxes occurred in the evening and even extended into 12- to 14-hour-long marathon sessions of cutting and assembling boxes.[6] Had the RDA taken on such a task it is likely that such work would have been completed by an outside contractor. Requiring the neighborhood to build the boxes resulted in an increased investment in the project, with some neighbors involved only with the construction, and not the gardening. In many ways, it is the presence of scarcity that breeds community because it creates reliance on others to give materiality to such a dream.

In addition to the city awarding a $50,000 grant, the Utah Arts Council also granted $50,000 to be used for portable art in the garden. Although the garden art has yet to be installed, all individuals who spoke about the art had reservations regarding the conceptual drawings, with descriptions ranging from "metal clip-art on sticks" to that of looking like a "McDonald's Play Place Center." It is interesting to note that both references refer to items that are mass-produced; both clip-art and McDonald's are anything but original. In addition, particularly in the case of McDonald's, images of capitalism spring to mind. This "impurity," in combination with the presence of the billboard, which permits the very existence of the garden in the first place, muddies the image of grassroots purity that is free of institutional or financial connections. For this garden to germinate and take root required institutional backing and support from non-profit organizations, a government agency, and the presence of a commercial billboard whose roots had more institutional weight than those of the humble peas and tomatoes.

My own analysis of the People's Portable Garden began in the spring of 2010 and is based on three sets of interviews: (1) interviews with gardeners; (2) interviews with the garden organizers; (3) and interviews with the non-profit organization overseeing the garden. In addition, there were two site visits to the garden location. During my time at the garden I took photographs of the garden beds and of the larger site the garden is situated in, and I also spoke with gardeners who were tending their nascent vegetable beds.

Bodies of Politics and Possibility: Redistributing the Sensible

The collision of bodies in space sparks changes. Encounters between an empty lot, human neighbors, and non-human bodies open a new space for the potential transformation of all involved bodies. Transcendent concepts like "imagination" and "possibility" collide with the material realm where immanent change occurs. In this space, the process of aesthetic resignification arises as a political act challenging the distribution of power, of what is acceptable, or, in Rancière's term, of what is "sensible." Aesthetics is part of this political struggle because it invokes a reimagining of what can be seen and heard in the realm of politics. The ability to be seen—to move from the invisible to the visible—changes the very image of society and culture. Such changes result not just in how a culture imagines itself, but also how the individual imagines herself. The woman who for the first time used power tools may have found the experience empowering and may challenge other social roles.

Although Rancière specifically refers to human bodies, it is important to remember that non-human bodies are also impacted by the political.[7] Thus, how we perceive the material world, the space we move through on a day-to-day basis, and the non-human encounters we have become both a political and aesthetic act. What bodies are seen? What bodies do we look away from? How do we move through bodies of space: Do our feet feel the contours of the ground beneath us as we walk with ease, or do we lock ourselves inside a shell of steel and glass that propels us forward but numbs the sensations in our feet? How does the outside world challenge my own body? The garden challenges how a space should be seen, experienced, and used. The inhabitants of the garden—the plants, the bugs, the birds, the microbes, the soil, and the worms—challenge who "belongs" in urban spaces.[8] The people of the neighborhood challenge what it means to live and form community in an area identified by the city's Redevelopment Agency as "blighted," a term that conjures up images of neglect, impurity, deterioration, and possibly violence.[9] These three spheres of bodies—the material space, the non-human, and the human—redistribute the realm of the sensible to bodies that have had no voice, who have not been seen, and whose political standing has held no sway. The garden creates the potential for a politics of aesthetics. Referring to the regime of aesthetics, Rancière writes:

> It is a delimitation of spaces and times, of the visible and invisible, of speech and noise, that simultaneously determines the place and the stakes of politics as a form of experience. Politics revolves around what is seen and what can be said about it, around who has the ability to see and the talent to speak, around the properties of spaces and possibilities of time.[10]

For Rancière, politics is liberated from the ballot box and Election Day, and now permeates acts of material, day-to-day living. Politics is material in the spaces where resistance can be staged. A garden serves as a stage for action and resistance.

Although this plot of land does not bear the radical history of places like the 1960s People's Park in Berkeley, it does challenge the notion of what ownership is and who claims it. The city has ultimate decision-making authority, but one can easily imagine this authority being challenged should residents experience a threat to both the literal and figurative roots established at that specific location. In turn, in a country that loves its suburbs, the gardeners themselves challenge normative views of where gardens should be grown. Although it is common to find community gardens in other metropolitan areas like Portland or Boston, such green spaces are still a relatively unusual sight in the Salt Lake Valley, which is acculturated to maintaining residences that can support large, individual families. In particular, the People's Portable Garden challenges the public understanding of the private and public due to its association with the Salt Lake Trax line, which runs immediately adjacent to the garden.[11] Commuters seeing the garden space are reminded that growing a garden is not necessarily something that only occurs in the privacy of one's backyard, but can also happen in the public sphere.

Not only does the garden challenge the physical space of the city, but also the simple acts of planting seeds, harvesting, and eating become highly political and imbued with fruits of opposition toward globalization and corporate agricultural powers like Monsanto and Cargill. The real shared commonality of gardening might become that of resistance toward capitalistic structures. These ruptures and spaces of resistance—like the People's Portable Garden—appear as moments of collective imagination. Collective imagination and resistance occur not just in human bodies marching on asphalt streets, but also in the very places where the multitude plants its feet—and its food—the soil we tread on but do not always register. Such acts of resistance become unfixed marks on the text of our urban landscape.

RESIGNIFYING THE SENSIBLE

Iterability and Deviation: The Theoretical Urban Landscape

Bodies transform old meanings by twisting and deviating from past patterns of being. In "Signature, Event, Context," Derrida asserts that through repetition language in different contexts can assume new meanings and is thus open to interpretation. Because no context is ever absolutely fixed, the meanings in those contexts will become polysemous: " . . . a context is never absolutely determinable, or rather in what way its determination is never certain or saturated."[12] Language is iterable and open to interpretation based on how it is used. Just as language can be used in different contexts that open the space for new meanings—or make its meaning open to interpretation—landscapes can also assume new meanings. Whereas a garden in a private backyard does not deviate from our standard expectations of where a garden should be, or what a backyard should be used for, a garden on the corner of an empty lot twists both our concept of "garden" and of "vacant lot." There is an iterability to space that opens up new possibilities. The People's Portable Garden is an example of an iterable space. The mixture of urban and agrarian, as well as rootedness and nomadism, has marked this corner lot since the garden's inception in 2009. What was once an "empty" lot with its own history is transformed into a garden. A city lot that was simply perceived as "vacant" and a spot for trash to blow or for tagging on city signs now supports life that highlights the non-human body: plants, a place for bugs, microbes, and birds. Neighbors who lived across from each other for twenty years and never spoke, an African-American family and a Mormon family, now engage in community potlucks in the garden. Other residents, who had been avoided because as transvestites they fell outside the realm of what was sexually "acceptable," were active in creating the boxes and now garden there. Race, religion, and sexuality collide in the public space of the garden, whereas in the past such spheres were kept safely enclosed within discrete houses and apartments. In the garden bodies collide, relationships are reconfigured, and meanings are open to change.

The Urban Palimpsest: Exploring Marks on the Land

For Rancière the written word of the text opens up a space that challenges hierarchies through play.[13] The written word should not be limited to black marks on a page, but rather should extend to marks on material space. With such an opening, the world becomes a text waiting to be both written and read, smelled, touched, and tasted. When considering the garden as a material body moving from the mundane, invisible urban environment into a political space, there are multiple ways of approaching the garden both as a text and as a framed space. Some of these texts have already been alluded to: an ignored city-owned lot now "owned" by the people who grow their food there. Indeed, the simple act of growing food becomes a political text subverting the status quo; even the vegetables themselves are texts revealing social stories and histories surrounding food.[14] The standard notion of aesthetics typically places it within the realm of the art world, inside of a museum where it is framed.

When it comes to expanding the realm of the sensible, it is far too limiting to assume that frames remain safely sequestered inside of museum walls. The garden also exists within frames. In addressing the frames surrounding the garden, there are both *literal frames*—like the frame of the window from a Trax train that passes by the garden, the frame of the fence surrounding the garden, or even the fame of the wooden, portable garden beds themselves—and there are the spectral frames. These spectral frames manifest themselves in the very soil where seeds put down roots to synthesize sunshine, air, and water: there is the political frame of land ownership and power that manifests itself in a deed of ownership; there are issues regarding control of food and corporate infusion into the soil by megacorporations whose copyright of genomes is a frame of capitalism and globalization; there are also people challenging the normative narrative of the status quo, who instead pick up a shovel and hoe as a frame of resistance. Aesthetics breaks free of the institutional walls of the museum and roams defiantly in the city streets.

The garden is a mark on our urban text, but within the garden you will find other marks. Some involve Rancière's somewhat fetishized written word. There are the gray garden boxes. Some bear no marks, where

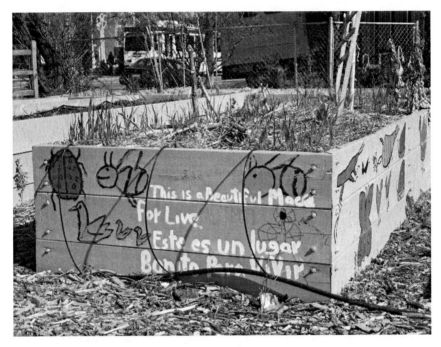

Figure 8.4 Both languages (English and Spanish) and animals collide. Photo taken by Natasha Seegert.

others are festooned with cheerful garden images of bees, butterflies, and birds, whereas others stake both a claim and a name to space (Figures 8.4 and 8.5). Adjacent to the garden sits another empty city-owned lot with numerous signs that instruct the public that this is not a parking lot, no dumping is allowed, and that there should be no loitering after 10:00 p.m.—some of these official signs are tagged with spray paint and contain marks that signify and challenge something else. Other marks in the garden may be made by non-human beings: Earthworms till soil and furrow their patterns within the garden beds, dandelions cheerfully disrupt pathways, while birds scratch the pathways in search of seeds or bugs. Just like coyotes who mark their territory with scat and urine, human animals also seem to have a need to mark space.[15] Perhaps a communal garden provides an outlet for markings, such as the painted flower beds, especially for individuals who do not fall within the standard categories of home ownership. The urban garden provides a new outlet of marking space that falls outside of capitalistic frames like home ownership, or more rebellious endeavors like graffiti. Such marks challenge whose "voices" can be heard.

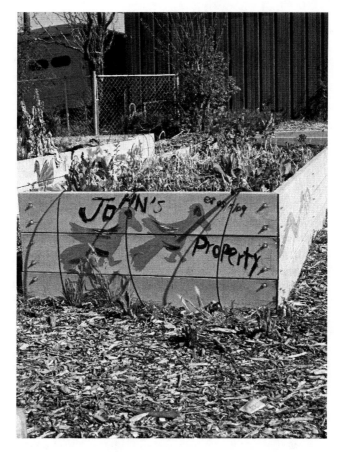

Figure 8.5   John claims property of an unconventional type.
Photo taken by Natasha Seegert.

Expanding the Conversation:
Hearing, Seeing, and Engaging the Invisible

When we consider the realm of the sensible and who is given a voice, the voices of the non-human world frequently fall into Spivak's notion of the subaltern—voices that try to speak, but because they fall outside of the realm of the sensible are not heard.[16] The non-human world most certainly speaks, but humans have forgotten how to listen or to understand what is being said. Yet, as landscape architect Anne Whiston Spirn points out, "The language of landscape is our native language. [. . .] Landscapes were the first human texts, read before the invention of other signs and symbols."[17] By inviting the non-human into our human-constructed urban environments, we are extending the conversation to those who have had no voice and thus no role in the political. Remembering that language extends to the non-human opens Bakhtin's concept of dialogue wider, guaranteeing the conversation will never end. The portable garden is a wonderful example of expanded dialogue as its nomadic structure guarantees that the conversation will extend to other city blocks and neighborhoods. By extending and then continuing this conversation, we remind ourselves of what it means to relate to a world outside of the human sphere. In addition, by taking the voices of the non-human world seriously, we come to re-learn the sweet scent of soil teeming with unseen life and thus know the difference between what is healthy and unhealthy; we pay attention to the wisps of clouds that write on the blue sky when the next rain shower will be; we note the absence of snow on the mountains, a lack that signals when we can plant our tomatoes. Spirn elaborates on this mode of literateness: "The language of landscape is a powerful tool. A person literate in landscape sees significance where an illiterate person notes nothing. [. . .] To know landscape poetics is to see, smell, taste, hear and feel landscape as a symphony of complex harmonies."[18] Inviting the non-human world into the anthropogenic urban environment provides opportunities to re-learn how to read, and relate to, a world that extends beyond humans.

Meanings are created only when words and languages are put in relationship to other words and languages. Bakhtin asserts, "The word in language is half someone else's. It becomes 'one's own' only when the speaker populates it with his own intention, his own accent, when he appropriates the word, adapting it to his own semantic and expressive intention."[19] Indeed, one could apply Bakhtin's concept of the "word" to material spaces, which becomes "one's own" only when engaged with other bodies, both human and non-human. This relational ontology highlights the encounter of bodies with other bodies, bodies that produce politics. It is important to note that such an extension of the conversation occurs in a material space and in time. The narrative of this neighborhood is now tied to both the corner lot and to the growing season. Bakhtin refers to the connection between space and time in language as the *chronotope* that grants materiality to something abstract like time:

> Time becomes, in effect, palpable and visible; the chronotope makes narrative events concrete, makes them take on flesh, causes blood to flow in their veins [. . .] Thus the chronotope, functioning as the primary means for materializing time in space, emerges as a center for concretizing representation, as a force giving body to the entire novel.[20]

Over the course of the growing season, events will take place in the garden that will drive the narrative and the identity of the neighborhood. A wedding will be attended by fellow gardeners, as tomatoes ripen there will be the threat of theft and discussion of establishing a neighborhood garden watch of the lot, relationships between humans and non-humans will emerge, and the conversation will extend and never end.

Like Bakhtin, Valentin Volosinov reminds us that discourse is inherently social: "Verbal discourse is a social event; it is not self-contained in the sense of some abstract linguistic quantity, nor can it be derived psychologically from the speaker's subjective consciousness taken in isolation."[21] Part of what makes us human is our participation with a world that is not anthropogenic. Just as utterances cannot be separated from social events or our own consciousness, our language itself cannot be separated from the non-human world we have evolved with. There are many forms of literacy and the ability to read the landscape is one such form that is frequently lost when the printed and spoken word takes primacy. When we remember that there is a story being told and that one of the roles of the listener/reader is to actually listen and not simply to decode but to respond, it changes the dynamic not only of how we perceive the non-human world, but also of how we engage with it. When sustenance relies upon the rays of the sun, or the rain from the sky, we acknowledge the heavens with an entirely different attitude and attention. No longer do we walk with our head down; we look upward and thank the sky for the presence of both moisture and heat.

Habitus Unfixed: Spaces of Becoming

The People's Freeway Community is not the suburbs. Looking at the neighborhood surrounding the People's Portable Garden you will find a mix of businesses, single-family homes, and apartment buildings. The population is relatively diverse given Salt Lake City's reputation for homogeneity. This area is also a neighborhood that the RDA refers to as "blighted," and "low income," not exactly the kind of neighborhood with a great deal of visibility or political currency. The empty lot on 900 S. and 200 W. not only became a space for creativity and imagination to take root and grow, but also created a political space for unheard voices to emerge. There is Jonnie Mae, the "mayor" of the People's Portable Garden, who is black. Jonnie Mae is black: race is made visible. There is the household of transvestites who were previously looked at with a sense of fear, but who now garden in skirts at the garden. Their sexuality is made visible. There is another woman who slowly gained a voice, and a support system, when her son committed suicide. Her pain and potential healing are made visible. The garden space itself begs the body to pause, look, and listen. Taking time to engage makes present not just the stories of the gardeners, but also the songs of birds, the scent of flowers, as well as the rush of traffic and the clang of light rail. The latter are sounds that we frequently naturalize in our urban setting but become acutely aware of when they are juxtaposed with sounds associated with the pastoral.

The garden defies our political expectation of the urban habitus. By challenging Bourdieu's notion of the habitus,[22] we dispute both the role of the "urban" and of the "natural." Spirn sees this new approach as a way of challenging myths of purity, and moving to a space of hybridity: "To call some landscapes natural and others artificial or cultural misses the truth that landscapes are never wholly one or the other."[23] The presence of urban agriculture challenges both the identities of urbanism and of the agrarian. Both terms experience a queering and come to resignify something new. It is important to note that this process is not simply a reconceptualization, but a transformation. In terms of Derrida's notion of iterability, both the urban and the garden are still connected to their historical meanings and understandings, but they now deviate from traditional meanings in a space of unfixed possibility and change. Following Rancière, this unfixed possibility is significant because a change in how language is circulated impacts the "social distribution of bodies" and thus of what is seen and heard within the realm of politics.[24] When the garden is considered in relation to other bodies, the political text stands out in multiple realms. There are the politics of whose voices are heard, both of human and non-human. There are the politics of what spaces are seen, and the politics of how we cannot simply reconceptualize these spaces but must instead actively *transform* them. A space (vacant city lot) for reclamation and change emerges if we claim what is considered to be abject or "blighted" and *resignify* it, to use Judith Butler's concept, into something new. The challenge is that of breaking out of our "common sense" habitus of the status quo, the realm that naturalizes relationships, like that of our expectations of the urban landscape and what is acceptable.[25] Such a break opens a space of resignification.

Aesthetic Resignification:
Transformed Bodies in Unfixed Space

Butler's concept of resignification, in tandem with Rancière's politics of aesthetics, provides a space of possibility that expands, rather than limits, modes of possibility and of imagination. Just as words thrown into the world are not sovereign, autonomous statements, but instead have roots that grow deeply and are entangled with historical and cultural meanings and implications, the same holds true for our physical spaces. Both repetition and Derrida's concept of iterability provide the potential for transformation so that speech acts, as well as physical spaces like the community garden, can take on new meanings. Derrida's notion of iterability of utterances is key to Butler because it provides the space to resignify practices; it thus opens up a process rather than closing it down. Rather than permitting language to "become sedimented in and as the ordinary" language enters into a realm of contestation where the invisible can potentially become visible.[26] These new meanings are what Butler refers to as resignification: "The resignification of speech requires opening new contexts, speaking in ways that have never yet been legitimated, and hence producing legitimation in new and future forms."[27]

The resignification of an urban lot can influence how we, as human animals, perceive and relate to the world we dwell in. The names we inscribe on the landscape, both figuratively and literally, imbue that space with its own subjecthood that can either elevate its status or diminish it. "Vacant lot" carries a very different image and meaning than "community garden." Both also demand something very different from us and from our encounter with that space. Because our encounter with the world demands something from our physical body, such as seeing and hearing, it can produce what Rancière refers to as a "community of sense" where a collective encounter produces a sense of "equality."[28] Rancière asserts that this community is "a form of a collective existence that will no longer be a matter of form and appearance but will rather be embodied in living attitudes, in the materiality of everyday sensory experience. The *common* of community will thus be woven into the fabric of the lived world."[29] Although Rancière's vision may appear a bit romantic, it is important to note that he is not advocating a utopic future graced with peace and harmony. Rather, much like the garden beds or the automobiles rushing to the freeway, this equality will always be shifting and nomadic. There is no fixed future for equality. The margins will always push against a center of what is considered "sensible" and shift this sensibility to new spaces.[30] The garden pushes against the urban landscape and thus challenges what is acceptable for both a garden and for a city. Due to the garden's portable nature, it guarantees that the landscape it travels through will never be fixed.

The Nomadic Garden: Organic Carnival

In November of 2012 the gardens will likely move to a yet to be determined location where new roots will be established. Although it is possible that residents will challenge the eviction of their garden, all agencies involved have stressed the temporary nature of the garden beds at their current location.[31] In anticipation of the future move, there are already plans to make the event a celebration with a parade of garden boxes through city streets to their new home. Such a parade conjures images of Bakhtin's carnival, where laughter breaks down boundaries and hierarchies. In this space, laughter has a dual nature of birth and death, happiness and sadness. Just as the loss of one location is something to mourn, its new location provides a space for celebration. The procession of boxes may conjure images of coffins and death, or they can spark images of homes where new plant and animal life will dwell. This dual nature does not reject the sadness of such a passing, but instead provides an opportunity to laugh and mourn simultaneously. Carnival expands the modes of interaction with a space and in the moment reminds us of the always moving, unfixed nature of our cultural relations.

The process of expanding and resignifying the sensible entails the constant act of renegotiating what is acceptable and normal and visualizing that the foundations and spaces we assumed were secure and fixed are actually always already in flux. The nomadic garden beds reveal that space is always in flux and ever-changing. Just as insects and caterpillars morph into other life forms, the physical space undergoes similar transformations. Bakhtin sees such changes as potential spaces for positive change: "Metamorphosis serves as the basis for a method of portraying the whole of an individual's life in its more important moment of *crisis*: for showing *how an individual becomes other than what he was*."[32] Not all metamorphoses undergo the same process of transformation. As a result, the exploration of resignified space and place will not always happen in the same way and will always be contingent upon an interrogation of the past and the relations that have been connected to that space over time. Such relationships are not constrained to human-to-human interactions but vitally involve more-than-human participants. Some spaces, like the People's Portable Garden, may provide a potential place for healing and hope and will change how we see a vacant lot (Figure 8.6). No longer is it empty, but it is instead a space of possibilities and potential becomings. The lot could be a space simply waiting to be filled with plants, sunshine, and wind, as well as the songs of birds whose names we had forgotten, but now find ourselves whispering as we plant seeds.

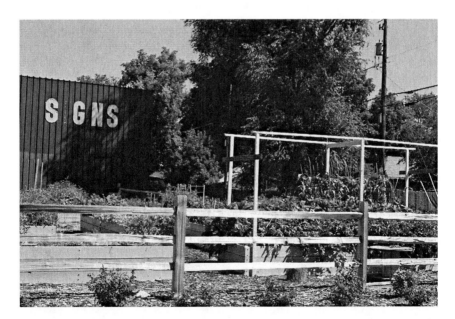

Figure 8.6 The incomplete "signs" reminds us that all signs are incomplete, and all resignifications are political acts of becoming. Photo taken by Natasha Seegert.

NOTES

1. Although the community in this area refers to itself as the "People's Freeway Community" in community meeting notes, the city refers to this area as the "West Temple Gateway Community." Both names conjure different images, but if one considers a freeway as a gateway to another location, perhaps this is simply an example of urban spin.
2. Jacques Rancière, *The Politics of Aesthetics* (New York: Continuum Publishers, 2004), 12.
3. The human animal, being highly visual and aural, frequently focuses on sight and sound. But other senses also come into play when encountering the realm of the sensible. We might see a garbage dump and hear the seagulls and tractors, but the primary signal will be the stench that we smell, or the grit on our skin. When it comes to the abject, we might be able to look away, but we can never "smell away."
4. Rancière, *The Politics of Aesthetics*, 40.
5. Beth Hinderliter et al., eds., *Communities of Sense* (Durham: Duke University Press, 2009), 11.
6. The funding was granted late in the gardening season in April, which resulted in the marathon production so they could meet the garden raising date of May 16, 2009. Perhaps this urgency for creation helped to cultivate a stronger sense of ownership among neighbors.
7. The recent oil spill in the Gulf of Mexico makes this painfully clear as the bodies of wildlife, the space of the ocean waters, the livelihood of humans, and the monolithic forces of corporations and political entities collide.
8. Indeed, during my own springtime visit to the garden, it did not take long for a gardener to notice my presence from her home, and then come over and challenge why I was in the garden. I did not belong, but I was welcome to stay and talk.
9. "Redevelopment Agency of Salt Lake City," Salt Lake City Corporation, accessed April 25, 2010, http://www.slcrda.com/.
10. Rancière, *The Politics of Aesthetics*, 13.
11. Appropriately enough, Trax itself challenges the notion of automobile ownership and the "private" act of commuting.
12. Jacques Derrida, *Margins of Philosophy* (Chicago: University of Chicago Press, 1982), 310.
13. Rancière, *The Politics of Aesthetics*, 55.
14. One gardener grew both okra and peanuts in her garden bed, both typical of southern cuisine where this gardener heralds from. It is worth noting that peanuts typically prefer a southern climate, but thrived in the People's Portable Garden. The gardener claims that it was due to her going to the garden each day to talk to her plants.
15. Consider, for example, the trails inscribed by off-road vehicles, the block letter "U" on the foothills behind the University of Utah, or the ancient Nazca Lines of Peru.
16. Gayarti Chakravorty Spivak, "Can the Subaltern Speak?," in *Marxism and the Interpretation of Culture*, ed. Cary Nelson and Lawrence Grossberg (Urbana: University of Illinois Press, 1988), 285.
17. Anne Whiston Spirn, *Language of Landscape* (New Haven: Yale University Press, 2000), 15.
18. Spirn, *Language of Landscape*, 22.
19. Mikhail Bakhtin, *The Dialogic Imagination*, ed. Michael Holquist (Austin: University of Texas Press, 1988), 293.

138   *Natasha Seegert*

20. Ibid., 250.
21. Valentin Volosinov, "Discourse in Life and Discourse in Art," in Valentin Volosinov, Neal Bruss, and I. R. Titunik, *Freudianism: A Marxist Critique* (New York: Academic Press, 1976), 105.
22. See, for example, Pierre Bourdieu, *Distinction: A Social Critique of the Judgment of Taste* (London: Routledge, 1984) and Pierre Bourdieu, *The Field of Cultural Production* (New York: Columbia University Press, 1993).
23. Spirn, *Language of Landscape*, 24.
24. Rancière, *The Politics of Aesthetics*, 55.
25. We frequently consider the sounds of traffic to be a natural part of the urban setting, so natural we no longer notice them. It is only when one pauses to hear the noise that it loses its naturalized, privileged status.
26. Judith Butler, *Excitable Speech: A Politics of the Performative* (New York: Routledge, 1997), 145.
27. Ibid., 41.
28. Jacques Rancière, "Contemporary Art and the Politics of Aesthetics," in *Communities of Sense*, ed. Beth Hinderliter et al. (Durham: Duke University Press, 2009), 38.
29. Ibid., 38.
30. Examples include the shift regarding gay rights as more cities and businesses grant benefits to gay employees and their partners. Looking to the non-human sphere, the country of Ecuador has granted constitutional rights to nature. Thus, the sphere of what is "sensible" has been expanded, but will most certainly not stop at such way stations.
31. The sign outside of the garden stresses both the portable nature of the garden boxes and their role in "revitalizing" the neighborhood and the "underutilized" property.
32. Bakhtin, *The Dialogic Imagination*, 115.

9 Lee Kyung Hae and the Dynamics of Social Movement Self-Sacrifice

Joshua J. Frye

"I do not ask the wounded person how he feels . . . I myself/become the wounded person . . ."

—Walt Whitman, "Song of Myself"

On September 10, 2003, fifty-five-year-old South Korean farmer-leader Lee Kyung Hae took his own life. As the Fifth World Trade Organization Ministerial Conference met in Cancún, Mexico for the first time since the notorious "Battle in Seattle" in 1999, Lee Kyung Hae scaled a barricade intended to keep protesters away from the deliberations, and then stabbed himself in the heart with his Swiss Army knife. Lee was rushed to the hospital but was declared dead later that afternoon. The announcement of Lee's death spurred invectives of "WTO Kills Farmers!"—the same message Lee Kyung Hae draped himself in with a sandwich board during the protest—from the thousands of protesters he left behind.[1] South Korean and international activists held a candlelight vigil outside of the WTO meetings in honor of Lee's sacrifice. His funeral later that month in Seoul was organized by the Korean Advanced Farmers Federation (KAFF) and attended by representatives of many global farmers' groups.[2] Lee's suicide grabbed momentary international media attention, but has immortalized him among South Koreans and peasant farmers the world over.

Farmers in several parts of Asia—notably India and South Korea—are killing themselves.[3] In a five-year period from 2002 to 2006, over 1,500 farmer peasants in Kerala, India committed suicide. A week after Lee Kyung Hae performed his social movement self-sacrifice, another Korean peasant farmer set himself on fire during a rally of seven hundred peasants in Seongju to honor Lee Kyung Hae. This trend is a most disturbing pattern when an entire professional demographic begins to enact such extreme protest choices. At first glance, this phenomenon seems to be an expression of desperation. Rhetorically, it is revealing to think through this phenomenon as a larger symbolic occurrence of *synecdoche*. A synecdoche uses the resources of symbolism to substitute a whole for a part, a genus for a species, or vice versa.[4] Asian peasant farmers killing themselves functions symbolically as substituting a part for the whole. To wit, farmers are killing themselves because farming itself (as it has been practiced for thousands of years) is dying. Individual peasant farmers from underdeveloped nations are losing ground in a world economy increasingly dominated by trade-liberalization policies that slant advantage to large, industrial-scale, chemicalized, genetically modified, export commodity farm operations. The traditional practices of farming, when understood as a cultural practice for sustenance and identity, are losing ground to high-tech, mechanized, and homogenized practices damaging to indigenous livelihoods, cultural identities, human health, biodiversity, and the environment. Farms are disappearing, and so too are the farmers whose identities are so strongly linked to a practice that has defined their way of life and productive capacity for as long as they can remember.

Scholarship examining certain instances of suicide as political, religious, or rhetorical is not abundant. Much of the literature examining these subjects seems to highlight a few historically significant patterns such as anti-Vietnam activists' use of self-immolation[5] and self-starvation in Northern Ireland.[6] Existing scholarship regarding protest suicide is helpful in advancing our understanding of definitions, motivations, interpretations, appropriations, and effects of such extreme acts. Nonetheless, disproportionate attention pertaining to protest suicide in the prior and tumultuous historical period of the 1960s rhetorically frames protest suicide as something of the past. Indeed, bracketed[7] within the notorious counterculture revolution of the 1960s, scholars run the risk of ossifying perceptions of protest suicide as a passé tactic, when in fact, politically motivated suicide is ongoing and has increased instead of diminished as an action in response to oppression.

Suicide as protest rhetoric has been called the ultimate form of nonverbal dissent. It differs from traditional suicide in that the act is intended as instrumental or as a form of rhetoric.[8] The protester intends his or her physical sacrifice to create any number of rhetorical, psychological, or sociopolitical effects. Suicide as protest rhetoric is arguably the most urgent act an activist can choose. Lee Kyung Hae's social movement self-sacrifice puts him in the legendary company of a select few, including Jesus, Socrates, Emily Wilding Davison, Norman Morrison, Terence James MacSwiney, Bobby Sands, Thich Quang Duc, and others. By definition, they are martyrs. They have *chosen* to die on behalf of a cause. They were spiritual leaders, philosophers, suffragists, pacifists, nationalists, and farmers. Social movement self-sacrifice is an expressly political act. As an expression, such an act is paradoxical. If protest suicide is intended as a gesture of hope—to trigger a movement or alter government policy—it is nevertheless ensconced in finality. As such, its expression ontologically negates its intended pragmatic outcome. This ultimate act precludes the ability of the agent to have intentional agency in the future. How can an act motivated out of what seems to be denunciation, eclipsing one's life, generate hope for the future in others? It is these types of conundrums that have driven psychological, philosophical, and religious analyses of self-sacrifice.

Protest suicide is not the same as suicide terrorism. Numerous instances of suicide as a form of attack (e.g., Kamikaze pilots during World War II, Tamil Tigers, suicide bombers) were intended to inflict physical harm upon others. They are distinct from protest suicide.[9] This chapter does not address the myriad issues surrounding suicide terrorism. Rather, this study highlights the case of Lee Kyung Hae's social movement self-sacrifice at the 2003 anti-WTO protest in Cancún, Mexico, and interrogates the definitions and dynamics encircling this most urgent selection of protest tactics.

Scholars from many fields, including psychology, philosophy, religious studies, and sociology, have debated definitions and classifications of suicide. Often these classifications focus on the motivations of the individual who commits suicide. Scholars in the field of rhetoric also have studied suicide, but with a focus on the intentions as well as the effects of suicide as a "symbolic inducement."[10] Questions exploring the functional differences between suicide, martyrdom, and heroism remain: What are the relevant criteria in distinguishing these classes and why does the classification matter? What are the dynamics at work that help to explain the expressive and instrumental selection of taking one's own life for a social cause? This chapter addresses these questions to illuminate and expand knowledge of this most extreme act.

THE WTO KILLS FARMERS!

Prognostications for a peaceful 2003 World Trade Organization (WTO) meeting in Cancún, Mexico fell short of accuracy. After the infamous 1999 Battle in Seattle, where a new model of social organizing in the anti-globalization movement disrupted trade talks, more civil unrest and confrontations between activists and establishment forces reached a crescendo in 2001 with the murder of Carlo Giuliani, a young Italian activist at the G8 summit in Genoa, Italy. Speculations for a mellower 2003 WTO meeting in Cancún followed. However, led by peasant farmers all over the world, resistance to trade liberalization policies continued to grow. In fact, through the 1990s and into the first decade of the twenty-first century, peasant farmers and transnational indigenous rights movements in Latin America, Asia, and Africa had become the chief adversaries of globalization.[11] For peasant farmers, trade liberalization policies resulted in the importation of devalued commodities from other parts of the world, and these importations resulted in price crashes in the value of domestically grown crops for domestic consumption and export.[12]

In many ways Lee Kyung Hae was a model social movement leader. Social movement leaders tend to be educated, articulate, and of comfortable economic status.[13] He had a college degree from a prestigious South Korean university.[14] He was a three-time elected member of a provincial assembly.[15] He served as an elected officer in the Korean Advanced Farmers

Federation (KAFF) and worked for many years with the Korean Organic Farming Association. Korean farmer leaders, including Lee Kyung Hae, organized KAFF in 1987 as a response to a move by America to open South Korea's rice markets.[16] Lee and his wife, while she was still alive, trained younger farmers on their land. He staged numerous hunger strikes and camped out in front of the World Trade Organization headquarters in Geneva[17] in previous years to sustain attention on the plight of South Korean peasant farmers losing ground to modernization programs, global agricultural trade policies, increasing debt, and falling prices for rice.

Lee's social movement self-sacrifice fits into a bigger picture of protest traditions within Korea. South Korea has a long history of a protest culture. From the 1960s onward, sustained confrontations culminated in rewriting the social contract.[18] Koreans innovated and adopted a wide array of protest tactics, including vigils, lie-ins, street theater, religious-derived rituals, band trucks blaring protest songs, caskets, mobile technology, protest costuming and attire, hunger strikes, and protest suicide. Overall suicide in Korea is higher per capita than every other country surveyed by the Organization for Economic Cooperation and Development (OECD). The latest available data reveal that out of 100,000 people, 21.5 Korean individuals committed suicide compared to 10.1 in the US and an overall OECD average of 11.1.[19] Protest suicide in particular has also gained ascendency in the Korean political culture of dissent. For migrant workers, temporary workers, students, and farmers, self-immolations, self-stabbings, and public self-hangings have rocked Korean social movements for several decades. These social movement self-sacrifices have been effective in a variety of ways. Sometimes the effect is martyrdom, as when in 1970 Chon Tae-il became a heroic figure for self-immolation on behalf of labor reform. Sometimes the effect is gaining the attention of the world, as when in 2003 Lee Kyung Hae stabbed himself at the anti-WTO protest in Cancún, Mexico. Sometimes the effect is a policy change, as when after the second protest suicide in 2004, the Hanjin Shipbuilding Company eliminated temporary workers from its workforce.[20]

Lee's social movement self-sacrifice also fits within a larger picture of his own deployments of agency. The most urgent act of Lee taking his own life did not occur as a spontaneous, irrational act. Lee's radicalization[21] occurred as a result of his perception of failed efficacy or lack of a consequential voice that was taken seriously. Lee had deployed numerous, less extreme tactics over the years leading up to his 2003 anti-WTO act of self-sacrifice. His legislative role in a provincial assembly and leadership with the Korean Advanced Farmers Federation are representative of his commitment to change the system from within. When economic globalization began to negatively affect the South Korean farming community, he escalated his tactics. His hunger strike in Geneva outside of the World Trade Organization headquarters earlier in the year was certainly more confrontational and contributed to further polarization between the peasant farming community and the transnational power elite. However, his voice did not register and his concerns went unheeded.[22] Finally, Lee's last stand—on the one hand participating in a legitimate protest rally and on the other climbing the police barricade and stabbing himself—is the pre-revolutionary tactic of Gandhi and guerrillas.[23]

FUNCTIONAL DIFFERENCES BETWEEN SUICIDE, MARTYRDOM, AND HEROISM

How society classifies the deliberate choice or willingness to end one's life matters. There are social, psychological, religious, and political reasons that matter. Whether we classify Jesus as savior, martyr, or suicide, Socrates as hero or suicide, or Lee Kyung Hae as suicide or martyr affects those left behind in sometimes subtle and sometimes profound ways. For example, socially, issues of legitimization and status are at stake. Psychologically, the memory of the deceased among those still alive as well as society's prevention, intervention, and reaction to such urgent acts are at stake. Religiously, ultimate salvation or damnation is at stake. Politically, how remaining social movement followers and the alleged oppressor respond is at stake. Many thinkers have explored some of this territory. Some foundational and relevant characterizations of their reflections and arguments follow.

Dostoyevsky's *The Devils*[24] characterizes the multiplicity of existential choices to enact freedom as manifestations of illusions of ultimate being. Tantamount to the fullness of sensual experience and expression in moral turpitude is the privileging of the self over the whole. Suicide is one instance of this "total self-assertion."[25] Suicide, according to Kierkegaard, is the negative expression of infinite freedom.[26] When freedom, goodness, truth, or beauty is asserted in the world through the auspices of individual agency, the other qualities perish due to the ontological fabric of an existence wherein disunion and tension exist between these auspicious qualities. According to the theologian Paul Tillich, this is the quintessence of the tragedy of selfhood.[27] Thus, when persons assert their total freedom by negating their existence, they ultimately assert their power through suicide.

Emile Durkheim was one of the earliest social scientists to examine suicide. Durkheim's definition of suicide is behavioral and intended to remove any contentious debate over the mentality or circumstances surrounding an individual's taking of his or her own life. Nevertheless, Durkheim cannot avoid the temptation to classify suicide as variable. He posits "egoistic," "altruistic," and "anomic" classes of suicide.[28] Zygmunt Adamczewski complicates the problem of criteria selection for defining suicide by recognizing differing individual motives for rejecting existence. He parses out categories of suicide into "aesthetic," "conscientious," and "heroic" suicide.[29] Aesthetic suicide is the case of an individual who perceives his or her life to be in store for immanent, unwelcome changes, and rather than adapt to the changes, ends his or her life. Conscientious suicide occurs when an individual decides he or she can no longer live with himself or herself due to remorse over misdeeds in the past. Heroic suicide is when an individual lays down his or her life for the welfare of others. Categorizing someone as a "suicide"—regardless of which variety—has a practical function of ascribing moral responsibility to the individual who has resolved to end his or her life, whether by the individual's own hand or by another agency.[29]

Suicide has traditionally and stereotypically been viewed by many as a socially deviant form of behavior. In the case of religious beliefs, suicide is semantically charged.[31] There are also many facets along which religious conceptions of suicide vary. Suicide can be taboo, non-redemptive, a worthy sacrifice, absolved, or the consequence of a boomerang effect resulting from dogmatic prohibition against the taking of one's own life. Among the world's major religions, certain schools of thought in Christianity, Hinduism, and Buddhism tend to emphasize co-active persuasion to solve worldly conflict, whereas Islam is more ideologically oriented toward conflict persuasion. In much Christian theology, suicide is considered an ungracious rejection of God's gift of life.[32] In Catholicism, it is an act committed by an irrational actor and the individual is thereby absolved of guilt.[33] Hindu doctrine treats it as a disruption in the cycle of reincarnation, and thus taboo. According to Ali Mazrui, Christian, Hindu, and Buddhist doctrines that emphasize pacifistic means to reconcile conflict—when fanatically embraced—can lead to a boomerang effect of religious-minded followers predisposed to suicide.[34] The Mahayana Buddhist tradition of self-immolation, a near millennial tradition, and suicide bombers stand in contrast to mainstream Christian, Buddhist, and Hindu doctrines, because they are religious-political hybrid performances[35] as well as extremist or fanatical manifestations.

Yet other criteria are relevant in classifying and illuminating the dynamics and effects of social movement self-sacrifice, and perhaps as worthy of reclassification as "martyr" or "hero." For instance, the *manner, context,* and *site* of the action matter. Often, but not always, social movement self-sacrifice is conducted in a manner that reflects the imagined or real suffering of the movement followers or those the agent is sympathizing with, as when in 1965 Norman Morrison, an anti–Vietnam War activist, Quaker, husband, and father, immolated himself in front of the Pentagon as a non-verbal parallelism or embodiment of empathy with those dying by napalm in Vietnam.[36] Also, the political context as perceived by the agent who sacrifices his or her life is central to understanding how to perceive and classify the action. A hero, for example, often puts himself or herself in a position of harm—even death—for the sake of values socially shared by the audience the hero is attempting to protect, assist, or save. Lastly, even if politically or ideologically motivated, an individual who chooses a private instead of a public setting for his or her ultimate act is arguably different. In 2010, Sai Kumar Meegada, a straight-A chemical engineering college student, hung himself in his dorm room in solidarity with an Andhra Pradesh separatist movement. He left a note stating, "My final and last request is take my body to the legislative assembly. Goodbye."[37] His message was clear, but no audience was present to witness the moment or manner of death. Unpacking these criteria of manner, context, and site is useful in better understanding the important symbolic and material differences in these different types of deaths.

The manner in which the act of intending one's own death is executed may be necessary but not sufficient grounds for distinguishing between suicide, martyrdom, and heroism. For instance, does the fact that one dies by one's own hand or the hand of another matter? Jesus, Socrates, and Terrence James MacSwiney were all resolved to die, even though the agency for their deaths was extrinsic. Jesus was nailed to a cross, Socrates was given hemlock to drink, MacSwiney starved to death in prison; their deaths were all dealt to them. This is the classic criterion of martyrdom: reveling in the supposedly appropriate transference of guilt, responsibility, and blame.[38] They unanimously relegated the responsibility for their death to others. The seemingly logical corollary, then, is that those that die by their own hand are suicides. This is less clear. Did Emily Wilding Davison intend to die when she ran out onto the track at Epsom Downs? Did Lee Kyung Hae intend to die when he stabbed himself in the chest at the anti-WTO protest in Cancún? The terminal motivation by the actor is private, and always will be. What seems to obtain across all of these cases, however, is the attribution of responsibility and blame to an external agent of oppression, regardless of whether they died by their own hand or that of another. Suicides do not, as a class, require the condition of attributing responsibility and moral culpability elsewhere as necessary to the ending of one's own life. Therefore, it seems that the manner (attitude) in which one intends the rejection of existence is a necessary but insufficient criterion, in a proper definition. Neither does heroism require the attribution of moral responsibility to an oppressor; in fact, heroes can and do emerge on both sides of a conflict because the hero reflects the political values for which he or she acts.

The second criterion necessary in distinguishing suicide, martyrdom, and heroism is the political context in which the individual dies. Most individuals who have lost their lives and are remembered as heroes fell in some form of combat with a foreign power. There are many mythic elements that compose the "hero" archetype. One of those elements is the hero that fulfills his quest by rejecting the responsibility to return to the world: " . . . the hero would be no hero if death held for him any terror; the first condition is reconciliation with the grave."[39] From earliest times blood was thought to be the vehicle of the soul and the heart its seat. The primitive warrior saw that as blood ran from the wounds of the fallen, the strength, and finally the life, also left the body. As the vehicle of the soul, blood carries with it the characteristics of its host.[40] The fallen hero is often a tragic one with whom it is easier to identify (as a noble loser) than perhaps the remaining victor. The audience psychology that is behind this tendency is due to the perception that the tragic hero retained his or her principles, values, and dignity in the face of a more powerful adversary.

Thirdly, the site of the act matters. As Kenneth Burke explains in his famous scene-act ratio, a scene can be expected to "contain" its action.[41] In other words, place or setting can influence the way actors act and how audiences make sense of those acts. The opposite holds true also: The same action executed by the same actor in different locations will be interpreted differently. But place is more potent than has been traditionally viewed within rhetorical theory. In addition to providing a backdrop suffused with material and symbolic opportunities and constraints, place is, according to Danielle Endres and Samantha Senda-Cook, "a performer along with activists in making and unmaking the possibilities of protest." [42] Thus, the specific place where a social movement protest action (in this case social movement self-sacrifice) occurs not only has descriptive value in helping audiences illuminate the meaning and significance of an action, but also can itself be rhetorical.

Viewing the phenomenon of taking one's own life from a rhetorical vantage provides a somewhat different frame than the social scientific and establishment media perspectives. Social movement self-sacrifice is a bodily performance and a rhetoric of resistance. Public performances of self-sacrifice have a distinctly rhetorical vector. They are rhetorics of display employing the body as a signifier. They also demand recognition[43] and evoke an immediate empathetic response.[44] Unlike taking one's life within a private space, social movement self-sacrifices performed in public, often in front of cameras, are distinctly dramatic acts that convey the urgency of a controlling exigence.[45] A private act of protest suicide could never achieve the same result of identification with the audience. It is perhaps one of the heights of identification that, along with other select profoundly powerful social experiences, publically performed social movement self-sacrifice reaches for and—due to its emotional resonance—perhaps grasps consubstantiality. Indeed, the other peasant farmers and activists attending the vigil for Lee Kyung Hae outside of the hospital where he was brought after he stabbed himself in the chest chanted "We are all Lee!"[46]

EXPRESSIVE AND INSTRUMENTAL DYNAMICS IN LEE KYUNG HAE'S SOCIAL MOVEMENT SELF-SACRIFICE

Expressive Dynamics

In death, Lee Kyung Hae has become immortalized. He is perceived by many Koreans and other peasant farmers from around the world as a patriot, a martyr, and a hero. But what are the expressive dynamics through which his chosen manner, political context, and physical place of death allowed others to frame him as something more than just a desperate, downtrodden, and irrational human being who committed suicide? Lee Kyung Hae fits the mold of a martyr more than a suicide and even expresses characteristics of the hero myth: He has fallen in battle before the war is won. As in the fallen hero myth, Lee Kyung Hae's journey involved a transnational journey away from South Korea that took him to Geneva, Switzerland and Cancún, Mexico. He did not return. Along the way, he met significant adversity, but this adversity was brought upon him in the form of a hunger strike and ultimately, a self-sacrifice.

The silent audience of hundreds of peasant farmers and other protestors from around the world held a vigil outside the hospital where Lee Kyung Hae had been rushed after he stabbed himself on the barricades outside the WTO meeting site. The expression of the will in the face of massive social or natural countervailing forces is a symbolic attitude or manner of death that befits the acquisition of the title of "martyred hero." It is the ultimate act of defiance in a controlling exigence or uncontrollable circumstance. It is the expression of what Jiddu Krishnamurti referred to as the power gained from renouncing one's own body and soul: "To give up is another form of acquisition."[47] Lee Kyung Hae's taking of his own life conveyed an expression of power against the seemingly all-encompassing existential powers of worldly institutions wielding economic neoliberalism with the effect of eliminating choice—if not agency—from multitudes of food laborers the world over.

The fact that Lee Kyung Hae wore a placard during the protest march that bore the message "The WTO Kills Farmers!" also factors into the rhetorical mix that constitutes the patriot, martyr, and hero attributions made by those who were present. Lee Kyung Hae died a patriot to his Korean counterparts because the economic plight of his fellow agriculturalists was couched in nationalistic rather than transnationalistic assumptions of economic security. His martyrdom is steeped in irony. A martyr needs to find an external source of blame and moral culpability (either direct or indirect) in the demise of those the target is oppressing. Lee Kyung Hae's message board was a clarion call to place blame on the WTO, thus exonerating him of his own death. A further aspect of the rhetoric of martyrdom that is relevant to this case is the psycho-religious belief that some sacrifice is needed for purification or good fortune to elevate the sacrificial lamb to the celebrated martyr. Interestingly, Lee Kyung Hae elevated himself *literally*— by scaling the barricade—with a consequence of being elevated *figuratively*.

Bruce A. Rosenberg observed that in the case of General Custer, the "legendizing" process happened spontaneously in oral communication and the newspapers.[48] Lee Kyung Hae's elevation to legendary status is a parallel case in terms of the instantaneous diffusion. This type of diffusion is classifiable as contagion.[49] In the case of such urgent acts as social movement self-sacrifice, the dramatic fervor surrounding the action ignites the emotions and imaginations in such a way as to promote a contagious diffusion process that, because of the fevered pitch and rapidity, lends itself to mythological framing (hero, martyr, patriot).

The location where Lee committed his social movement self-sacrifice was on top of a fence that was erected as a temporary barricade set up by the police to contain thousands of protestors so that the WTO ministerial meeting could proceed as planned. Because Lee chose the most urgent act in a public place of contested legitimacy, Lee's act was rhetorically forceful. Lee Kyung Hae's action of stabbing himself on top of a temporary fence keeping some of the world's poorest of the poor far removed from international power elites is ripe with significance. Both the symbolic and physical elements of that place are ephemeral.[50] The fence where Lee Kyung Hae initiated his social movement self-sacrifice no longer exists; it was a temporary physical structure erected by the establishment to instantiate that whereas some are on the "inside" of brokering a global economic order, others are indeed on the "outside." Lee Kyung Hae chose the apex of this temporary, physical-symbolic transnational border zone to make his ultimate statement. Yet, because this terminal action occurred in a place that has all but disappeared because of the very fluidity of place, it is perhaps more challenging for accurate public memory of such extreme power disparities and their organized resistances in the twenty-first century. If, however, Lee Kyung Hae devotees decided to hold regular vigils at the place of his ultimate act on the street in Cancún where he had scaled temporary police barricades, they would be choosing to engage in a rhetoric of "repeated reconstruction" and thereby would be exercising the agency of living activists in the continuous meaning-making of place.[51]

Instrumental Dynamics

Lee's dramatic self-sacrifice is considered one of the primary causes for the collapse of the trade liberalization discussions at the WTO meeting in Cancún.[52] The first major stoppage since the collapse of the WTO meetings during the 1999 Battle in Seattle, Lee Kyung Hae's social movement self-sacrifice in 2003 during the WTO meeting in Cancún helped to compel the collapse of the trade talks. After his dramatic death, days of peasant farmer marches, Korean-led confrontations with the police, and the first formal communiqués in four years to an international audience broadcast on pirate radio from the Zapatistas spurred the protest.[53] The intensified protests following Lee's death led several delegates, ultimately followed by Mexico's foreign minister, to leave the talks. This resulted in the second collapse of attempted multilateral neoliberal trade agreements since Seattle.[54]

Before the collapse of the Cancún meeting, however, there was another brief, but significant, effect of Lee Kyung Hae's action: an official moment of silence.[55] Silence has typically been understood as the opposite of speech and as a form of passivity. Some scholars, however, have cast silence as an active and even performative gesture.[56] A moment of silence invoked by an official body of powerful transnational decision-makers is symbolic. In fact, it may profitably be understood as an "event."[57] Cross-cultural meanings of silence are many, but there can be little doubt that, in this context, it functioned as a gesture of respect for Lee Kyung Hae. The "moment of silence," a performative event, was called for by religious and political officials alike, thus demonstrating civil religious incarnations at the WTO meeting in Cancún.

Lee Kyung Hae's social movement self-sacrifice was followed by Korean peasant farmers organizing a rally in Seoul to honor and mourn Lee. They hoped Lee's self-sacrifice would function as a triggering event for the anti-globalization movement.[58] Social movement self-sacrifice is a powerful mode of social influence. It often functions as internal rhetoric[59] to incite true believers to further escalation. Sometimes the sacrifice may even convert those sympathetic to the plight of the smitten, thereby gaining ideological adherents and swelling the enlistment of movement followers. There is potential for compassion to be transformed into action through the empathetic response of those who viewed or learned of the spectacle of Lee's urgent protest action. As Susan Sontag maintained, it is easy for people to be indifferent when they feel safe.[60] The action of killing oneself during a protest

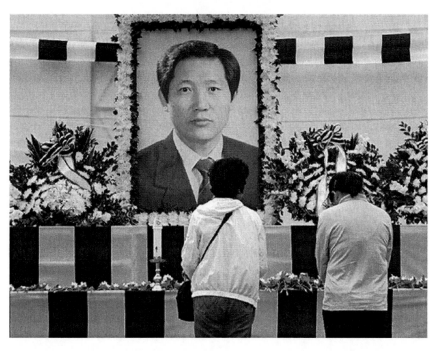

Figure 9.1   Lee Kyung Hae memorial hall. Photo used by permission of the Korean Advanced Farmers Federation and the Asian Farmers Association for Sustainable Rural Development.

in front of thousands of people is a gruesome performance. It symbolically and simultaneously carries the power of desperation and decisiveness to those left behind and insinuates that complacency is merely deferred defeat.

In addition to the numerous planned vigils, memorials, and rallies in honor of Lee Kyung Hae's sacrifice, a virtual memorial hall has been erected for Lee Kyung Hae.[61] Extending the reach of martyred heroes is the Internet's capacity to broadcast the message of the martyr to potentially all computer-users in the world. The virtual memorial hall provides some background information about Lee's activism, publishes the archived petition Lee Kyung Hae wrote to the WTO, and displays a variety of protest photographs featuring Lee Kyung Hae's activism. These photographs of Lee, the dead martyr-hero, have the instrumentality of promoting agency and sustained civic engagement.[62]

CONCLUSION

The identity politics of indigenous peasant farmers worldwide have dead-locked against a brave new world of democratization, economic liberalization, and decentralization. Peasant farmers whose identities are rooted in previous structural conditions and cultural practices are faced with vexing strategies to renegotiate issues of representation, resources, and rights.[63] Those who are unable or unwilling to adapt to such disparities between transnational powerful elites and those swept up in the incoming tide of international trade policy reforms may feel anger, utter voicelessness, and despair. From a rhetorical perspective, however irrational social movement self-sacrifice may appear to unsympathetic bystanders, both expressive and instrumental power exists in an intentional taking of one's own life, particularly when the confluence of the criteria of manner, context, and site result in transforming a seemingly voiceless peasant into an international martyr-hero. It is an act of freedom from controlling exigency. The act tends to immortalize the agent of the act, providing a legacy, often fitting into the rhetorical mold of mythic constructions. Protest suicide often functions as a triggering event for a movement that is losing ground: retreat to advance. In some instances, social movement self-sacrifice can even serve as effective advocacy for policy change. In the case of Lee Kyung Hae's 2003 social movement self-sacrifice at the WTO ministerial in Cancún, a rip current of sympathetic protestors mobilized to carry the trade talks, drifting out to sea. According to some commentators, the second collapse of WTO trade talks in five years revealed that, aside from the WTO, the second most powerful entity in the world is global civil society— the power of the people. The radical agency of the human spirit of sacrifice for the greater good can be the rhetorical fuel to perpetuate the struggle in the face of such gross power disparities.

Even though it is analytically useful to distinguish between instrumental and expressive effects of social movement self-sacrifice, these functions are complex, interrelated aspects of the *gravitas* of bodily suffering and extinguishing the light of life as rhetoric of resistance. Social movement self-sacrifice involves an indisputable element of public performance and a selection of a means to influence target audiences. Embodied in the protest action of Lee Kyung Hae was the inherent expression of suffering. Lee stabbing himself in the chest in front of his primary audience of likeminded anti-WTO protestors potentially embodied emotional expressions and responses of compassion, guilt, anger, empathy, and resurrection of urgency as evidenced in the myriad motives and consequences of Lee Kyung Hae's social movement self-sacrifice.

As Young-Cheon Cho articulated, "insofar as a body may make a public statement, it requires a context and significant symbols (most typically words) to explain its actions."[64] Thus, social movement self-sacrifice rhetoric is one of highly charged expressiveness instrumentally affecting audience attributions of meaning to the message. Lee's termination of his physical ability to create messages electrified the corporeal body politic to pick up the slack and amplify his message to the authorities. If the body is essentially mute in communicating pain,[65] then the activist can elect to accompany his deadly performance with language, signs, and other symbols that contextualize the meaning and lend salience and significance to his message—as Lee Kyung Hae did. If the activist does not clarify his purpose then the audience present, the media, and other social actors left behind will ascribe culpability and infer motive and meaning. But the logic and linearity of traditional, formal modes of public argumentation are not nearly as adept at harnessing identification. When social movement self-sacrifice is enacted as a nonverbal parallelism to the suffering of the represented, those present at the performance are all the more likely to be engulfed by the emotional resonance of the performance. When social movement self-sacrifice is conducted in a public site in a manner that embodies conjoined suffering with an empathetic audience within a politically charged and antagonistic context, it is a performance par excellence and the conditions for transmogrifying a "suicide" into a "martyr" or "hero" are met. Socially, contagious diffusion occurs. Psychologically, the one who takes his or her own life is perceived and remembered as a martyr or hero. Rhetorically, deeply emotional audience identification, message amplification, increased mobilization, and punctuated, momentary, dramatic, political change may become possible. What movement there is in this case is a result of the unplumbable agency of the human spirit of freedom and sacrifice against the machinations of a corporate transnational trade system.

ACKNOWLEDGMENTS

The author would like to thank Theron Verdon, Michael Bruner, and the anonymous reviewers for their helpful comments and suggestions during earlier versions of this chapter.

NOTES

1. Nick Mathiason, "Daughter Waits for the Real Harvest from Her Father's Suicide," *The Observer*, July 29, 2007, 7.
2. "South Korean Suicide Farmer's Funeral to Be Held in Seoul September 20," BBC's *Summary of World Broadcasts*, September 17, 2003, LexisNexis Academic.
3. Mathiason, "Daughter Waits," 7; Jose George and P. Krishnaprasad, "Distress and Farmers' Suicides in the Tribal District of Wayanad," *Social Scientist* 34 (2006): 70–85.
4. Richard A. Lanham, *A Handlist of Rhetorical Terms*, 2nd ed. (Berkeley: University of California Press, 1991), 148.
5. For example: Ali Mazrui, "Sacred Suicide," *Transition* 21 (1965): 10–15; Cheyney Ryan, "The One Who Burns Herself for Peace," *Hypatia* 9 (1994): 21–39; Michelle Murray Yang, "Still Burning: Self-Immolation as Photographic Protest," *Quarterly Journal of Speech* 97 (2001): 1–26; Young-Cheon Cho, "Empathy, Compassion, and the Body in Pain: The Politics of Suffering in Self-Immolations" (paper presented at the annual meeting of the International Communication Association, New York, NY, May 2009); Barbara Reynolds, "In Witness of Man's Oneness," *Christian Century* (1966): 81; Sallie King, "They Who Burned Themselves for Peace," *Buddhist-Christian Studies* 20 (2000): 127–50.
6. For example: Carroll Edwards, "Hunger Strike: Protest or Suicide?," *America* 144 (1981); Kevin O'Gorman, "The Hunger Strike of Terence MacSwiney," *Irish Theological Quarterly* 59 (1993): 114–27; Terence M. O'Keeffe, "Suicide and Self-Starvation," *Philosophy* 59 (1984): 349–63; Jim Smyth, "Unintentional Mobilization: The Effect of the 1980–81 Hunger Strikes in Ireland," *Political Communication and Persuasion* 4 (1987): 179–90.
7. Bruce E. Gronbeck, "The Rhetorics of the Past: History, Argument, and Collective Memory," in *Doing Rhetorical History: Concepts and Cases*, ed. Kathleen J. Turner (Tuscaloosa, AL: University of Alabama Press, 1998), 51.
8. Cheryl R. Jorgensen-Earp, "Toys of Desperation: Suicide as Protest Rhetoric," *The Southern Speech Communication Journal* 53 (1987): 83; O'Keeffe, "Suicide and Self-Starvation," 358.
9. An interesting rhetorical difference between suicide terrorism and suicide protest rhetoric is that agents employing suicide terrorism as a tactic kill themselves in order to kill, maim, or otherwise destroy others' property. Suicide protest rhetoric involves the killing or sacrifice of oneself (no one else) with the symbolic transference of blame for the death. There is a key difference in the relationship between political action and the attribution of responsibility. In one case, an individual kills others and himself or herself in the process and takes the credit. In the other, an individual kills himself or herself and seeks to displace the nature of agency.
10. Richard B. Gregg, *Symbolic Inducement and Knowing: A Study in the Foundations of Rhetoric* (Columbia: University of South Carolina Press, 1984), 119.
11. Dorothy L. Hodgson, "Introduction: Comparative Perspectives on the Indigenous Rights Movement in Africa and the Americas," *American Anthropologist* 104 (2002): 1037–49; Andrea Muehlebach, "What Self in Self-Determination? Notes from the Frontiers of Transnational Indigenous Activism," *Identities: Global Studies in Culture and Power* 10 (2003): 241–68; James Petras, "Globalization: A Critical Analysis," *Journal of Contemporary Asia* 29 (1999): 3–37.
12. Petras, "Globalization," 8–10.

13. See Joshua Frye, *The Origin, Diffusion, and Transformation of "Organic" Agriculture* (Saarbrucken: VDM, 2009), 126; Charles J. Stewart, Craig Smith, and Robert Denton Jr., *Persuasion and Social Movements*, 4th ed. (Prospect Heights, IL: Waveland, 2001), 105.
14. Mathiason, "Daughter Waits."
15. James Brooke, "Farming Is Korean's Life and He Ends It in Despair," *New York Times*, September 16, 2003, 6.
16. Mathiason, "Daughter Waits."
17. "Agency Gives Details of South Korean Suicide Farmer's Background," BBC's *Summary of World Broadcasts*, September 11, 2003, LexisNexis Academic.
18. Gabriele Hadl, "Korean Protest Culture," *Kyoto Journal* 60 (2005): 44–49.
19. Organization for Economic Co-operation and Development, *OECD Indicators* (OECD Publishing, 2009), doi: 10.1787/health_glance-2009-en.
20. Hadl, "Korean Protest Culture," 44–49.
21. John Wilson, "Social Protest and Social Control," *Social Problems* 24 (1977): 469–81.
22. Walden Bello, "The Meaning of Cancún," *Yes! Powerful Ideas, Practical Actions*, Positive Futures Network, Winter 2003–2004, http://www.yesmagazine.org/issues/whose-water.
23. John W. Bowers et al., *The Rhetoric of Agitation and Control*, 3rd ed. (Prospect Heights, IL: Waveland, 2010), 48.
24. Fyodor Dostoyevsky, *The Devils*, trans. David Magarshack (New York: Penguin, 1953).
25. Mikhail Blumenkrantz and Lucy Daniels, "From Nimrod to the Grand Inquisitor: The Problem of the Demonisation of Freedom in the Work of Dostoevskij," *Studies in East European Thought* 48 (1996): 240.
26. Soren Kierkegaard, *Either/Or II*, ed. and trans. Howard V. Hong and Edna H. Hong (Princeton, NJ: Princeton University Press, 1987), 246.
27. Paul Tillich, *The Dynamics of Faith* (New York: HarperCollins, 1958).
28. Emile Durkheim, *Suicide*, trans. George Simpson and John A. Spaulding (New York: The Free Press, 1979), 44.
29. Zygmunt Adamczewski, "Reflections on Suicide," *Chicago Review* 14 (1960): 59.
30. Suzanne Stern-Gillet, "The Rhetoric of Suicide," *Philosophy & Rhetoric* 20 (1987): 160–70.
31. Olufunke Adeboye, "Death Is Preferable to Ignominy" (paper presented at the Harriet Tubman Seminar, Toronto, Canada, October 24, 2006); Darwin Sawyer and Jeffery Sobal, "Public Attitudes toward Suicide," *The Public Opinion Quarterly* 51 (1987): 92–101.
32. Adamczewski, "Reflections on Suicide," 46.
33. Ryan, "The One Who Burns Herself," 25.
34. Mazrui, "Sacred Suicide," 10–15.
35. Yang, "Self-Immolation," 9.
36. Reynolds, "In Witness," 81.
37. Lydia Polgreen, "Suicides, Some for Separatist Cause, Jolt India," *New York Times*, March 31, 2010.
38. Mazrui, "Sacred Suicide," 10–15; Stern-Gillet, "The Rhetoric of Suicide," 160–70.
39. Joseph Campbell, *The Hero with a Thousand Faces* (Princeton, NJ: Princeton University Press, 1968), 356.
40. Bruce A. Rosenberg, "The Legend of the Martyred Hero in America," *Journal of the Folklore Institute* 9 (1972): 121.
41. Kenneth Burke, *A Grammar of Motives* (Berkeley: University of California Press, 1969), 3.

42. Danielle Endres and Samantha Senda-Cook, "Location Matters: The Rhetoric of Place in Protest," *Quarterly Journal of Speech* 97 (2011): 258.
43. Ryan, "The One Who Burns Herself," 29.
44. Cho, "Empathy, Compassion, and the Body in Pain."
45. Jorgensen-Earp, "Toys of Desperation," 91.
46. "Suicidal Protest over WTO," *The Mercury*, September 12, 2003, 24; Kenneth Burke, *A Rhetoric of Motives* (Berkeley: University of California Press, 1969), 21.
47. J. Krishnamurti, *Commentaries on Living*, ed. D. Rajagopal (New York: Harper & Row, 1956), 162.
48. Rosenberg, "The Legend," 129.
49. Doug McAdam, "Cross-National Diffusion of Movement Ideas," *The ANNALS of the American Academy of Political and Social Science* 528 (1993), 56–74.
50. Endres and Senda-Cook, "Location Matters," 263.
51. Tim Cresswell, *Place: A Short Introduction* (Malden, MA: Blackwell Publishing, 2004).
52. "South Korean Suicide Farmer's Funeral," BBC's *Summary of World Broadcasts*, September 17, 2003, LexisNexis Academic.
53. John Vidal, "Farmer Commits Suicide at Protests," *The Guardian*, Thursday, September 11, 2003, accessed August 22, 2011, http://www.guardian.co.uk/world/2003/sep/11/wto.johnvidal.
54. Charlotte Denny, Larry Elliott, and David Munk, "Brussels Urges Shakeup of 'Medieval' WTO," *The Guardian*, Tuesday, September 16, 2003, accessed August 22, 2011, http://www.guardian.co.uk/business/2003/sep/16/europe-anunion.wto.
55. Bello, "The Meaning of Cancún."
56. Kris Acheson, "Silence as Gesture: Rethinking the Nature of Communicative Silences," *Communication Theory* 18 (2008): 535–55; Bernard Dauenhauer, *Silence: The Phenomenon and Its Ontological Significance* (Bloomington: Indiana University Press, 1980).
57. Calvin O. Schrag, *Communicative Praxis and the Space of Subjectivity* (West Lafayette, IN: Purdue University Press, 2003).
58. Stewart, Smith, and Denton, *Persuasion and Social Movements*.
59. Charles J. Stewart, "The Internal Rhetoric of the Knights of Labor," *Communication Studies* 42 (1991): 67–82.
60. Susan Sontag, *Regarding the Pain of Others* (New York: Farrar, Straus and Giroux, 2003).
61. The virtual memorial hall for Kyung Hae Lee can be found by visiting http://cancun.jinbo.net/maybbs/list.php?db=cancun&code=enews&page=.
62. Yang, "Self-Immolation," 21.
63. Hodgson, "Introduction: Comparative Perspectives," 1040–41.
64. Cho, "Empathy, Compassion, and the Body in Pain," 13.
65. Hannah Arendt, *The Human Condition* (Chicago: The University of Chicago Press, 1958), 310.

10 *Let's Move*
The Ideological Constraints of Liberalism on Michelle Obama's Obesity Rhetoric

Abigail Seiler

Two competing discourses have dominated the discussion of rising obesity rates and unhealthy eating habits in the American context, one focusing on individual behavior modification and personal habits and the other emphasizing systemic prevention and environmental determinants of obesity. These divergent responses to the prevalence of obesity are reflective of their respective underlying ideologies, one grounded in neoliberal individualism and the other in post-structuralist social reproduction. In her position as First Lady, a non-elected representative of the president's administration, Michelle Obama is at the crossroads of these two discourses. Through her *Let's Move* campaign, does she articulate the material and social conditions that engender American eating habits? Or does she continue to promote what has become since the 1980s the more dominant narrative, that of individual responsibility and self-discipline?

Providing deeper understanding of the relationship between thought, structure, and discourse serves as the basis for my analysis of the ideologies that compete in Michelle Obama's rhetoric, as well as the potential implications of her discursive performances. The competing discourses about where responsibility for food choices lies collide in the discourse of *Let's Move*, constituting a rhetorical performance shaped by a powerful discursive regime. I argue that throughout her *Let's Move* speeches Michelle Obama alludes to the existence of systemic causes of obesity; however, her explanations of such phenomena are hampered by the hegemonic status of liberal ideology in American culture, the powerful language of individualism, and the lack of alternative ways of publicly discussing these issues.

CHARACTERIZATION OF OBESITY IN THE US

Rising obesity rates became a matter of national concern in the US in the late 1970s and 1980s. The discourse surrounding obesity and healthy eating that emerged at that time characterized obesity as an inability to control one's impulses, a physical manifestation of an individual's deficiencies as a person.[1] A federal government–sponsored campaign begun in the late 1970s attempted to "extirpate" obesity from America. The tone of the campaign was that of admonishment and personal responsibility.[2]

Changing economic and social conditions coupled with increasing food choices and the rising availability of convenience and fast food during this period contributed to a widening nutritional disparity between the rich and poor. Those who could afford to spend and eat well readily devoted time and money to dieting and cutting calories, whereas those with less income relied on social supports for food or purchased new types of food that were cheap and available, but often nutritionally deficient.[3] This nutritional gap persists today and is associated with both class and race. For example, a 2008 study by the Centers for Disease Control found that obesity rates among African Americans were 51 percent higher than white Americans and 21 percent higher among Hispanics.[4] The history of obesity in America, therefore, is one riddled with class-based and racial inequalities.

More recently, the phrase "obesity epidemic" has been used to characterize America's rising obesity rates and to draw attention to them. This recent move illustrates Tim Lang's assertion, "Nutrition, like any study concerning humans, is inevitably framed by social assumptions."[5] The discursive use of such terms and phrases both illustrates and invites a medicalized understanding of the phenomenon, thus ignoring the array of contributing social influences, collective histories, and political dimensions. Such paradoxical and narrow conceptions of weight, obesity, consumption, and personal responsibility have hampered efforts to improve the health of America's population,[6] and it is in this context that Michelle Obama's *Let's Move* campaign is situated.

THE INDIVIDUALIZING RHETORIC OF LIBERALISM

Since the Reagan era, which strongly coincided with the rise of obesity in the US, discussion of the so-called "obesity epidemic" has been dominated by narratives of self-discipline and individual responsibility,[7] and the influence of the individualizing nature of liberal and neoliberal thought is undeniable. In an effort to understand the origin of these narratives, we can look to Foucault's genealogical account of Western styles of government.

Foucault's work showed that after an era of feudal governance buoyed by the Christian church the modern era of government became "centered on the ideal of personal autonomy—a composite notion including . . . ideas of personal independence, rationality and responsibility" that he referred to as "governmental rationality."[8] Foucault argued that both economic and familial processes became disembedded from their social and economic interconnections,[9] resulting in the perception of an individual as acting more or less in isolation and of his or her own accord. Liberalism moved these beliefs beyond the doctrine of governance, engendering a "way of thinking" that we are rational, autonomous individuals—a way of thinking that has come to permeate many aspects of American life. Foucault recognized the centrality of discourse in the propagation of such a viewpoint. Thus the development of this ideology and its articulation through discourse are fundamental to our understandings of personal responsibility and assumptions about the causes and solutions of obesity.

As Foucault contends, truth, as we come to know it, is produced through "discursive regimes," which are themselves produced within systems of power.[10] Scientific discourse in particular is produced and transmitted under the control of a select few economic and political apparatuses. Medicine, as it has developed during the Enlightenment era and since, is bound up in certain ways of speaking and seeing, an "ensemble of practices" that has transformed the way we conceive of and talk about the body.[11] Thus, contemporary discourses surrounding healthy eating are constituted through the formation of truth born out of the historically rooted and mutually producing relationship between language and power. As such, it is the language of power that is most readily available for use by rhetors. Alternative discourses and truths about the nature of obesity in the US are not as easily accessed and are therefore not as commonly articulated.

"Truth," however, must be understood not just as a mere *product* of discourse, but also as a *means* for capitalism and social structures to be reproduced. In the neoliberal era, market principles and economic schemata have been transposed onto social spheres, and social domains have been encoded in economic terms. A model of "rational-economic action" acts as a justification for limited government intervention and is emblematic of an epistemological shift that has expanded the "objects addressed by the economy"[12] to include nearly all forms of human behavior and action, including health and eating.[13]

Governmentality, then, can be expressed as "technologies of the self" or forms of self-regulation. Thomas Lemke posits that neoliberal governments such as the US have "developed indirect techniques for leading and controlling individuals without at the same time being responsible for them,"[14] freeing themselves of the responsibility to address social risks and ailments. Instead, a model of self-care is put forth, placing responsibility squarely in the domain of the rational individual and framing individual actions and their consequences as "free will."[15] This perspective is typical of the government programs that have traditionally tackled obesity rates and, as we will see, surfaces in the discourse of Michelle Obama as well.

That the primary interest of the neoliberal government is the economic, rational, thinking individual has profound implications for the relationship between governance and the health of a population.[16] Under this model, the individual's civic obligation is to "moderate the burden of risk which he or she imposes on society, by participating, for example, in preventative healthcare programs."[17] Thus, this paradigm constitutes a reversal of the welfare state, demanding that the individual act in a manner that promotes the stability and security of the state rather than the state working to ensure the security of the individual. In other words, "social duty" is understood as the "duty of a man in society" rather than a "duty of society."[18]

These values, with origins in the Enlightenment period and modern governance, have carried over into contemporary discourses, especially in regard to health. Monica Greco extends Foucault's discussion of the rationality of pathology and medicine born out of liberal ideals into what she calls "healthism."[19] In this interpretation, health becomes conceptualized as the primary enterprise of oneself, thus positing a "faculty of choice" in preserving one's own health. Inasmuch as the economic individual has a civic duty to take responsibility for his own well-being, Greco argues that under this paradigm, disease is a function of an individual's moral failures, a failure to care for one's self through "the regulation of life-style, the modification of risky behavior and the transformation of unhealthy attitudes through sheer strength of will."[20]

The problem of obesity has been firmly entrenched in such narratives of personal lifestyle and individual risk reduction. Despite the prevalence of obesity in the US, it remains a stigmatized condition; to be obese is to have failed in one's food choices, and as such, is not the responsibility of society at large. Healthism and its historical antecedents are powerful regimes that those arguing for structural explanations and solutions to rising obesity rates must overcome. The liberal ideas conceived in the age of Enlightenment seem only to be strengthened in this current era of neoliberal conservatism.

PUBLIC HEALTH AND SOCIAL DETERMINANTS

The articulation of alternative paradigms for understanding health and obesity is aided by theoretical concepts that enable us to view eating habits and choices as not based solely on individual preferences, but also integrally related to socialization, social structure, and cultural markers such as race and class. Thus, we turn to sociological, rather than psychological, understandings of behavior, and utilize concepts such as habitus, taste, choice, chance, and lifestyle.

In his notion of *habitus* as a set of durable and predominantly unconscious dispositions that are derived from social structures and embodied by the agent, Bourdieu provides an alternative way of understanding habits and actions.[21] Habitus is "history turned into nature," produced by "different modes of generation . . . [that] cause one group to experience as natural or reasonable practices or aspirations which another group finds unthinkable or scandalous."[22] Using the notion of habitus, we can view food choices and habits as shaped by social structure and participation in social networks, and view individuals as both produced by and reproducers of collective history. One's preferences or taste, therefore, are reflective of class position, placing socioeconomic class structure at the heart of the issue and highlighting the need to attend to the historical structures and dynamics of collectivity that give rise to eating behaviors.

The post-structural perspectives presented here contrast with the liberal schema of individual responsibility and discipline in food choices by acknowledging various constraints on choice that truncate people's behavioral options. The notion of chance suggested in Max Weber's description of lifestyle is offered as a counterpoint to choice. Although recognizing that preferences and choices become embodied in patterns called lifestyles, Weber highlighted the "dialectical interplay between choice and chance."[23] Individual choice is constrained by one's chances, which can be defined as "the crystallized probability of finding satisfaction for interests, wants and needs, thus the probability of occurrence of events that bring about satisfaction."[24] As William Cockerham et al. explain, "chance is socially determined, and social structure is an arrangement of these chances."[25] Thus social structure and one's participation in various status groups underlie the choices that are available to us with regard to lifestyle, including our food choices.

The significant increase in available food options in the post-modern world can be seen in the proliferation of new products in grocery stores and advertising media that are designed to help us "eat better." This greater diversity, however, has not diminished the influence of social structure in constraining choice and creating unequal sets of chances. As John Mirowsky and Catherine Ross argue, because upper- and middle-class people experience more life chances or, to use Weber's definition, a greater likelihood of satisfaction, they develop a stronger sense of control over their lives.[26] This sense of agency generates an expectation that planning and effort will usually give rise to the desired result. To the contrary, lower-income people experience fewer chances for satisfaction and, consequently, do not develop this same sense of control. This perceived lack of agency can result in a mindset whereby one's health is considered to be beyond one's control; thus fewer actions to improve health are undertaken. The greater diversity of options that has come about as a result of post-modernity has created an illusion of the possibility of greater choice for all, and this has been taken up in liberal arguments for individual responsibility in personal choices related to food and lifestyle.

Furthermore, Anthony Giddens argues that lifestyle can be understood as a cluster of habits that have a degree of unity, providing an individual with a sense of "ontological security" in the increasingly choice-laden post-modern world. He asserts that we have "no choice but to choose," and thus we enact lifestyle behaviors appropriate for our group, be it characterized by class, race, gender, nationality, location, or a convergence of these categories.[27] In other words, our food choices are informed not only by a cultural history of eating patterns and tastes, but also by the socially determined options available to us, and a disposition toward unity and coherence in the post-modern world.

COMPETING DISCOURSES AROUND
OBESITY AND HEALTHY LIFESTYLES

Because of the dominance of liberal individualism in our discourse, public health campaigns have been successful in "transferring the health values of the upper-middle class to society at large" without acknowledging the systemic reasons why persons of lower classes may not be able or likely to adopt the same lifestyle.[28] These campaigns, constructed out of our larger understandings of health and responsibility, have led to a more consumer-ist model of health that benefits those with more resources and life chances for healthy life choices.[29] The inadequacies of this tendency are becoming increasingly evident, especially in the case of poor nutrition, making the First Lady's decision to enter the debate all the more noteworthy. We shall see, however, that she too is constrained by this choice-based orientation.

Public health theory has come to acknowledge the tension between divergent approaches to addressing obesity in the US. The two prevailing policy approaches, "medical" and "public health," surrounding obesity and healthy lifestyles reflect divergent understandings of the nature of the problem and its causes.[30] The *medicalized approach* concentrates on the treatment of obesity, framing it as a matter of individual behavioral choices and responsibility. This approach assumes an informed, independent agent capable of making health-conscious choices, a characterization born out of liberal ideals and crafted through governmentality. Consequently, the resulting interventions focus on providing educational information about obesity, healthy eating, and exercise, as well as promoting motivation to help individuals act responsibly. The *public health approach,* on the other hand, focuses on the prevention of obesity, emphasizing the influence of environmental factors that lead individuals to make health-damaging behavioral choices. This perspective reasserts the idea that social structures and social norms have a greater impact on behavior than individual agency and should therefore be given primacy. Thus, "public health"–based inter-ventions center around broad policy changes and altering community or environmental surroundings. Such competing discourses surrounding obe-sity reflect the tensions that exist between conflicting notions of individual empowerment and victim blaming.

These tensions are manifest in the rhetorical landscape of obesity dis-course. In an effort to reveal alternative frameworks for understanding, Lawrence Wallack and Regina Lawrence deconstruct the liberal language surrounding obesity.[31] Their work posits that the "first language" of the US is that of *individualism*, creating an absence of alternative language.[32]

Fostering more adequate language for discussing the health of populations would require proliferation of the secondary American language, that of *community*, a discourse already used by some in the field of public health.[33] They argue that in order to advance the public health approach, rooted in core social justice values, we must invigorate the language of community. Although public health scholars and practitioners widely acknowledge the impact of societal forces on health, the dominance of narratives about personal responsibility, which accompanied the emergence of liberalism in the nineteenth century, has meant that most intervention approaches still target individual behavioral changes.[34]

In the *Let's Move* campaign, Michelle Obama has taken on the health of the nation's families as her primary cause and has assumed a central role in this public discussion.[35] The impact of discursive regimes on contemporary thinking about obesity and their relation to competing understandings of human behavior is the focus for analyzing this campaign. These perspectives are essential to understanding the ideological assumptions, articulations, and framings of obesity presented in the discourse of *Let's Move* and ultimately to understanding the potential of her campaign to bring about change.

THE RHETORIC OF *LET'S MOVE*

Michelle Obama's discourse as she campaigns to reduce childhood obesity and improve the eating habits of Americans represents a cross section of the ideological perspectives dominating health issues. Although she acknowledges that the causes of our poor diet are often systemic, she suffers from society's inarticulateness on such issues and does not provide a thorough or politicized explanation of these causes and how they came about. Similarly, the solutions advocated by her *Let's Move* campaign attempt to address environmental causes, but do not address the power structures that underlie these environmental contributors. These notable absences are perhaps the most significant characteristic of her rhetoric. Reading the silences of the First Lady, perhaps even more than her words, sheds light on the nation's inability to discursively engage with social problems. To analyze her rhetoric and identify the ideological implications, I examine Obama's discussion of the four primary solutions she proposes as the keystones to her campaign: (1) extensive educational campaigns targeting parents, (2) improving the nutritional quality of school lunches, (3) eliminating food deserts, and most recently, (4) corporate partnership. Through an exploration of this discourse, I argue that although Michelle Obama's rhetoric at times addresses the structural elements that greatly determine lifestyle choices, her rhetoric is constrained by the more pervasive, familiar, and depoliticized language of individualism.

Parental Awareness Campaign

The initiatives connected with parent-targeted, nutritional awareness raising proposed by Obama are the most overtly individualized aspect of her
campaign. These proposals presuppose an autonomous, rational individual—the liberal ideal—and take a single focused approach to food habits.
In her discussion of these programs, she emphasizes the responsibility of
parents in making food choices for their children, echoing the liberal expectation of self-discipline and moral ramifications of failing to live up to these
obligations. To improve their decision-making abilities, she advocates that
we "offer parents the tools and information they need . . . to make healthy
choices for their kids."[36] This language implies that if given the "right"
information, parents will naturally make healthy choices. One of these proposed "tools" is to "make our food labels more customer-friendly."[37] In this
conception of healthy eating, the individual consumer is responsible for
checking the label and acting accordingly; given the necessary information,
he or she should make the rational choice. Furthermore, the word "tool"
implies a narrow and instrumental approach to the problem of eating habits, ignoring the social derivation of taste through *habitus* and the adoption
of class or status group preferences. Instead, Obama presents the issue in
this way: The problem is a quantifiable lack of information and the solution is to make this information more accessible. Questions regarding what
systemic barriers might prevent the successful use of these newly available
tools are not mentioned in her speeches, a void that reflects a discursive
regime guided by liberalism, which makes articulating systemic inequalities difficult and unappealing. This approach obfuscates structural problems with access to healthy food and sufficient resources, such as time and
money, problems that may prevent parents from taking the actions deemed
appropriate by health promoters.

Further reflecting the ideology of individualism, Obama's public awareness rhetoric ignores the importance of considering the cluster of habits
that compose lifestyles more generally. Instead, she adopts a more medicalized approach, such as the provision of "prescriptions" for better health by
pediatricians. According to her address at the launch of *Let's Move*, she
and her supporters are proposing a program that will "ensure that doctors
not only regularly check children's BMI, but actually write out a prescription detailing steps parents can take to keep their kids healthy and fit."[38]
In this scenario, the only actors are the doctor and the parent, once again
making the assumption that if parents are given the appropriate knowledge
about good health, they will know how to use it, and will be motivated and
able to do so. In her address at Philadelphia's Fairhill Elementary School,
she further explained that pediatricians would "write a prescription to
families when they identify a problem with a step-by-step sort of process
for what they can actually do."[39] Such an explanation depicts doctors and

parents working largely in isolation from the rest of society to address the problem after it has been manifested and to fix the problem with the use of individualized, instrumental methods for correction. Thus, the rational, autonomous individual is envisioned once again.

Several loud silences are noticeable in Obama's parental awareness campaign. She fails to present or describe any external variables ranging from the quality of the doctor-patient relationship to environmental and financial deterrents that may interfere with this ideal transfer of knowledge to action. Her speeches also ignore the impact of cultural norms on an individual, the entrenched nature of one's *habitus*, and the futility of singling out a particular behavioral pattern that is part of a larger lifestyle. Although the actual policy may work to address these confounding issues, Michelle Obama's rhetoric does not reveal these complexities. Thus, we begin to see the limitations of her discourse in promoting substantial structural change in American food culture.

School Lunches

Michelle Obama identifies the second task of *Let's Move* to be the nutritional improvement of school lunches. Her approach in this regard attempts to address some of the environmental factors that prohibit healthy eating habits among school children, yet her discourse remains largely apolitical.

Her remarks at the School Nutrition Association Conference in March 2010 identified the important role school lunch providers play, saying to conference participants, "You're shaping their habits and their preferences, and you're affecting the choices that they're going to make for the rest of their lives."[40] In this instance, we see awareness on the part of Obama of the longevity and habitual nature of food choices, much more in accordance with Bourdieu's theory of *habitus*. Thus, Obama's discourse contains shades of post-structural thought in her depiction of eating. What her discourse lacks, however, is an explanation of how these habits develop from the preferences, lifestyles, and economic structures of the communities in which they are embedded and suggestions of structural change that might create other possibilities.

The limited and universalized scope of her attribution of habit formation can be seen throughout her discussion of school lunches and the *Let's Move* campaign. In the same speech to school lunch providers, she noted, "We've seen healthy habits falling away, replaced by habits of convenience and necessity. You know, parents want to buy healthy food for their kids, but they're sometimes tight on money and can't afford it. Or they're tight on time because they're juggling extra jobs, extra shifts, and they just can't swing those home-cooked meals anymore."[41] In this quotation, Obama paints all of America's children with the same brush, as if they all carry the same collective history and have been socialized in the same status groups, which is a clear misrepresentation. Her discussion of school lunch reform portrays the problem as universally experienced by American children, failing to point out the severe inequality within the public schooling system, an inequality that largely correlates with the racial segregation of the nation's schools. It seems likely that Michelle Obama is aware of the deeply political and racially charged nature of school disparities, yet her rhetoric fails to acknowledge these entrenched differences.

In this and other speeches on school lunches, Obama articulates some of the external factors that can impact and dictate our nutritional choices and the ways in which these inhibitors are affecting large groups of people. On the other hand, Obama rarely explicitly states how these barriers have come to be, never identifying the power structures and policies that have given rise to inequality and diminished "life chances." Instead, she blames the vague and abstract "pressures of today's economy and the breakneck pace of modern life."[42] The lack of a systemic critique in these quotations is emblematic of Obama's *Let's Move* discourse. Although many public health scholars have identified systemic and environmental factors as significant causes of today's rising obesity rates, it is clear that Obama is not engaging in such complex and challenging conversations.

Food Deserts

The third component of *Let's Move* that directly aims to change America's food habits is the goal to eliminate food deserts, defined by Obama as "communities without a supermarket," within seven years.[43] Obama's presentation of this ambitious goal is the most overt in its identification of the social environment as a major contributor to unhealthy eating, yet once again we see no mention of racism, income disparity, discriminatory urban planning, or any other contributing factor to today's abundance of food deserts. She praised the "collective stand"[44] that community members and policymakers took in Philadelphia to reduce the severity of their city's food deserts. She said to her Philadelphia audience, "You could have decided that these problems were just too big and too complicated and too entrenched and thrown your hands up and walked away."[45] Through this comment, Obama hints at the complexity that undergirds America's food systems. At the same time, however, she argues that a small group of committed community members have enough agency to counteract these entrenched dynamics, a claim others would dispute or qualify. Thus, her successful characterization of food deserts as bound up in structural inequalities is undermined by her focus on individual actors. Being primarily articulate in the language of individualism, she reverts back to that more comfortable and less politically contested discourse. Although not intending to diminish Philadelphia's fight against food deserts or to judge its success, Obama's language nonetheless is constrained by the ideological obstacles entrenched in America's commitment to neoliberal thought.

In her speeches, Obama advocates a model similar to Philadelphia's, including state investment and partnership with private businesses, to bring fresher and more diverse and nutritious food choices to underserved communities. She said, "And when we bring fresh, healthy food to communities, what do we learn? People will buy it, right? People will buy it. These stores are turning a profit."[46] However, it remains unclear what exactly people are buying and if their food choices are changing simply by making better foods more available. Are their socially derived preferences and tastes changed so quickly? I am not critiquing bringing supermarkets to nutritionally deprived communities. However, I suggest the need to challenge the idea that is presented through Obama's rhetoric: that the establishment of supermarkets in underserved communities will fundamentally change how and what people eat within a generation, the stated goal of *Let's Move*. Through discourse that promotes a simplified understanding seemingly devoid of attention to race and class, Obama may be doing a disservice to those working to change the food system at more structural levels and in ways that do not rely as heavily on private businesses to address issues of food and social justice. Yet Obama goes even further in aligning her campaign with commercial interests in the fourth area of her campaign.

Corporate Partnership

The most recent efforts of the *Let's Move* campaign have targeted the food industry, calling on them to provide healthier options, reduce the amount of sugar, salt, and trans fats in their products, and become part of her nation-wide movement to reform America's eating. Whereas the benefits of corporate involvement can be debated, Michelle Obama's discussions of these joint ventures are overwhelmingly positive and clear the industry of much of the blame that others attribute to it. Furthermore, integrating industry in this way follows the same reasoning articulated in her other initiatives—the model of increased access and options leading to rational choice. She stated, "Efforts like this show us that yes, we can improve how we make and sell food in this country. We can do that. And we can feed our kids better."[47] Given the dominant portrayal of eating and health as largely a matter of access to healthy foods, this statement is seemingly unproblematic. Yet upon closer inspection, it neglects the myriad of other factors that influence how, why, and what we eat, factors such as cultural traditions embodied in *habitus*, lifestyle and taste, constraints on choice, and the role of powerful discursive regimes. Instead Obama gives her audience the easy answer—provide healthier food, and they will eat it. Some might see her discourse as evidence of political savvy or shrewd rhetorical choice, but it is striking that the First Lady, the most prominent, and arguably powerful, popular voice in today's debate about healthy food, is confined to these simplistic and individual-oriented discussions of eating habits.

In specific speeches, Obama has portrayed the food industry in a very favorable light. Her remarks at the announcement ceremony of Walmart's Nutrition Charter act to humanize the industry, characterizing CEOs "not just as executives who care about their company's bottom lines, but as parents and as grandparents who care about our nation's children."[48] This rhetorical move no doubt makes for more amenable relations when working with business leaders and seems an obviously smart political maneuver. Yet the predictability and unproblematic nature of this characterization reaffirm the dominance of consumerist and choice-based models for improving eating habits. Such portrayals of superficial and easy explanations demonstrate the pervasiveness and power of a discursive regime rooted in neoliberal individual responsibility.

Ideological Underpinnings

Michelle Obama's rhetorical portrayal of the *Let's Move* program, regardless of the degree to which it acknowledges environmental and systemic determinants, gives the sense that the solution to curb obesity rates in the US is based in the availability of appropriate information and healthier food options. Once these choices are provided, the logic follows that individuals will know or quickly learn how to change their eating practices, resulting in lower rates of obesity and healthier lives. It is this logic that is presented in her speeches and therefore reinforced through her discourse. This linear sequencing of causality relies on liberal notions of the "modern autonomous individual" and "rational-economic action" as elaborated by Foucault, notions that dominate the current discursive regime surrounding health. These ideologies of the Enlightenment are pervasive in Obama's discourse and percolate throughout, limiting and silencing her even as she endeavors to give credence to environmental factors.

In the opening of many of her addresses, she states, "to get to where we want to go, we need to first understand how we got here."[49] This objective is never fulfilled, however. Instead, she provides her audience with a narrative about her own childhood and the differences between then and now. In her narratives she recalls, "In my home, we weren't rich. The foods we ate weren't fancy. But there was always a vegetable on the plate. And we managed a pretty healthy life."[50] In another speech she says, "And back then we ate sensibly. We had many more home-cooked meals. That was the norm. And much to our dismay, there was always something green on the plate. Fast food and dessert was a special treat. You had it but you didn't have it every day, and the portion sizes were reasonable."[51] In both of these recollections and in others, Obama is describing a different set of norms, a different set of cultural preferences, a different lifestyle. But what was it about life in those days that gave rise to those norms and what is different today? These are the systemic questions left unarticulated and unanswered by Obama and by *Let's Move* more generally.

IMPLICATIONS

Efforts to address the obesity issue, as well as other food-related health problems, have largely relied on prescriptive messages, and to some extent Michelle Obama's campaign follows in that tradition. Others argue that integrated approaches to nutrition would be more effective, and fortunately these are becoming increasingly prominent in the field of public health.[52] However, as this chapter suggests, the more easily digestible and hegemonic narrative of individual responsibility has made it difficult to promote socially rooted and environmentally sensitive public health initiatives more widely.

Michelle Obama's rhetorical efforts to curb obesity rates and promote healthier eating habits are constrained by the reified language of individualism, even as alternative perspectives attempt to gain traction. This rhetorical constraint is evident in the way her efforts to characterize obesity as a community and societal issue easily slip into narratives of individual behavior. Wallack and Lawrence attribute this phenomenon to the deficiency in language available for discussing social determinism among the general public. They contend that even those who support community-centered social welfare programs or public health projects often lack the vocabulary to explain why, whereas those who oppose such programs draw easily from the language of individualism.[53] This argument is an extension of cognitive linguist George Lakoff's thesis that conservative rhetoric is predicated upon a central metaphor of government as a "Strict Father," valuing individual responsibility over community support. This "package" of metaphors used in conservative and, more generally, individualist language is rooted in widely accepted American moral values,[54] whereas the language of community and social justice can sound foreign and uncompelling to the American ear in comparison.[55] Furthermore, our individualist conceptualization and articulation of obesity mirror our political values and are therefore less politically contested. Thus, it is no surprise that even many public health professionals revert to a language of individual behavior modification for lack of more convincing or acceptable alternatives.

Media framing of public health issues, including obesity and poor diet, compounds this phenomenon. Sei-Hill Kim and Anne Willis examined how the media frames issues of responsibility with regard to rising rates of obesity in the US and argue that the heavy emphasis on individual responsibility has led to an imbalance in the attribution of cause.[56] They point to the media coverage of obesity as the primary source for the framing of these issues, noting the media's tendency to oversimplify the root causes of obesity by adapting their messages to fit the sound-bite style of reporting that has become commonplace.[57] Environmental and social causes, which are more complex and more challenging to understand, are often ignored in favor of more digestible presentations of the problem. Although Michelle Obama's *Let's Move* initiative does strive to embrace a more nuanced understanding of the causes of obesity, critical analysis reveals it does so with only limited success.

CONCLUSION

The rhetorical perspective brings to this discussion a sense of agency in speaking that a purely structuralist discussion would diminish. However, through the discourse of Michelle Obama, we can see how the limiting nature of the language of individualism is enacted or imposed, even on powerful agents. Although she endeavors to change the "national conversation" about obesity in America, Obama's message is constrained by an inadequacy in language for the explanation of social conditions, and the subsequent media circulation of her rhetoric may perpetuate and reinforce this phenomenon. The prominence of her position within the discussion of a topic of increasing national concern magnifies this potential constitutive effect and shines a spotlight on our culture's inability to fully articulate a language of community. Although her recent extension into the legislative and food industry arenas provides a possible path for deeper changes in our food systems, without a discourse that articulates the inequalities and injustices that belie and corrupt this system, changes will most likely be minimal and superficial. She, like others, remains trapped in the discursive regime passed down from the age of Enlightenment, a regime that stifles our language and, thus, our actions.

The extent to which Michelle Obama will and can challenge the current hegemonic discursive regimes may largely depend on her willingness to deviate from political and cultural expectations. The mere fact that questions of systemic causes of obesity are being raised by such a highly visible and influential person points to the cracks in liberalism's historically hegemonic dominance. Scholars of public health and sociology will no doubt be tracking the progress of initiatives started by *Let's Move* and will be the ones to ultimately reveal the programmatic success. Although I argued that Michelle Obama's discourse is still bound up in the language of individualism and struggles to accurately identify the social conditions underlying today's obesity rates, but her highly publicized attempts at changing the popular discourse may help kick-start a trend toward deeper examinations of American food systems and cultures that can slowly alter the process of social reproduction that has led to such disparities in nutritional health.

NOTES

1. Harvey Levenstein, "Paradoxes of Plenty," in *Paradox of Plenty: A Social History of Eating in Modern America* (Berkeley: University of California Press, 2003), 237–55.

2. Ibid., 237–55.
3. Ibid., 237–55.
4. CDC, "Differences in Prevalence of Obesity among Black, White, and Hispanic Adults—United States, 2006–2008," *MMWR* 58 (July 17, 2009): 740–44.
5. Tim Lang and Michael Heasman, *Food Wars: The Global Battle for Mouths, Minds and Markets* (London: Earthscan, 2004), 104.
6. Levenstein, "Paradoxes of Plenty," 237–55.
7. Lang and Heasman, *Food Wars*, 98–125.
8. Colin Gordon, "Governmental Rationality," in *The Foucault Effect*, ed. Graham Burchell, Colin Gordon, and Peter Miller (Chicago: University of Chicago Press, 1991), 1–52.
9. Graham Burchell, "Peculiar Interests," in *The Foucault Effect*, ed. Graham Burchell (Chicago: University of Chicago Press, 1991), 119–51.
10. Michel Foucault, "Truth and Power," in *The Foucault Reader*, ed. Paul Rabinow (New York: Pantheon, 1984), 51–75.
11. Ibid., 51–75.
12. Thomas Lemke, "'The Birth of Bio-politics': Michel Foucault's Lecture at the Collège de France on Neo-liberal Governmentality," *Economy and Society* 30 (May 2001): 197.
13. Vijay Kumar Yadavendu, "Social Construction of Health: Changing Paradigms," *Economic and Political Weekly* 36 (July 2001): 2784–95.
14. Lemke, "The Birth of Bio-politics," 201.
15. Ibid., 190–207.
16. Gordon, *The Foucault Effect*, 1–52.
17. Ibid., 1–52.
18. Ibid., 1–52.
19. Monica Greco, "Psychosomatic Subjects and the 'Duty to Be Well': Personal Agency within Medical Rationality," *Economy and Society* 22 (August 1993): 357–72.
20. Ibid., 361.
21. Pierre Bourdieu, *Outline of a Theory of Practice*, trans. Richard Nice (Cambridge: University of Cambridge Press, 1977), 72.
22. Ibid., 78.
23. William C. Cockerham, Alfred Rütten, and Thomas Abel, "Conceptualizing Contemporary Health Lifestyles: Moving beyond Weber," *The Sociological Quarterly* 38 (Spring 1997): 321.
24. Ibid., 325.
25. Ibid., 325.
26. John Mirowsky and Catherine E. Ross, "Education, Personal Control, Lifestyle and Health: A Human Capital Hypothesis," *Research on Aging* 20 (July 1998): 415–49.
27. Anthony Giddens, *The Constitution of Society: Outline of the Theory of Structuration* (Cambridge: Polity Press, 1984), 82.
28. Cockerham, Rütten, and Abel, "Conceptualizing Contemporary Health Lifestyles," 333.
29. Jean Baudrillard, *Selected Writings*, ed. M. Poster (Stanford, CA: Stanford University Press, 1988).
30. Nancy E. Adler and Judith Stewart, "Reducing Obesity: Motivating Action While Not Blaming the Victim," *Milbank Quarterly* 87 (March 2009): 49–70.
31. Lawrence Wallack and Regina Lawrence, "Talking about Public Health: Developing America's 'Second Language,'" *American Journal of Public Health* 95 (April 2005): 567–70.

32. For more on the languages of individualism and community, see Robert Bellah et al., *Habits of the Heart: Individualism and Commitment in American Life* (Berkeley, CA: University of California Press, 1985).

33. Wallack and Lawrence, "Talking about Public Health," 567–70.

34. Ibid., 567–70.

35. Mary L. Kahl, "First Lady Michelle Obama: Advocate for Strong Families," Communication and Critical/Cultural Studies 6 (September 2009): 316–20.

36. Michelle Obama, "Remarks of First Lady Michelle Obama: Let's Move Launch," released by the Office of the First Lady, February 9, 2010.

37. Ibid.

38. Ibid.

39. Michelle Obama, "Remarks by the First Lady at the Fresh Food Financing Initiative," released by the Office of the First Lady, February 19, 2010.

40. Michelle Obama, "Remarks by the First Lady at the School Nutrition Association," released by the Office of the First Lady, March 1, 2010.

41. Ibid.

42. Ibid.

43. Obama, "Let's Move Launch," 2010.

44. Obama, "Fresh Food Financing Initiative," 2010.

45. Ibid.

46. Ibid.

47. Michelle Obama, "Remarks by the First Lady during Let's Move! Walmart Announcement," released by the Office of the First Lady, January 20, 2011.

48. Ibid.

49. Obama, "Let's Move Launch," 2010.

50. Ibid.

51. Michelle Obama, "Remarks by the First Lady to the National Governors Association," released by the Office of the First Lady, February 20, 2010.

52. Lang and Heasman, *Food Wars*, 98–125.

53. Wallack and Lawrence, "Talking about Public Health," 567–70.

54. Wallack and Lawrence draw specifically from George Lakoff, *The Political Mind* (Chicago: University of Chicago Press, 1996).

55. Wallack and Lawrence, "Talking about Public Health," 567–70.

56. Sei-Hill Kim and L. Anne Willis, "Talking about Obesity: News Framing of Who Is Responsible for Causing and Fixing the Problem," *Journal of Health Communication* 12 (June 2007): 359–76.

57. Ibid., 359–76.

11 Spatial Affects and Rhetorical Relations

At the Cherry Creek Farmers' Market

Justin Eckstein and Donovan Conley

> There are moments in this life that I recall not as visual snapshots but as tastes and fragrances. They make sense to me, to who I am, in ways that I suppose are profoundly rooted. At the same time they are blessedly involuntary; for I cannot control when they spring up within me and take over. They are truly re-membered, that is, those moments seem as deeply etched into the matter of my body now as anything can be.
>
> —Gary Paul Nabhan[1]

There have always been farms in the US and there have always been markets, but in the past few decades, especially the past few years, the "farmers' market" articulation has become much more than a space where producers and consumers exchange money and goods. Like the Lyceums and Tent Chautauquas of the nineteenth century, farmers' markets have become mixed spaces of social leisure, civic training, and political hope. Here private pleasure is fused with public morality, and the delights of everyday consumption are aligned with the political urgencies of cosmopolitan citizenship. Today political magazines like *The Nation* publish a special issue on the role of farmers in "Food and Democracy," documentaries like *Food Inc.* receive an Academy Award nomination for touting local markets, and First Lady Michelle Obama takes communal gardening to new heights of national political importance.[2] As Michael Pollan, the leading voice of this new food movement, puts it:

> Farmers' markets are thriving, more than five thousand strong, and there is a lot more going on in them than the exchange of money for food. Someone is collecting signatures on a petition. Someone else is playing music. Children are everywhere, sampling fresh produce, talking to farmers. Friends and acquaintances stop to chat. One sociologist calculated that people have ten times as many conversations at the farmers' market than they do in the supermarket. Socially as well as

sensually, the farmers' market offers a remarkably rich and appealing environment. Someone buying food here may be acting not just as a consumer but also as a neighbor, a citizen, a parent, a cook. In many cities and towns, farmers' markets have taken on (and not for the first time) the function of a lively new public square.[3]

This quotation captures our entire argument in a nutshell. Pollan is citing the powerful semiotic *and* somatic dynamics through which consumer-citizens assemble themselves amidst the weekly pleasures of the local market.

Let us consider the farmers' market, then, as a rhetorically charged civic space. In what follows we shall consider one market in particular, Denver's upscale urban destination, the Cherry Creek Farmers' Market (CCFM). Our analysis is grounded in the politics of place, which describes the constellations of material affects that undergird a location and enable different kinds of relations and movements. In seeking to explain the civic value of the farmers' market our project deliberately moves beyond the predominance of the visual and the symbolic in spatial rhetorics to address other senses such as the olfactory, auditory, and gustatory. As Karen Barad explains,

[T]he relationship between the material and the discursive is one of mutual entailment. Neither is articulated/articulable in the absence of the other; matter and meaning are mutually articulated. Neither discursive practices nor material phenomena are ontologically or epistemologically prior. Neither can be explained in terms of the other. Neither has privileged status in determining the other.[4]

Incorporating a broader spectrum of sensory information provides a more robust and detailed discussion of how relations are cultivated in particular spaces, and thus how movements and communities begin to take shape. Our goal is not to affirm a pointless dichotomy between semiotics and somatics, but rather to showcase the full rhetorical power of affects in everyday spaces. A greater attention to the ways bodies are organized spatially produces a better understanding of how communal formations are preconditioned. Our main claim is that the spatial affects of the CCFM "prime" subjects to foster novel forms of relationality. In this respect the market serves as an incipient space of community.

The analysis unfolds in three stages. We first describe the field of analysis, the market itself. Seeking to ground our claims in the empirical details of the place, we attempt to explain the allure of the CCFM as an urban destination. This section identifies the trope of "dirt" as a common element among three explanations for why farmers' markets have recently become favored spaces of social and civic investment. Second, we turn our attention to the rhetorical politics of the everyday. Here we draw on the concept of "micropolitics" to describe how embodied subjects are rhetorically arranged through spatial affects. Micropolitics provides a nuanced critical vocabulary to better describe the "taxis" of bodies in material space.[5] With this conceptual framework in place, we then turn, third and finally, to the particular spatial affects and rhetorical relations at the CCFM. This section offers detailed accounts of three specific non-visual senses—smell, sound, and taste—to demonstrate the fine grain of affects at the CCFM. It thereby illustrates how the CCFM rhetorically "primes" subjects and thus conditions the possibility of civic renewal by fostering new forms of relationality. The material space of the farmers' market is a space of incipient communalism, a "becoming-common," which we offer in conclusion through a discussion of a politics of the virtual.[6]

DIRT IS THE NEW BLACK

The Cherry Creek Farmers' Market (CCFM) is located in the heart of Denver's most expensive shopping district, Cherry Creek. Named after the small, wandering creek that forms the district's southern border, this densely populated region is home to the Cherry Creek Mall, Cherry Creek North, the Denver Country Club, and the Cherry Creek bike path. The CCFM is located in the mall's west parking lot and nestled next to the addendum shops and in the middle of "the Rocky Mountain region's premier shopping environment."[7] The CCFM occurs bi-weekly, Wednesday and Saturday, from 8:00 a.m. until 2:00 p.m., from May until October (the Wednesday market is significantly smaller). To the west of the market, across University Boulevard, is the exclusive Denver Country Club, the oldest country club west of the Mississippi.[8] Giving the mall a lovely green, western border, the country club is outlined by old brick walls that slightly cover the trunks of the towering trees. Directly north of the mall is Cherry Creek North. Covering an expansive 320 acres, this lifestyle center includes gourmet restaurants, a Whole Foods, boutiques, spas, and high-end galleries.[9] The CCFM is even described as the "cadillac of farmers' markets among nearly 50 markets throughout Colorado."[10] The CCFM is, in other words, a privileged space of urban leisure.

The CCFM presents a unique rhetorical challenge. Given the abundance of commercial options in the area, how does this particular space manage to attract such lively interest? In fact the question is the answer; rhetorically, the market stands out precisely because of its redundancy and abundance. At Cherry Creek, more is more, especially when more has the dirty, rustic look and feel of "less." Shoppers can easily purchase many of the same products within a square block of the market, often times at a cheaper price. Bhakti Chai, Love Grown Granola, and Udi's Breads are just a few of the brands shared by both the CCFM and the adjacent Whole Foods store. Richard Tomkins, writing about farmers' markets in England, examines the relationship between the farmers' market and the modern-day grocery store. He observes, "Once, you paid extra if you wanted only the best quality vegetables, carefully trimmed, thoroughly washed and properly packaged. Now, you pay extra if you want your vegetables authentically bruised, rotten and misshapen."[11] Indeed, customers willingly pay more for inferior-looking products, like weather damaged lettuce or odd misshapen tomatoes. Rustic, it seems, has become chic. Dirt has become the new black, to borrow an expression from the fashion world. Customers willingly pay more for "lesser" products because the added value signified by "dirt" is the promise and reassurance of an ethics-based system of production. Dirt is "green," with all the dolphin-safe, pasture-raised, anti-ethanol connotations that term carries. The difference between chai from the CCFM and Whole Foods is not a question of substance—it's the same chai in both markets—but rather a question of resignified value. This resignification in turn becomes a matter of spatial affects and rhetorical relations, of how products are located in a particular assemblage of goods, bodies, and sensations.

Why do people willingly pay more money to go to a farmers' market?[12] What explains the allure of this space? We believe the answer contains at least three salient, overlapping valences: ethics, the myth of the eternal return, and somatics. For present purposes, ethics describes how subjects form obligations that influence their decisions and behaviors. In particular, the ethical valence helps explain how subjects feel bound to pay more money for a particular product because it aligns with their personal values. Reading the mission statement of Colorado Fresh Markets (CFM), the CCFM's parent company, reveals three ethical topoi at play in the farmers' market: community, environment, and health. The CFM boasts:

> [T]he average piece of produce travels 2000 miles before it reaches you and with each day loses more of its nutritional value. Shopping at Colorado Fresh Markets helps local family farmers stay in business, preserves quality local food sources for Colorado while using less resources, and most importantly, provides you with access to the freshest and most nutritious produce available.[13]

In this statement we see appeals to each of the three ethical topoi. The CFM informs its customers that shopping at the CCFM helps the local community. Consumers ought to feel well disposed toward spending a little extra money because they are helping out their neighbors, "local family farmers." Also, the products are environmentally friendly because they did not travel far. Farmers' markets are able to boast smaller "carbon footprints," the reigning index of ethical consumption, which justifies an increased price. It is a measure of just how globalized our everyday lives have become that many today are willing to pay more for nearness itself. And finally, at the end of its statement CFM refers to the health benefits of shopping at the CCFM, an increasingly urgent public concern.[14] Quite apart from the truth-value of its claims, the CFM displays the rhetorical machinery of ethics that animates contemporary consumers' desire to visit the market.[15]

"Community," "environment," and "health" function rhetorically as an axis of social justice.

Second, the appeal of farmers' markets also lies in a promise of wholeness, which we can trace through Mircea Eliade's "myth of the eternal return."[16] The contemporary moment, as scholars of post-modernity insist, is characterized by anxiety and dislocation. Subjects find themselves increasingly fragmented, and thus struggle to find themselves at all.[17] Subjects are entangled in a multi-layered, multi-textured reality, occupying many spheres of engagement simultaneously.[18] The speed of capital flows and the constant folding of time-space through different communication technologies leave the prospects for contemporary subjectivity in a precarious situation. Greg Dickinson writes that "for the subject to come to 'know' itself in some more or less coherent way depends on an ability to 'locate' itself, while the subject's ability to locate itself depends in part on the ability to create a coherent subjectivity."[19] To locate and thus "fix" ourselves is the search for wholeness; it is the odyssey of the modern subject.

Eliade theorizes that one important way we create coherent subjectivities and thus "fix" ourselves is through myth. Communities re-articulate events in the parlance of myth: War becomes coded as an epic struggle between good and evil, while famine is framed as God's punishment.[20] Myth operates as a vehicle to escape the anxiety of the contemporary moment. What the farmers' market offers is a nostalgic return to the time of the mythic yeoman. Here again, dirt signifies deeply cherished sentiments of a long-lost, simpler time, of small farms and small towns, honest physical labor, and family-based communities held together by bonds of order, morality, and self-sameness. Going to the market is a way of participating in rituals of a "simpler time" that provide a temporary outlet from the fragmented, banal drudgery of the present conjuncture. In visiting a resonant space like the farmers' market, shoppers are rhetorically "fixing" themselves through a fantasy of dirty localism.

Finally, what knots these valences together is a unique and powerful somatic experience. Strolling through the aisles visitors become tangled in a web of sensations. Smells intersect with the images that accompany tastes, which in turn reference sounds and temperatures. Situated in the open air, patrons are drawn to the market to smell the fresh food being cooked, to hear local musicians and talk with vendors, to touch and physically evaluate the products, and to sample an array of local specialties. Attending a farmers' market is an acutely resonant, physically immersive experience. A palpable, invigorating, dirty immediacy characterizes one's time here. And as it is felt, so it becomes understood. The somatic slides into the symbolic as affects become coded into different narratives and hence different "lines of flight." Emerging from the somatic, then, are new arrangements of civic relations, where blooming practices of community agriculture and "co-ops," rhetorics of "sustainability" and "organic" and "localism" and "slow food," and a "Do It Yourself" ethos of grass roots social production are gaining mass appeal as an emerging *food formation*.[21] Because of its rich empirical texture and incipient political power, we explore the somatic grain of the market space in a separate section ("Affective Resonances")— for to better understand the rhetorical composition of the farmers' market is to investigate the affective dimensions of space. This move in turn requires that we first explore the relations between rhetoric and everyday-ness, which we do next through a discussion of micropolitics.

RHETORIC AND THE EVERYDAY

Rhetorical scholars of the everyday have focused recently on "texts" rang-ing from architecture to museums and memorials to cinema and the body.[22] "Place making," Jessie Stewart and Greg Dickinson explain, "is a distinctly communicative practice, for it is through a series of (often nonverbal) forms and signs that places make a claim to placeness. More than communicative, place making gestures are always rhetorical."[23] Place thus *becomes* space through a particularized network of symbols, formations and lived rela-tionships; that is, through a specific assemblage of moving bodies. Thus far, rhetorical scholarship on space has tended in one of two general directions: first, toward spaces of communal and/or national identification, like muse-ums and memorials; and second, toward the unassuming, banal, mundane spaces of the everyday, like grocery stores, tattoo parlors, and shopping malls.[24] Call these space studies in the major and minor mode.

Our project moves in the second direction to examine the quotidian spaces that subjects traverse in often semi-conscious and fleeting ways, those spaces that may at first blush seem insignificant and devoid of political value. The CCFM is one such space, replete with the banal, mundane, and routine details that characterize the everydayness of actual assemblages. Places like health food stores, tattoo parlors, coffee shops, leisure centers, and shopping malls are not simply the background of our "real" lives; they play a part in forming who we are and how we live. Subjects are ordinary bodies moving through ordinary space. What arranges bodies and spaces, rhetorically, is affects. There is much that happens, and much that matters, at a farmers' market that pushes past the realm of words or images to the deeply material terrain of affect.[25] In an effort to garner a richer under-standing of this process, we next conceptualize the politics of the everyday as a *micropolitics*. Doing so helps us move beyond visual representations to investigate a broader spectrum of spatial affects that condition the arrange-ment of bodies and communities.

Micropolitics

Broadly speaking, micropolitics describes a politics crafted around the con-tingency of the present. It is interested in how the potentiality of a given situation can be both activated and conducted. It is grounded in the realm of affect, of the somatic, which is both distinct from and related to emotion. Brian Massumi defines emotion as "a subjective content, the sociolinguistic fixing of the quality of an experience which is from that point onward defined as personal."[26] Affect refers to a pure intensity occurring outside of language (and often perception), whereas emotion occurs when the intensity is incorporated into the symbolic order (language), personalized and narrativized. This disjunction is illustrated by the difference between eating a delicious meal and attempting to explain it. The act of eating is unmediated and exists entirely in the moment. As any foodie will attest, mere words cannot capture the rich sensual details of eating: the pangs, the aromas, the textures, the involuntary jolts and shudders and euphoria.[27] These are all affects. Linguistic representation can approximate these sensations, but can never fully capture or re-present them. Emotion, then, occurs retroactively, when an embodied moment is codified into language ("surprising") and placed within a narrative framework ("pan-Asian").

At the most abstract level, affect materializes consciously when the body "bumps" up against an event or happening, like an aroma or a taste. When such an event occurs it forces the incorporeal parts of the body, namely consciousness, to become aware of the materiality of the body. It literally jolts the body into different positions and states of readiness. These "bumps" are microperceptions. "Microperception," Massumi explains, "is not smaller perception; it's a perception of a qualitatively different kind. It's something that is felt without registering consciously. It registers only in its effects."[28] Massumi uses the concept of "shock" to explain the relationship between a microperception and a corporeal response. "Shock" captures the disjunctive nature of microperception, an interruption that signals the transition from one state to another. These become *points of departure* as the body transitions from one capacitation to another. A microperception can be ignited by a flicker in the corner of one's eye, the sounds of children splashing in water, or the lingering aroma of citrus in the air.

At the CCFM the comforting tone of the vendor's voice in conjunction with the tart, citrus smell emanating from Noosa Yoghurt's booth captures the notice of some passing customers. As they walk by, hints of fresh-cut lemon hang in the air. You will observe the customers perk their ears, pause suddenly, turn toward the booth, and investigate the source of this appeal. They are likely not thinking about why they stopped right here, right now, beyond one customer's simple response: "It's because it is delicious!" The affects of smell and taste organize bodies as a queue forms in the direction of the newest yoghurt flavor, fresh lemon curd. Then, as patrons wait for their sample, they start talking. Looking at a clear grocery bag held by the man in front of her, a young woman strikes up a conversation by asking where he got his "delicious looking sausages." Experiences are shared and savored, knowledge of the market is transmitted, and the connections within the assemblage are multiplied. Recall Michael Pollan's comment, cited in the introduction, that shoppers have ten times as many conversations at a farmers' market than at a supermarket. The difference is rooted in affect. Although these queuing-up moments are fleeting, the bumps and shocks of smell, taste, and sound excite conversations and thereby establish new relations between strangers. This is how new formations and movements emerge, first through microperception and then through shared semiotic reflection.

This configuration of affect and semiotic repetition produces new forms of relationality that are both organically rendered and externally conducted. Affects are organically internalized through the subjective associations of sensations with an event: A family outing becomes glued to the smell of fresh coriander, the taste of lavender cupcakes excites the memory of a first date, or the canvas smell of a tent provokes paralyzing anxiety. Likewise, the farmers' market conditions subjects on how to feel about certain products. On the symbolic level, the market articulates one's affective experience with buzzwords like "fresh," "local," "grass-fed," "pasture-raised," and "sustainable." Each time these words are used, memories of the market are solicited. Each affect contorts and orients the body. In a deeply material way, affects produce the very platform upon and through which communication, and community itself, takes shape.[29] Our project thus joins a chorus of critical scholars invested in the material dimension of rhetoric.[30] Moving beyond the predominance of the symbolic, we hope to make sense of how affect rhetorically co-produces the assemblage of bodies and spaces. In the next section we attempt a descriptive analysis of the CCFM's affective texture.

Affective Resonances

Given everything we have established thus far, accounting for the material and symbolic texture of the CCFM becomes a slippery task. There is not enough space in this project, or enough words in our vernacular, to capture the multi-dimensional richness of the market. Plus, it is not possible to "capture" a living, breathing assemblage. Minimally, to begin this task is to examine other senses beyond the visual. Accordingly, we turn our attention to the three "lesser" senses: smell, hearing, and taste. Of course, any linear categorization of the senses is inherently problematic, as they operate simultaneously and in crosscurrents of varying intensity. William Connolly explains how an image of a tomato requires an intersensory memory of texture, smell, and taste for us to understand the object.[31] That is, meaning is produced not only from the image's semiotic code, but also from pulling on past material experiences with prior tomatoes. Connolly's observations are augmented by recent discoveries in neuroscience.[32] This section discusses the senses separately, not because we subscribe to a functionalist view of the senses, but simply to highlight their individual operations and the critical vocabulary engendered through doing so.

Smell

Perhaps the most outstanding affective signature of the market is its smell. The market emits its products throughout Cherry Creek, inviting customers to come explore. Indeed, the CCFM is a web of different smells: the maple, smoky aroma of sizzling bacon emanating from Dolly's Omelets converging with the rich, tangy scent of rosemary coming from the Denver biscuit company; The Greatful Bread Company's buttery, sweet cinnamon rolls floating alongside the salt and saffron in Le Central's paella. Walking from the parking lot into the market proper, one is confronted with this aromatic matrix, some smells easily discerned, others faintly suggested. The outer fringes of the parking lot are demarcated by the heavily smoked presence of bacon. Nearing the entrance of the market, the smells start to blend into a kind of affective collage—notes of Kaladi's rich, earthy coffee intermingling with the Soap Lady's soft lavender, mixing with Pinche Taco's smoky, paprika-filled, sizzling chorizo.

Here, smell functions in three different ways: (1) It gives space a certain texture; (2) It folds and extends a subject's conception of space and time; and (3) It activates desire. But how does olfaction organize space? Located near the top of the nasal cavity, the olfactory bulb is the only part of the human nervous system that has direct contact with the external world. [33] Sometimes olfaction is consciously registered as smell; other times it determines our mood, or even, as Teresa Brennan adds, "how we 'feel the atmosphere.'"[34] Smell, for example, accounts for the feeling of excitement before a concert or a sporting event. Brennan theorizes that when people congregate in a single location, they emit different pheromones that provoke bodies. These smells impinge upon interpersonal interactions, defining the parameters for relationality. Smell allows us to feel another's presence behind us and explains how someone "rubs us the wrong way." This cocktail of chemicals also explains a space's palpable feeling of excitement, or its viscous tension. As bodies gather, different chemicals coalesce and create a place's distinctive signature. Bodies start to organize themselves in different formations as they decode the pheromones and release new ones. A kind of feedback loop is generated that defines intersubjective interactions. It is this "self-organizing" phenomenon that Brennan locates as the cause of "mob mentality," because these different chemicals enter the body and influence "the mood of the other."[35] That is, affects do not exist within *a* subject, or *the* group, but somewhere in-between, in this recursive mixing and mingling of different chemicals.

Bodies thus become circuits within the larger assemblage of the CCFM. As the nose internalizes smells, it emits its chemical reaction that in turn affects others. A kind of chemical dialogue is induced between bodies, bending flesh, coloring perceptions, and thereby inducing new forms of relation. Dina Marie Zemke and Stowe Shoemaker found that manipulating scent could have significant effects on how people interact by tweaking how a space "feels." Specifically, they found that filling a space with a pleasant ambient scent, like lavender, "can have a positive effect on increasing social interaction behaviors of participants in an environment where the participants are strangers."[36] Smell is thus capable of lubricating social interactions and reassembling bodies. As smells penetrate the body, the subject becomes part of the "smellscape." Fresh flowers, crispy fried comfort foods, hot grass and trees, and earthy skin products are not simply topics of conversation; they are low-level conductors of memories, moods, and interactions. Likewise, patrons emit their own chemicals in a kind of affective "conversation" that blurs the distinctions between bodies, semiosis, and space. For Brennan smell is invisible, pervasive, and the primary way that bodies communicate. It operates on a micropolitical plane of invisibility—that is, affect—that can significantly alter how we feel, think, act, and congregate.

Sound

As previously noted, the CCFM is located in the middle of Denver. The surrounding sounds of the city are both ubiquitous and calamitous—car horns and tires, collective chatter, and music all envelope the market. The roar of cars speeding down the busy, adjacent streets, the loud screaming of the bus as it stops next to the market, and the buzz of vendors and patrons are common sonic elements of this space. There are numerous street musicians positioned throughout the bazaar. One can hear anything along the musical spectrum, from blues to Celtic music. Over there is Katherine, the twenty-something recent University of Denver music school graduate, playing folk songs on her guitar. The ambient noise from the patrons and vendors alike constructs distinct "walls," so as bodies pass from one musician to another they encounter a new "stage" of sound. Moving from Katherine's location to the only sitting area in the market, right next to the Cowboy Catering Cart (a move of only a few booths), there is a band made up of four older, middle-aged gentlemen playing bluegrass. Bluegrass is the unofficial official farmers' market genre; the rootsy, plucky, twangy music is a sonic expression of "dirt."

Music intersects with the sounds of the booths. At any given moment one hears the cheerful haggling of customers, the pop and hiss from Snow Creek Ranch's grill, or the loud pounding of plantains from the arepa stand. The sounds merge and blend, creating a distinctive "soundscape" that intermingles with the previously described "scentscape." Ubiquitous noise can act as a "subtext from which conscious thought, feeling and discursive judgments draw some of their substance."[37] This is because, like scent, sound affects subjects below the plane of awareness. "Consider the experiment with organ music in which vibrations that excite the skin below the level of audibility are first retained in a church performance and then blocked," Connolly observes, adding, "the evidence suggests that sub-audible responses to the first set of vibrations find expression in feelings of awe and wonder that are lost when the sub-audible vibrations are dampened."[38] Falling within the realm of micropolitics, soundscapes activate certain kinds of subjective states and (re)define patterns of relationality.[39]

To describe the power of aural affects in the movement of bodies, Massumi uses the term "priming." He argues that priming describes how the body is trained, through repetition, to react to certain events. "The *trace* of past actions, *including a trace of their contexts*," Massumi argues, is "conserved in the brain and in the flesh, but out of mind and out of body understood as qualifiable interiorities, active and passive respectively, direct spirit and dumb matter."[40] When a subject is startled, he or she literally jumps and moves. The jump is not a consciously perceivable decision, but rather the startling represents a "shock" that moves the body. In the space between the startle and corporeal movement, the body has two concurrent but mutually exclusive potentialities, fight or flight. Ultimately the body chooses one of these potentialities, which manifests itself in bodily movement. It is only *after* the body has moved that the event begins to register in the psyche. The traces impressed upon the body act as a blueprint for subjectivity and relationality. It outlines the catalogue of traits and responses the body may choose from. Priming creates a map of incipiency or a catalog of potentialities that may yet actualize.

Massumi's observations are useful in explaining the way that the aural space of the CCFM affects the bodies assembled there. The patrons of the market are immersed in signals of warning and welcome. Standing in the middle of the market a subject is confronted with the screech of tires, the ever present reality of crunching and crashing metal, the pop and swoosh of busses, the gurgle of foaming milk, the hiss of Cowboy Catering's griddle, the wailings of a small child, the barking of a little dog, the twang and thump of an old bluegrass band—thousands of bodies all talking, shuffling, and swirling around themselves. The tonality and frequencies of these sounds change throughout the course of the day, the adjacent streets becoming busier and noisier. The market thus provides a "safe space" away from the din and hurly-burly of the city. The noises of warning emanate from the market's borders, while inside the folksy music and the bright hum of laughter fill the space with a sense and meaning all its own. Iain Chambers notes the importance of sound in producing a body's orientation in space. He writes that sound "participates in rewriting the conditions of representation: where 'representation' clearly indicates both the semiotic dimensions of the everyday and potential participation in a political community."[41] This point reminds us that outside the CCFM we find aural conditions of metal cacophony representing a world filled with ambiguous danger, emergency, and strangeness. By contrast, inside the CCFM we find aural conditions of fleshy exuberance—talking, laughing, singing, dancing—forming a gathering of dirty togetherness.

Taste

We know that taste matters because the fast food industry spends billions annually on flavor research. "Flavorists," as chronicled in the *New Yorker* article "The Taste Makers," spend their workdays combining exotic chemical compounds to create, say, that authentic whiff of citrus consumers enjoy when they bite into their "lime" tortilla chips.[42] Eric Schlosser famously reported on the largely invisible business of food flavoring in *Fast Food Nation*, noting that in 2002 the fast food giants spent $1.2 billion to create appealing taste experiences for their customers.[43] Indeed, the world-conquering triumph of the McDonald's french fry is ultimately a story of a laboratory's ability to replicate the essence of beef tallow when the company switched to a healthier cooking oil. This laboratory creation is known simply as "natural flavor."[44]

Taste has always mattered. The ability to discern sweet from bitter, edible from inedible, was one of the ways our ancestors navigated an uncertain environment of potentially dangerous edible goods. From our origins as a species, taste has been built into the very fiber of our daily lives, as a navigator of space, a selector of goods, and thus a mediator of social relations. Then along came culture.[45] Perhaps no historical example better expresses the conjointly material and semiotic power of taste than the ancient spice trade that was largely responsible for establishing a global network of commercial and cultural exchange. As Tom Standage writes in *An Edible History of Humanity*, spices have played the uniquely historical role of connectors. Alluring and fascinating by themselves, spices became intensifiers of the links in the chains of cultural transmission. When we think of curry, we think of the coming-together of several unique flavors to create some new and wonderful taste assemblage. Standage argues that spices have worked this way historically not only on the plate but also at the level of global trade. Because spices are so deeply entwined in the regionalisms of a given culture, they carry and connect not just flavors but also, as Standage reminds us, a semiotic-material cocktail of ideas, practices, technologies, and diseases from distant lands.[46] The point here is that what is often considered the basest of senses, physical taste, in fact plays a deeply significant role in the composition of our social, cultural, and political worlds. Taste is absolutely crucial in the material makeup of daily life, often because it is most ordinarily associated with "mere" consumption. We readily assume that, as eaters, subjects possess either no choice whatsoever or nothing but choice when it comes to their taste preferences.[47] So why bother thinking about taste at all?

One reason is that taste itself is a significant driver of what else happens at the farmers' market. We shall avoid any attempt to identify what accounts for the deliciousness of the goods at farmers' markets beyond noting that it has much to do, once again, with dirt and nearness. It has to do with the intensification of natural flavors. What you often hear after patrons sample the products at farmers' markets are exaltations of *more-ness*: Tomatoes taste "tomato-ier," chickens taste "more chickeny," and so on. You often hear implicit theories of affect, when shoppers proclaim that the taste of local produce simply cannot be described in words. It is almost like the words that escape them are the very phrases that describe their groundedness. One way subjects negotiate locality, Dickinson theorizes, is through the ingesting of something natural.[48] Yet, unlike Dickinson's globalized coffee, the CCFM offers up various tastes of the local soil. At the corner of the Palisades Fruit stand, like many of the stands at the CCFM, is a small, Styrofoam plate with peach slices. Customers swarm to this stand, often bumping into one another, to taste the product. Sometimes people cycle back multiple times to grab a sample and continue walking. There are stands where patrons can purchase rocky ford cantaloupe, palisade peaches and pears, and Turquoise Mesa wine. In an odd but real way, eating these products allows patrons to literally ingest the fruits of Colorado, and thus Colorado itself. The tasting of the soil and the place allows shoppers to connect themselves, literally and emotionally, to their surrounding community. To enjoy fresh local berries is to participate in the pride of place.

"Terroir" was originally a French term used to describe the place-specific qualities of different wines. More generally the term describes the hyper-particular signature of a place as expressed through its wines, cheeses, produce, and animals. Terroir is realized through the converged forces of soil, rain, sun, wind, worker hands, technology, chemicals, history, and so on. It is, very simply, the accumulated expression of place located in what we call taste. These mutual concerns with taste and place are propelling forces behind the farmers' market assemblage. Bodies arrange themselves, often explicitly and knowingly and rapturously, because *this* is the juiciest peach to be found anywhere in Colorado or because *that* is the single best tomato stand on the planet. Farmers' market patrons are often fanatical about taste and texture; it is often the very reason shoppers will drive long stretches each weekend to stock up on fresh, dirty products.[49] The indescribable qualities of deliciousness on offer become the reason to gather alongside and intermingle with others from the community. In this way, taste literally drives the arrangement of bodies through space and amplifies the links through which new civic relations may take hold.

CONCLUSION

Our goal has been to reach beyond an overly linguistic view of space to consider how the deep grain of materiality conditions the prospects of civic life. This agenda has involved a turn to the study of affect. Yet as demonstrated, affects are messy and unruly.[50] They reside in the space between the knowable—that which can be codified into language, translated into emotion, and/or registered as meaningful—and the flux of life itself. Attempts to taxonomize affect will necessarily fail. We cannot expect to harness the terrain of affects for the purposes of replication or recommendation. What we may hope to attain, however, is a better understanding of the combinatory capacities of the bodies and spaces we encounter every day. We may hope to attain greater sensitivity to the skins of sensuousness through which communal relations emerge and take shape.

Our analysis shows how smell, sound, and taste converge to assign meaning and texture to geography. Yet to say that the space impresses only upon bodies would be incorrect. As different micro-shocks bump against our skin, the world is re-created, re-made, and new durations begin.[51] These micro-processes are far from stable and symmetric. As phenomenological experience changes, the body acts, emits chemicals, and contorts, all of which impact relationships within the market. As Erin Manning reminds us, "space and body are in continuous shifting dialogue."[52] That is, we cannot divorce a space from the bodies that occupy it. The CCFM does not pre-exist its patrons and vendors; it is only when this unique configuration of bodies enters the Cherry Creek parking lot that the market begins to assemble anew. Space is always relational and is itself an assemblage between body and place.[53] Indeed, revisiting the market for successive observations reminded us of Heraclitus's maxim that you can never dip your foot in the same river twice. Nevertheless, we offer a few general comments.

Through the course of taking notes and talking with peers familiar with the market, we could not ignore the market's elite quality. The CCFM is one of the most exclusive farmers' markets in Colorado. To say that the CCFM looks nothing like a "real farmers' market" would be a reasonable accusation. After all, the market is populated with more corporations than farmers and has more prepared food than produce stands. The clientele is noticeably wealthy. It is common to see local celebrities, new Land Rovers, and Rolexes. We have attended other markets in Missouri, Illinois, California, and Washington that look and feel more "authentically" rural. Yet, this is no reason to abandon the CCFM. We should not get caught up in what the market *is*, because the present is always contingent. Instead, we should investigate the halo of potentiality that encircles the space. Or, put differently, we should locate the CCFM within the "politics of the virtual."[54]

A politics grounded in affect is concerned with the contingency of the present.[55] As such, we are less concerned with ontic statements (the market *is* x or y) than with velocities, trajectories, and becomings. In short, we are interested in the potentialities of the market. To gain a register on a politics of contingency Lawrence Grossberg distinguishes between the possible and the virtual. The former describes abstract theorizing and utopian thinking whereas the latter is anchored within empirical reality. That is, a politics of the virtual is grounded within the present moment and looks at all the possibilities that may arise. It believes "reality is making itself and it will continue to, and that therefore there is a contingency about the world that opens up possibilities."[56] Attending to the virtual within the actual allows us to raise specific alternatives tailored to place. So, what are ways we can reimagine relationality that enable a becoming community? Grossberg instructs us not to look at just what is possible but also what potentialities the present moment provides. Micropolitics provides a useful language to uncover a politics of the virtual. It investigates how different impressions and traces are left upon the body that may be excited to activate agency. It takes as its central assumption the potential of a situation, instead of its actualization. It investigates the number of potential subjectivities and relationalities that may exist in any given moment. We believe this view may open up space for evaluating maps of incipiency.

What is the map of incipiency drawn from our experience in the market? We believe that the CCFM harbors potential for a becoming-common among its patrons. We envision a market that is conducive to a spirit of collectivity knitted around the shared consumption of local ingredients. The market scaffolds attachments to the community as one enters. Customers are reminded of the local affiliation of the market and the other customers as neighbors. The market may spawn philanthropy like the non-profit Colorado Farm to Table and/or produce the camaraderie between street food providers evidenced in the Justice League of Street Food, and/or the excitement of Hush Denver's pop-up restaurant scene. The CCFM contains the connecting power for such assemblages. Some patrons may be unaffected or even soured by the experience. They may dislike the bourgeois feel of the space, resent how much money they are spending, and/or care nothing at all for dirty food. But the CCFM also contains the potential of a becoming-common. Patrons can gain a sense of immediacy and a being-with-other that is fresh and newly resonant, which could prime subjects to recognize the inherent humanity of fellow shoppers. Indeed, the simple act of consuming food among strangers, we believe, encourages community. Gary Paul Nabhan writes that "food should be valued less for its caloric content and more for what it expresses about our relationships."[57] More than anything else, the affective texture of the CCFM promotes civic renewal simply because it accelerates the processes by which new social relations come into themselves. Smell, sound, and taste drive the relations that drive the renewal of community.

NOTES

1. Gary Paul Nabhan, *Coming Home to Eat* (New York: W. W. Norton & Company, 2002), 17.
2. See the special issue "Food for All: How to Grow Democracy," *The Nation*, September 21, 2009, accessed September 29, 2011, http://www.thenation.com/issue/september-21–2009. See Michelle Obama's website for her *Let's Move* campaign to end childhood obesity, accessed September 12, 2011, http://www.letsmove.gov/.

3. Michael Pollan, "The Food Movement, Rising," *The New York Review of Books*, June 10, 2010, accessed September 28, 2011, http://www.nybooks. com/articles/archives/2010/jun/10/food-movement-rising/?pagination=false.

4. Karen Barad, "Posthumanist Performativity: Toward an Understanding of How Matter Comes to Matter," *Signs: Journal of Women in Culture and Society* 28 (2003): 822.

5. We are deliberately invoking Nathan Stormer's piece, "Articulation: A Working Paper on Rhetoric and Taxis," *Quarterly Journal of Speech* 90 (2004): 257–84.

6. On "becoming-common," see Donovan S. Conley and Lawrence J. Mullen, "Righting the Commons in Red Rock Canyon," *Communication and Critical/Cultural Studies* 5 (2008): 180–99.

7. "Get the 411," *Cherry Creek Shopping Center*, accessed November 2, 2010, http://www.shopcherrycreek.com/visit/about_the_mall.

8. "Club Information," *Denver Country Club*, accessed November 3, 2010, http://www.denvercc.net/club/scripts/public/public.asp?NS=PUBLIC.

9. "About Cherry Creek North," *Cherry Creek North*, accessed November 3, 2010, http://cherrycreeknorth.com/about/.

10. "About Colorado Fresh Markets," *Colorado Fresh Markets*, accessed November 3, 2010, http://www.coloradofreshmarkets.com/about.html.

11. Richard Tomkins, "Farmer's Markets? No Thanks. That's Sheer Snobbery," *The Financial Times*, January 11, 2005, accessed June 22, 2011, http://www.ft.com/intl/cms/s/0/648bf6ec-6375–11d9-bec2–00000e2511c8. html#axzz1Q1XNFH5K.

12. For example, a recent price comparison found that a similar sized eggplant cost $4.25 at the CCFM but only $3.29 at the adjacent Whole Foods. Similarly, the popular Noosa Yoghurt costs $2.50 per single serving at the CCFM (or two for $4.00), compared to $1.79 at the nearby *Sun Flower* supermarket.

13. "About Colorado Fresh Markets," *Colorado Fresh Markets*, accessed November 3, 2010, http://www.coloradofreshmarkets.com/about.html.

14. *Let's Move* campaign website, http://www.letsmove.gov/.

15. Recent work on ethical consumerism includes Tania Lewis, "Transforming Citizens? Green Politics and Ethical Consumption on Lifestyle Television," *Continuum: Journal of Media and Cultural Studies* 22 (2008): 227–40; and Isabelle Szmigin, Marylyn Carrigan, and Deirdre O'Loughlin, "Integrating Ethical Brands into Our Consumption Lives," *Journal of Brand Management* 14 (2007): 396–409.

16. Mircea Eliade, *The Myth of the Eternal Return* (New York: Princeton University Press, 1974), 2.

17. For more on the topic of fragmentation and the post-modern condition see, for instance, Michael Calvin McGee, "Text, Context, and the Fragmentation of Contemporary Culture," *Text and Performance Quarterly* 54 (1990): 274–89; Greg Dickinson, "Joe's Rhetoric: Finding Authenticity at Starbucks," *Rhetoric Society Quarterly* 32 (2002): 5–27.

18. Many of us exist in "telecocoons," able to maintain "intimacy" at a distance while immersed in a constant stream of mediated information. For more on this concept see Kazys Varnelis and Anne Friedberg, "Place: The Networking of Public Space," in *Networked Publics*, ed. Varnelis and Friedberg (Cambridge: MIT Press, 2008), 15–42.

19. Dickinson, "Joe's Rhetoric," 7.

20. These arguments are also explained in Barry Brummet's discussion of apocalyptic framing: Barry Brummett, "Premillennial Apocalyptic as a Rhetorical Genre," *Central States Speech Journal* 35 (1984): 85–93.

21. We are deliberately invoking Lawrence Grossberg's notion of a "rock formation" in *We Gotta Get Out of This Place: Popular Conservatism and Postmodern Culture* (New York: Routledge, 1992).

22. For a good example of museum criticism see Greg Dickinson, Brian Ott, and Eric Aoki, "Memory and Myth at the Buffalo Bill Museum," *Western Journal of Communication* 69 (2005): 85–108. For the study of memorials see Carole Blair and Neil Michel, "Commemorating in the Theme Park Zone: Reading the Astronauts Memorial," in *At the Intersection: Cultural Studies and Rhetorical Studies*, ed. Thomas Rosteck (New York: Guilford Press, 1999), 29–83.

23. Jessie Stewart and Greg Dickinson, "Enunciating Locality in the Postmodern Suburb: FlatIron Crossing and the Colorado Lifestyle," *Western Journal of Communication* 72 (2008): 283.

24. Ibid., 280–307.

25. For more on the extra-linguistic quality of affect and "structures of feeling," see Lawrence Grossberg, "Affect's Future: Rediscovering the Virtual in the Actual," in *The Affect Theory Reader*, ed. Melissa Gregg and Gregory J. Seigworth (Durham: Duke University Press, 2010), 313–18.

26. Brian Massumi, *Parables from the Virtual* (Durham, North Carolina: Duke University Press, 2002), 28.

27. Marcel Proust famously illustrates the complex and detailed relations between the sensual and the symbolic in his portrait of the "petit madeleines." For an analysis of this episode, see Conley, "Taste-Power," forthcoming in *Pre/Text*.

28. Brian Massumi, "Of Microperception and Micropolitics: An Interview with Brian Massumi, 15 August, 2008," *Inflexions: A Journal for Research-Creation* 3 (2009): 4.

29. We agree with Michael Warner's account of how publics are created and extended through discourse itself, but he neglects the material dimension of how bodies come into and receive new textual stimuli. There is more to be said about what arranges publics textually, and we think it is to be found in the spatial affects of linguistic bodies. See Warner, *Publics and Counterpublics* (Brooklyn: Zone Books, 2002).

30. It should be noted that "material rhetoric" has at least three different meanings in this discipline. We are interested in the particular line of inquiry that investigates how communication also has material affects. A good review of this literature can be found in Carole Blair, "Reflections on Criticism and Bodies: Parables from Public Places," *Western Journal of Communication* 65 (2001): 288. For a sampling of other critical-rhetorical writings on materiality, see Debra Hawhee, *Moving Bodies: Kenneth Burke at the Edges of Language* (Columbia, SC: University of South Carolina Press, 2009); Dana L. Cloud, "The Materiality of Discourse as Oxymoron: A Challenge to Critical Rhetoric," *Western Journal of Communication* 58 (1994): 141–63.

31. William E. Connolly, *A World of Becoming* (Durham: Duke University Press, 2011), 34.

32. For examples, see M. Luisa Demattè, Daniel Sanabria, and Charles Spence, "Olfactory Discrimination: When Vision Matters?," *Chem Senses* 34 (2009): 103–9. Also see Daniel W. Wesson and Donald A. Wilson, "Smelling Sounds: Olfactory-Auditory Sensory Convergence in the Olfactory Tubercle," *The Journal of Neuroscience* 30 (2010): 3013–21.

33. "How Does Our Sense of Smell Work?" *The National Institute on Deafness and Other Communication Disorders*, July, 2009, accessed January 17, 2011, http://www.nidcd.nih.gov/health/smelltaste/smell.html#smell_02.

188　*Justin Eckstein and Donovan Conley*

34. Teresa Brennan, *The Transmission of Affect* (Ithaca: Cornell University Press), 9.
35. Ibid., 10.
36. Dina Marie V. Zemke and Stowe Shoemaker, "Scent across a Crowded Room: Exploring the Effect of Ambient Scent on Social Interactions," *Hospitality Management* 26 (2007): 936.
37. As quoted in Charles Hirschkind, *The Ethical Soundscape: Cassette Sermons and Islamic Counterpublics* (New York: Columbia University Press, 2006), 83.
38. Connolly, *A World of Becoming*, 31.
39. The military has keenly understood the "persuasive" implications of this point, as it has even weaponized sounds. For more information see Steve Goodman, *Sonic Warfare: Sound, Affect, and the Ecology of Fear* (Cambridge: MIT Press, 2010); also see Greg Goodale, *Sonic Persuasion: Reading Sound in the Recorded Age* (Chicago: University of Illinois Press, 2011).
40. Massumi, *Parables from the Virtual*, 30.
41. Iain Chambers, "The Aural Walk," in *Audio Culture: Readings in Modern Music*, ed. Christoph Cox and Daniel Warner (New York: Continuum, 2010), 101.
42. Raffi Khatchadourian, "The Taste Factory," *The New Yorker*, November 23, 2009.
43. Eric Schlosser, *Fast Food Nation* (New York: Perennial, 2002), 124.
44. Ibid., 125.
45. Roland Barthes theorizes that taste is also a way to discern classes. He argues that tastes, like bitter, are the product of certain cultural training associated with the elite. For more information see Roland Barthes, "Toward a Psychosociology of Contemporary Food Consumption," in *Food and Culture: A Reader*, ed. Carole Counihan and Penny Van Esterik (New York, Routledge, 1997), 21.
46. Tom Standage, *An Edible History of Humanity* (New York: Walker, 2009), 75.
47. For recent work on how taste is manipulated by the food industry, see David Kessler, *The End of Overeating: Taking Control of the Insatiable American Appetite* (New York: Rodale, 2009). For a discussion on the relationship between taste and the cultivation of eating habits see J. Amy Dillard, "Sloppy Joe, Slop, Sloppy Joe: How USDA Commodities Dumping Ruined the National School Lunch Program," *The Oregon Law Review* 87 (2008): 221–58.
48. Dickinson, "Joe's Rhetoric," 11.
49. It needs to be acknowledged that not all products on offer at farmers' markets are strictly local, especially large-scale operations like the CCFM.
50. For an excellent discussion of affect's unruly nature see Gregory J. Seigworth and Melissa Gregg, "An Inventory of Shimmers," in *The Affect Theory Reader*, ed. Gregg and Seigworth, 1–25.
51. For a more in-depth discussion of the concept of duration and its corresponding importance for world-making see Gilles Deleuze, *Bergsonism*, trans. Hugh Tomlinson and Barbara Habberjam (New York: Zone Books, 1991); also see Michael Hardt, *Gilles Deleuze: An Apprenticeship in Philosophy* (Minneapolis: University of Minnesota Press, 1993).
52. Erin Manning, *Relationscapes: Movement, Art, Philosophy* (Cambridge, MA: MIT Press, 2009), 18.
53. The relationality of space is a key issue in Doreen Massey, *For Space* (Thousand Oaks: Sage, 2005).
54. Grossberg, "Affect's Future," 318.

55. For an excellent discussion of the folding of the virtual into the actual, see Matthew Bost and Ronald Walter Greene, "Affirming Rhetorical Material-ism: Enfolding the Virtual and the Actual," *The Western Journal of Com-munication* 75 (2011): 440–44.
56. Grossberg, "Affect's Future," 318.
57. Nabhan, *Coming Home to Eat*, 18.

12 Revolution on Primetime TV

Jamie Oliver Takes On the US School Food System

Garrett M. Broad

"The USDA (United States Department of Agriculture) has got to evolve and change, and support communities that want to change. If you've got everyone in the world that wants to cook the food from fresh, but they can't buy the food from fresh, that's a problem . . . Maybe I can use my influence to ask the USDA to make special allowances. But maybe the USDA needs to make special allowances for everyone."[1]

There are many reasons to criticize the industrialized, market-based system of American food production and distribution. Buttressed by US governmental and multinational food policy, the current practices of multinational agricultural business conglomerates are ultimately environmentally unsustainable, inhumane to animals, and marginalizing to local farm economies and workers.[2] Food distribution and retail networks have historically been inequitable and characterized by racist patterns of disinvestment in low-income and minority communities, while the highly processed foods sold to consumers have been connected to a variety of chronic diseases.[3] Together, these criticisms stand as the foundation for many of the contemporary (if decentralized) US movements that work to construct a healthier and more sustainable food system. For years, however, these oppositional arguments were largely confined to circles of academics, farmers, urban agriculturalists, policy wonks, and anti-hunger advocates. Over the last several decades, conscious consumers have joined the conversation as well, and their consumer voices have been heard most clearly in the burgeoning market for local and organically grown foods.[4] Conscious food consumers have been implored to "vote with their wallet three times a day" for health and sustainability, a neoliberal mantra that has placed the consumer in direct control of her own well-being as well as of the well-being of her physical and social environment.

The quote at the top of this chapter should resonate with those who believe it is necessary to move beyond the neoliberal ethos of consumer solutions in order to fix the food system. With the use of the term "neoliberal," I work from theorists who have outlined how the hegemonic theory of neoliberalism proposes that human well-being is best achieved in a global capitalist system that eliminates state intervention in social and institutional life in favor of a commitment to entrepreneurial freedoms, market-based solutions, and the power of consumer choice.[5] This opening statement, however, takes a different tack, as it seems to call for significant political pressure that would encourage state intervention within the food system; that is, intervention that would also transform the government and multinational priorities from those that favor the interests of transnational agri-business corporations to prioritize instead the health of the nation's citizens. Yet, the quotation does not come from an avowed critic of neoliberalism, not an academic, anti-hunger activist or farmer, but rather from a British chef and a highly successful television entertainer, Jamie Oliver. Moreover, the celebrity chef's criticisms of the USDA were featured in a venue to which food system activists, academics, and agroecologists have rarely, if ever, been given access—primetime network television. *Jamie Oliver's Food Revolution*, first broadcast on the ABC network in the early months of 2010, detailed the chef's efforts to transform the school food system of Huntington, West Virginia by replacing its cafeterias' unhealthy, frozen, processed foods with fresh fruits, vegetables, and healthy meals cooked from scratch.

This chapter uses the case of *Jamie Oliver's Food Revolution* as a way to think through the issues that arise from the recent intersection between progressive food system initiatives and the world of popular consumer culture. What was once an active constellation of movements with little to no media visibility has seen a rapid surge in attention in just a few short years. This chapter attempts to make sense of what this complex visibility means, how it functions, and what opportunities it presents for progressive food movements at large. Focusing on the first season of the program, I argue that *Jamie Oliver's Food Revolution* is rife with contradictory discourses that are put on display, as potentially radical food politics are presented through the lens of commercial reality television. *Food Revolution* and Oliver's persona are in many ways the product of the commercial, neoliberal state, and yet, given our current political and economic situation, such outgrowths of neoliberalism and popular culture represent an important opportunity for progressive food system movements to advance efforts toward long-term food system change. Indeed, Oliver's rhetoric demonstrates the ways that neoliberalism itself has bred a variety of oppositional movements that still maintain significant elements of that neoliberal frame, but remain a potentially useful piece of the broader food system struggle.

I was one of many people, personally invested in food system issues, who nervously awaited the premier of *Jamie Oliver's Food Revolution*, not quite sure how the genre of reality television would depict the complex issues associated with school food. What happens when the school food system—one of several primary foci of progressive food system initiatives—is

192 Garrett M. Broad

subjected to the constraints of network commercial television? How are the problems presented, and what types of solutions are offered? Most importantly, what, if anything, does this piece of popular culture mean for the future prospects of school food change and food system transformation?

In the pages that follow, I first highlight the state of the school food system and current efforts that are in progress to improve its glaring deficiencies. I then briefly discuss popular media portrayals of food and nutrition, and situate the history of Jamie Oliver and ABC's *Food Revolution* within this conversation. Next, I present a textual analysis of the program, make reference to the reactions of progressive food system advocates, and conclude with thoughts on the program's potential contribution to food system change within the context of neoliberalism.

THE SCHOOL FOOD CRISIS

Over the course of the last several decades, a variety of distinct but interconnected progressive food system initiatives have developed as a means to counter the detrimental social and ecological impacts of the status quo in the industrial food system. Within these initiatives, the topic of school food has emerged as one of the primary battlegrounds. Advocates' concerns with the current state of school food are many, and it is well beyond the scope of this chapter to detail their critiques and recommendations. As a brief and incomplete summary, the modern National School Lunch Program (NSLP) began with the National School Lunch Act of 1946, which provides cash subsidies and donated commodities from the USDA for each meal a school serves. In 1966, Congress passed the Child Nutrition Act, which created the School Breakfast Program, established a food service equipment assistance program, and increased funds for meals served to needy students. Today, approximately 94,000 public and private schools offer the NSLP, feeding more than thirty-one million children on a typical school day, while the School Breakfast Program is available in 84,500 schools and serves more than ten million children on a typical day. Through these programs, students can purchase free or reduced price lunches on a sliding scale based on their household income.[6]

All school lunches must meet applicable recommendations from the USDA's 1995 Dietary Guidelines for Americans, but schools are able to decide the specifics of the meals they serve and how they prepare them. These dietary guidelines themselves are extremely problematic, most concretely because they are so heavily influenced by the lobbying of corporate agri-business and their colleagues in the USDA. More conceptually, the guidelines rely on a rhetoric of quantification that ignores notions of culture, taste, or even nourishment, and instead prioritize an interpretation that focuses not on foods, but on the nutrient components of foods. This focus leads to a situation in which highly processed, unhealthy foods from the USDA are used heavily by schools in order to meet these "nutritional standards"—for instance, french fries become an acceptable serving of vegetables.[7] Nonetheless, in return for their participation in the NSLP, schools get cash reimbursements for each of the meals sold, as well as donations from the USDA of excess industrial food commodities (including meats, cheeses, vegetables, fruits, and juices).[8] School food has increasingly been treated by administrators as an arena that must economically break even and ideally should become one of the prime profit-making initiatives for schools and districts. This economic bottom line has led schools to rely on heavily processed USDA meals and commodity donations, as well as on vendor contracts for unhealthy corporate food products, which, along with a number of other factors, have contributed to the striking rise in diet-related disease among American children.[9]

In response, progressive food system advocates have proposed policy recommendations and have initiated projects to improve the school food environment.[10] For instance, a number of farm-to-school (FTS) programs have been created that link locally grown fruits, vegetables, and other products to cafeterias, often through direct links to local farmers or gardens on school grounds. These programs tend to arise as a result of hard work and logistical coordination between concerned parents, school administrators, healthy food and anti-hunger advocates, and local farmers, among others. With that said, FTS must work within the same nutritional and economic confines that typify the current school food system. Patricia Allen and Julie Guthman have argued that these entrepreneurial programs, while of good intent, tend to produce detrimental neoliberal forms and practices all over again—that is, forms that devolve responsibility from higher levels of government to local actors, marketize and privatize public resources, and overly benefit the well-organized and economically advantaged.[11] In response to this critique, scholars and FTS practitioners have argued that while FTS is not socially or economically feasible for all at this point in time, it does offer an important alternative to the status quo, one that has the potential to be refined and scaled up in time.[12]

THE FOOD SYSTEM IN POPULAR CULTURE

Food and cooking have a storied history in American television and popular culture, one that has generally been presented through the lens of the celebrity chef or food aficionado. Indeed, the big issues with which progressive food system activists are engaged have not historically been a part of these depictions. Instead, these food celebrities have maintained a focus on a consumer-oriented approach to food television, in which stylized advice about preparation and consumption is provided to the viewer.[13] It is only through the recent work of a number of authors, activists, public officials, and filmmakers that concerns related to the industrial food system have been brought into the popular culture arena. Perhaps most notably, journalists Eric Schlosser and Michael Pollan wrote bestselling books that took aim at "big agriculture" and the worlds of fast and processed foods, in which they criticized the environmental and health impacts of the contemporary food system. Their works were then repackaged and eloquently presented in the Academy Award–nominated film *Food, Inc.*[14] When it came to offering solutions to the myriad of problems they outlined, however, their rhetorical strategy seemed to mirror the consumer-oriented, un-systemic tendencies of television's celebrity chefs. The closing credits of *Food, Inc.* asserted: "You can vote to change this system . . . Three times a day . . . You can change the world with every bite." Critics have argued that these types of rhetorical moves place all responsibility for food choice and dietary health on the backs of individual decision-makers; they do not shed light on the systemic and policy solutions that are needed in order to transform the institutions of the global food system.[15] Indeed, this narrowing process of "individualization" is a hallmark of neoliberal approaches to societal and environmental improvement.[16]

Given this history of food in popular culture and television, *Jamie Oliver's Food Revolution* represents a new development for progressive food system initiatives. Broadcast on major network reality television, Oliver's work was sure to reach a broad-based audience that has grown accustomed to the approach of conventional celebrity chefs, and had not been reached in full by the critiques like those depicted in *Food, Inc.* But what could be expected from a reality television show about food? Several researchers have asserted that it is unlikely that advertisers would ever sponsor shows that seriously address any of the problems with contemporary food production and consumption.[17] Further, in reality television, the neoliberal state has found a very effective mouthpiece by which to assert the value of individualization. Laurie Ouellette and James Hay have described how reality television functions to circulate techniques of governmentality "through which individuals and populations are expected to reflect upon, work on and organize their lives and themselves as an implicit condition of their citizenship."[18] A show that focuses on unhealthy eating and its impacts on obesity, for instance, demonstrates that healthy bodies are still an important public value and political objective, but the onus is on the individual and on the market—and not on public institutions—to ensure that health is achieved.[19] With this in mind, how revolutionary could the *Food Revolution* possibly be?

FROM NAKED CHEF TO MBE

Jamie Oliver's career merging cooking and the world of entertainment spans over a decade, beginning in 1999, when the twenty-three-year-old's first series, *The Naked Chef*, debuted on the BBC and later on the

US Food Network. His style resonated with viewers, and his television success was followed by a European bestselling cookbook and a multi-million-dollar endorsement deal with Sainsbury's, one of Europe's leading grocery chains.[20] Several other television shows followed, including *Jamie's Kitchen*, in which Oliver trained a group of fifteen disadvantaged teens, with the promise that they would be given jobs at his restaurant, "Fifteen," if they completed the course. He achieved even greater prominence with the production of *Jamie's School Dinners*, aired in Britain in 2005, in which he highlighted the prevalence of unhealthy, processed junk foods at a typical British school. He worked with the school cooks to introduce fresh, healthy meals, and launched the "Feed Me Better" campaign to apply pressure on the British government to improve school food standards.[21] Oliver is often credited with forcing the government's hand in making changes to the school food system—in reality, school food reform had been on the ruling Labour Party's agenda for several years, and certain reforms were already in the works, but Oliver certainly helped raise awareness about the issue and his influence may have helped initiate some novel proposals.[22]

Oliver's interesting blend of entertainment food programming and dietary health advocacy continued in Britain with the production of *Jamie's Ministry of Food* in 2008, in which he traveled to Rotherham, South Yorkshire, to attempt to improve the food culture of the town of approximately 250,000.[23] Around the same time, Oliver also produced several documentaries that investigated the abysmal state of contemporary factory farming processes in Europe. 2008's *Jamie's Fowl Dinners* and 2009's *Jamie Saves Our Bacon* were critical of industrialized meat production's impact on animals, farmers, the environment, and human health. Treading a line between calls for systemic reform and individualization, a promotion on the Channel 4 website for *Bacon* trumpeted: "Once again, he wants to help consumers make better-informed choices about the food they eat by showing exactly how pigs live and die to put pork, ham and bacon on our plates."[24]

In light of his efforts, Oliver was awarded an MBE (Member of the Order of the British Empire) in 2003 and the prestigious Technology, Entertainment, Design (TED) prize in 2010, among other honors. Of course, his work has hardly been just a labor of love, as he has carefully crafted a highly successful international corporate portfolio that has reaped him significant economic benefits, including a net worth estimated at one time around $65 million.[25] At times, however, Oliver's advocacy has come into conflict with his corporate image, including incidents that involved his first and biggest sponsor, Sainsbury's. The grocery chain was not happy, fairly early in their corporate relationship, when Oliver remarked, "For any chef, supermarkets are like a factory. I buy from specialist growers, organic suppliers and farmers."[26] Several years later, after an Oliver tirade against junk food packed in students' lunches from home, Sainsbury executive Justin King took issue with the criticisms: "While I agree with Jamie's drive to get children eating healthily, his attack is neither correct nor the best way to achieve a change . . . There is no such thing as bad food—just bad diets."[27] They came into conflict again in 2008 when Oliver criticized the supermarket chain for not publicly supporting his campaign against battery-cages for chickens. With his contract in jeopardy, Oliver apologized and appeared in a Sainsbury advertisement that promoted the "higher-welfare chickens" sold by the grocery chain.[28]

AND NOW, THE *FOOD REVOLUTION*

Oliver's work had put him in a position in which he had to balance several sometimes conflicting roles—chef, entertainer, educator, health advocate, and corporate mouthpiece. As he made the transition to mainstream American television, this balancing act would once again be put to the test. While Oliver had achieved modest success in the US with Food Network productions, *Jamie Oliver's Food Revolution* was his breakout opportunity, broadcast in primetime on the ABC network. By all accounts, the first season of the show was a solid performer for the network, especially early in its run. Over 7.5 million viewers tuned in for its first episode in its regular Friday, 9:00 p.m. timeslot, second only to the NCAA men's basketball tournament that evening. The numbers dipped to around 4–5 million viewers for the remainder of the six-episode series, but it finished either first or second in its timeslot each broadcast.[29] The episodes were also available via online video websites like Hulu.com, where it received hundreds of viewer comments and was likely watched by thousands of additional viewers. Oliver took part in a heavily scheduled promotional tour, with appearances on *Oprah*, *The Late Show with David Letterman*, *Larry King Live*, and *Good Morning America*, to name a few.

The first season of the program consisted of six one-hour episodes, and took place in the town of Huntington, West Virginia. The city came to the attention of Oliver and the show's producers when an Associated Press story reported that, on the basis of 2006 data from the Centers for Disease Control, Huntington was the fattest and unhealthiest city in the US. More than half of its adult population was classified as obese, the worst percentage in the nation, and they also had the worst outcomes on several other measures, including incidence of heart disease, diabetes, and percentage of elderly people who had lost all of their teeth.[30] As it turned out, that analysis was actually based on data for a five-county metro area, which included parts of Ohio and Kentucky, but because Huntington was the largest city in the area, it received the brunt of the attention and was continually referred to as the unhealthiest city in America throughout the *Food Revolution* production.

Food Revolution combined elements from several of Oliver's previous shows as he attempted to improve the food environment of Huntington's schools, as well as to connect to individuals and families within the broader Huntington community. His biggest mission was to reduce the amount of heavily processed, "heat-and-serve" foods being fed to students, and to replace them with scratch-cooked meals of fresh vegetables and meats. The first several episodes followed his exploits in a local elementary school, where Oliver was appalled to see a steady diet of processed pizza, chicken nuggets, and sugary flavored milk served for both breakfast and lunch. He was met with resistance from the school cooks, who complained that their current system of serving processed food worked well enough, and suggested that Oliver's methods for cooking fresh foods would be too time-consuming and costly.

Oliver began to learn about the federal nutrition standards for school lunches set by the USDA, and he butted heads with Rhonda McCoy, the district's director of Food Services. He came to understand that frozen pizzas and processed french fries passed USDA muster, while several of his fresh-cooked meals did not meet the federal nutritional requirements and would be un-reimbursable. A few days in, he achieved modest success getting the young students to eat his fresh meals but was grossly over-budget. McCoy informed him that he could continue his program on a temporary basis, but would need to figure out ways to get the kids to eat his food, and he had stay within the school's financial constraints.

Food Revolution was full of the dramatic conventions, story arcs, and spectacular events that have come to typify reality television fare. In the first season's final episode, Oliver came back to Huntington after several months away promoting the upcoming television program. Before he left, a local hospital had offered $80,000 to retain the food service provider Sustainable Food Systems to keep the healthy meals in the school. As he returned, he found out that McCoy planned to reintroduce some processed foods into the school lunch, as a vast amount of USDA commodity donations had stockpiled with no other place to go. He also found that more students were opting out of the school lunch, and instead were bringing brown paper bags filled with all sorts of junk foods and candy from home.

In a conversation with McCoy and the district superintendent in the final episode, it was clear that, although a number of local schools had integrated healthy food into their lunches, the long-term sustainability of the program was at serious risk. Oliver noted, "By the sounds of it, it's down to me to negotiate with the USDA to allow them to get a hold of the fresh foods that they need. So, look, this ain't a happy ending."[31] His time in Huntington ended on a cautiously optimistic note, as Oliver spoke to a crowd of parents, teachers, students, and other Huntington residents: "I really think we can change things, we really can . . . All of you need to make sure that this works. It's really important that everybody does their bit. You don't have to do a lot, but if you do your bit, change in every school in the country can happen, it really can." In the final moments, Oliver spoke directly to the camera: "We are at a tipping point right now, it can go either

way. This is the first generation of kids expected to live a shorter life than
you. You guys can start kicking some ass, and expecting more, demanding more, wanting more. Why? Because you deserve more. It's over to you
now, guys, it can't just be my fight anymore. This is not the end. This is the
beginning."[32]

INDIVIDUALIZATION AND SYSTEMIC CHANGE
IN *FOOD REVOLUTION*

The following section takes a closer look at several scenes from the final
episode of the first season of *Food Revolution* to further investigate the
possibilities and constraints of reality television with respect to progressive
food system change. After several weeks away promoting *Food Revolution*,
Oliver returned to a Huntington elementary school that had instituted his
healthy food program. He found that more and more students were bringing unhealthy, brown bag lunches from home—which were not subject to
any nutritional regulations—and the cameras followed him asking elementary school students if he could peruse their packed lunches. After looking
through a young girl's meal, he observed: "That is not a lunch—potato
chips, potato chips and candy. If she had that lunch every school day of her
life, that is child abuse." He continued walking angrily around the cafeteria, but each time he had anything negative to say about a particular food,
the brand names were audibly and visibly censored. "There's going to be
blurs and bleeps all over this scene." Oliver continued, "At the moment,
we've got parents betraying this energy and love and care and effort going
into the fresh food . . . by giving their precious little kids lunch boxes completely barren of any decent nutrition." Moving forward two scenes in the
program, Oliver conducted a cooking demonstration, along with several
school cooks, for local residents at his "Boot Camp" to try to raise more
support for the healthy school food initiative. As he prepared a sample
school food meal, the camera panned in on a close-up of "Green Giant"
brand Niblets Corn and a "100% natural" claim on the label. "The great
thing about the frozen veggies," Oliver said, "Is they freeze them within a
number of hours and they lock in the nutrients. So, actually, nutritionally
speaking—really, really good." In the original broadcast, a Green Giant
commercial—complete with storybook views of a pastoral farm landscape—was aired immediately after this segment.

   This example highlights some of the clear drawbacks of a reality television depiction of food system issues, and also underscores the tensions
between Jamie Oliver's conflicting roles as a healthy food advocate and
a corporate entity. Among all types of advertisements seen by children
of all ages, food is the largest product category, and the vast majority of
these ads are for candy, snacks, sugary cereals, and fast foods.[33] Networks
like ABC must retain a healthy relationship with these primary sponsors,

so "bleeping and blurring" is a necessity. Meanwhile, food-based reality shows offer food corporations—like Green Giant—a prime opportunity to seek product placements that work to build associations with health and environmental stewardship. Owned by the corporate food behemoth General Mills—which also owns countless unhealthy cereals and snack foods—Green Giant is hardly the type of vegetable producer associated with a more localized, petro-chemical reducing, sustainable food system.

Similar to his Sainsbury's *mea culpa* of the past, Oliver seemed to know when he had to tone down his own beliefs about food production practices and tout the products of his corporate sponsors. Indeed, Oliver's strategy for transforming Huntington's school food products did not include working directly with local farmers, as many farm-to-school initiatives do. Rather, he sought to decrease (and hopefully eliminate) the schools' volume of heavily processed foods while he increased the volume of fruits, vegetables, and "fresh" meats. Of course, these meats were more than likely the products of environmentally destructive and inhumane factory farming techniques, while the fruits and vegetables surely came from industrial agricultural practices that relied heavily on oil-based pesticides and herbicides. With that said, it *was* a step in the right direction if Oliver could urge a Huntington resident or a television viewer to eat Green Giant vegetables instead of snacking on unhealthy processed foods, or if Oliver could move a school from relying on these processed foods to fresher vegetables and meats. However, it was *also* a step with clear ethical ambiguities from the perspective of advocates for progressive food system change.

The cafeteria scene described earlier speaks directly to neoliberal notions of individualized self-improvement that are present in many reality television programs. By insisting that parents had "betrayed" the efforts that went into the preparation of the fresh school food, Oliver asserted that the preservation of a child's health could be ensured by parental food consumption decisions. While he was critical of the processed foods, those products went unnamed and remained obscured. However, he was able to speak directly to the parents of Huntington—and the viewing public—to let them know that it remained their responsibility to keep the unhealthy foods out of the brown bags. This admonition individualized the problems and the solutions for dealing with unhealthy foods, and challenged the viewer to take control of her health, her child's health, and the health of her community by *choosing* the *correct* foods to eat. It is this type of consumer moralism in discussions about food in US media that, according to authors like Toby Miller, "has led to a doctrine of personal responsibility, militating against both collective identification and action."[34]

Despite these instances of corporate protectionism and neoliberal individualization, *Food Revolution* did indeed show flashes of broader food system thinking and action, as well as subtle critiques of neoliberalization in school food, which should be encouraging to advocates for a more progressive food system. In the final episode, Director of Food Services

Rhonda McCoy brought Oliver into the district's food storage freezer to show him their excess of donated USDA commodities. With brown boxes piled high full of processed apricot cups, chicken nuggets, french fries, and other junk food products, McCoy noted that the commodity deliveries had not stopped, and that, in order to ensure that they would have food for the following school year, they decided to put in another, albeit marginally smaller, order for next year: "Some of it only costs like $3.90 a case. I mean, it's really cheap." Caught in his "nightmare scenario," Oliver spoke directly to the camera as he clearly laid out the problem to his audience: "The problem is, cheap junk food is just too good to be true, that's what Rhonda's saying. The USDA have given us so much of this cheap, cheap junk food, we can't resist it. You'd be mad not to. So, we can't sell the USDA food—it's illegal—we can't give it away either, you know, you know we can't do anything else with it. We're in an impossible situation."

One would be hard-pressed to find an instance in which a primary structural deficiency of the school food system—and in particular of the USDA's role in that system—was marked out in such an accessible narrative with the potential for broad cultural reach. By taking aim at the USDA and outlining the "impossible situation" placed on the shoulders of individual actors working to improve the school food environment, Oliver countered his own tendency, and the broader tendency of reality television, of placing the responsibility for change solely on the shoulders of the neoliberal subject. System change, and not just individual consumer habits, was implicated as part of the solution to improve the nation's health and well-being. This rhetorical contradiction should not be totally surprising in the context of activism in a neoliberal age. As David Harvey has argued, "Neoliberalization has spawned within itself an extensive oppositional culture. The opposition tends, however, to accept many of the basic propositions of neoliberalism . . . It takes the neoliberal rhetoric of improving the welfare of all and condemns neoliberalization for failing in its own terms."[35] Indeed, no one on *Food Revolution* went as far to question the neoliberalization of school food itself—rather than asking why US school cafeterias should be subject to the whims of the market at all, they instead argued that the neoliberal system was simply not providing the full range of services it had promised. In its critique of the school food system, *Food Revolution* at once propagated and challenged the generally unquestioned hegemonic neoliberal doctrine.

CONCLUSION

Jamie Oliver's Food Revolution, as well as Oliver's personal appearances on a variety of media outlets, led to a great deal of discussion in the mainstream press, on the Internet, and in local communities throughout the US. This conversation was particularly charged among food system

activists—it was a topic of interpersonal discussions as well as online discussions in countless blog posts and commentaries on food-related list-
servs. A number of food system advocates were simply irritated by the
program's presentation. They saw Oliver as arrogant, disrespectful, manipulating, and ill-informed about the American food system, and too concerned with individual choices as opposed to systemic issues. The online
news site *Alternet* featured an eviscerating editorial along these lines, titled
"How TV Superchef Jamie Oliver's 'Food Revolution' Flunked Out." As
evidence, the author cited a survey that showed that students in Huntington were unhappy with Oliver's meals, participation in the lunch program
had dropped, and that Oliver's work was over-budget and failed to meet
the federal nutrition standards.[36] Although Oliver might have ultimately
had altruistic aims, advocates from this perspective argued that because he
consented to be used by a reality television show, he was beholden to the
types of corporate advertisers that were the biggest problems in the food
system to begin with. To them, this made his efforts ineffectual and useless
for the broader movement.

Not all of the reactions demonstrated this type of condemnation, however. Another segment of food system advocates were more hopeful about
the show's prospects, but were ultimately disappointed by his lack of knowledge about the school food system and his failure to highlight the good
work already being done by practitioners and advocates in school food
around the country. They were annoyed that he repeatedly referred to "his"
food revolution, while the fact that Oliver knew little about the USDA at
the start of the program showed that he "didn't do his homework." Diane
Chapeta, a public school food service director, said she received countless
phone calls from angry parents after the first episode aired, and she noted
that the show "set off a tidal wave of misinformation sprinkled with well-
meaning intentions . . . What Jamie Oliver failed to take note of is that a
food revolution in the school lunch program already exists."[37] Although
they were disappointed in Oliver and the production overall, there was
still some hope among these healthy food advocates that *Food Revolution*
might lead to some marginal benefits for their cause.

Finally, there were a number of progressive food system advocates who
were energized and excited by Oliver's work and its potential to strengthen
the movement. This is not to say that they did not have problems with certain aspects of the production—indeed, they voiced many of the same concerns expressed earlier—but to them, the important thing was that Oliver
had given a boost to the conversation about school food and the food system in a way the movement had never seen before. As an activist remarked
in a personal conversation, "One thing about the 'good food' movement—
we're so myopic and so tiny. We lose sight of the fact that the average
person rarely gives these issues a thought at all . . . What Jamie Oliver put
on people's radar is just how deeply things are linked to our agricultural
system."[38] Few, if any, of such advocates felt that Jamie Oliver himself had

enacted much change at all; in fact, they felt that he could never be *expected* to do much at all. But they did believe that his work would assist them in advancing their own efforts by helping them get their foot in the door to start conversations with everyday citizens, policymakers, and other power- ful private and public sector entities. In short, they were excited by their new level of visibility, but they were sure that the increased visibility alone would do nothing for them. It was time for them to take advantage of the media conversation as an opportunity to point out what Oliver got right, what he got wrong, and what personal, political, and economic changes could be enacted in order to work toward an equitable, sustainable food system for all. These advocates recognized the inherent contradictions of oppositional movements in the neoliberal age, and took it upon themselves to extend the systems-level perspective hinted at by Oliver but constrained within the medium of commercial reality television.

Online and on television, Oliver continually reiterated that, if everyone worked together and did "their bit," parents, students, teachers, cooks, and administrators could help change every school in the country. It is easy to argue that *Food Revolution* reverted to the same neoliberal individualiza- tion and entrepreneurship that have characterized the proffered solutions of much of the reality television genre. In many respects, these criticisms are spot-on. At the same time, an analysis of *Food Revolution* does dem- onstrate a tension between individualized and systemic solutions. Calls for true food system change were indeed made more visible than ever before. Do individualized, consumer solutions retain the spotlight? Yes, indeed. Does this strip the program of its value for the movement? Only if activists and advocates leave it at that.

In many ways, *Food Revolution* mirrors the tensions that are ever-pres- ent in progressive food system initiatives, and in a variety of other oppo- sitional movements within contemporary neoliberalism. Should the focus be on challenging macro-level neoliberal structures that reinforce poverty, or should the focus be on building a broader movement by empowering communities through entrepreneurial program development? The answer, as unsatisfying as it might be, must be "yes" to both. Without continually confronting the structural inequities within the current economic system, progressive food system initiatives will provide a service to only the privi- leged classes of our society. But without engaging aspects of the neoliberal market, the movement will never develop and refine the tools necessary to construct an equitable, sustainable food system. The foundations of neo- liberalization have so permeated contemporary life that broad-based oppo- sitional movements will almost certainly borrow frames of reference from the very neoliberal system they seek to transform.

With Oliver and others as celebrity spokespersons, advocates for pro- gressive food system change can expect to continue to see food system issues discussed in the arena of popular culture. For all of the drawbacks and constraints of celebrity advocacy, activists would be remiss if they did not engage with these portrayals—applauding where it is deserved, correcting where it is necessary. Most importantly, *Food Revolution* (and other products of popular culture) can spur conversations that need not be as constrained as they are on reality television. Henceforth, advocates must work hard to articulate that it is not Oliver's food revolution, after all. It is a revolution that has already been long in the works, populated by people from different perspectives, professions, and cultures. It is a revolution that faces resilient and powerful institutional barriers. It is a revolution that has a place for conscious consumption, but must use concerted collective action as its driving force. And it is a revolution that will take time to see through—the current food economy was not built in a day, and health, equity, and sustainability will not be quick fixes either.

NOTES

1. "Jamie Oliver's Food Revolution—Episode 6," *Hulu*, April 23, 2010, accessed March 5, 2012, http://www.hulu.com/watch/144640/jamie-olivers-food-revolution-episode-6
2. See, for instance, Mark Gold, "The Global Benefits of Eating Less Meat," Compassion in World Farming Trust, 2004, accessed August 29, 2011, http://www.ciwf.org.uk/includes/documents/cm_docs/2008/g/global_benefits_of_eating_less_meat.pdf; Joan D. Gussow, "Dietary Guidelines for Sustainability: Twelve Years Later," *Journal of Nutrition Education* 31 (1999): 194–200; Jack Kloppenburg et al., "Coming in to the Foodshed," *Agriculture and Human Values* 13 (1999): 33–42; Marion Nestle, *Food Politics: How the Food Industry Influences Nutrition and Health* (Berkeley: University of California Press, 2007); Raj Patel, *Stuffed and Starved: The Hidden Battle for the World Food System* (New York: Melville, 2008); David Pimentel et al., "Environmental, Energetic, and Economic Comparisons of Organic and Conventional Farming Systems," *BioScience* 55 (2005): 573–82; Stephanie A. Robert, "Socioeconomic Position and Health: The Independent Contribution of Community Socioeconomic Context," *Annual Review of Sociology* 25 (1999): 489–516.
3. See, for instance, Michael Pollan, *In Defense of Food* (New York: Penguin Press, 2008); Amanda Shaffer, "The Persistence of L.A.'s Grocery Gap: The Need for a New Food Policy and Approach to Market Development," *The Urban and Environmental Policy Institute*, 2002, accessed August 29, 2011, http://departments.oxy.edu/uepi/publications/the_persistence_of.htm; Shannon Zenk et al., "Neighborhood Racial Composition, Neighborhood Poverty, and the Spatial Accessibility of Supermarkets in Metropolitan Detroit," *American Journal of Public Health* 95 (2005): 660–67.
4. Carolyn Dimitri and Catherine Greene, "Recent Growth Patterns in the US Organic Foods Market," in *Organic Agriculture in the US*, ed. Alison J. Wellson (New York: Nova Science Publishers, 2007), 129–90.
5. David Harvey, *A Brief History of Neoliberalism* (Oxford: Oxford University Press, 2005).
6. National Farm to School Network, Community Food Security Coalition and School Food Focus, "Nourishing the Nation One Tray at a Time," 2009, accessed August 28, 2011, http://www.foodsecurity.org/Nourishingthe-Nation-OneTrayataTime.pdf.

7. Jessica Mudry, *Measured Meals: Nutrition in America* (New York: SUNY Press, 2009); Pollan, *In Defense of Food*; Janet Poppendieck, *Free for All: Fixing School Food in America* (Berkeley: University of California Press, 2010).
8. "National School Lunch Program," 2009, accessed August 29, 2011, http://www.fns.usda.gov/cnd/lunch/AboutLunch/NSLPFactSheet.pdf; Nestle, *Food Politics.*
9. National Alliance for Nutrition and Activity, "National Health Priorities," 2010, accessed August 29, 2011, http://www.cspinet.org/new/pdf/cdc_briefing_book_fy10.pdf; Nestle, *Food Politics.*
10. Mark Vallianatos, "Healthy School Food Policies: A Checklist" (working paper, Center for Food and Justice, Urban and Environmental Policy Institute, 2005), accessed August 27, 2011, http://departments.oxy.edu/uepi/cfj/publications/healthy_school_food_policies_05.pdf.
11. Patricia Allen and Julie Guthman, "From 'Old School' to 'Farm-to-School': Neoliberalization from the Ground Up," *Agriculture and Human Values* 23 (2006): 401–415.
12. Jack Kloppenburg and Neva Hassanein, "From Old School to Reform School?," *Agriculture and Human Values* 23 (2006): 420.
13. Cheri Ketchum, "The Essence of Cooking Shows: How the Food Network Constructs Consumer Fantasies," *Journal of Communication Inquiry* 29 (2005): 217.
14. Eric Schlosser, *Fast Food Nation: The Dark Side of the All-American Meal* (New York: Houghton Mifflin, 2001); Michael Pollan, *The Omnivore's Dilemma: A Natural History of Four Meals* (New York: Penguin, 2006); *Food, Inc.*, directed by Robert Kenner (2008; New York, NY: Magnolia Pictures, 2009), DVD.
15. Julie Guthman, "Can't Stomach It: How Michael Pollan et al. Made Me Want to Eat Cheetos," *Gastronomica* 7 (2007): 264.
16. Michael Maniates, "Individualization: Plant a Tree, Buy a Bike, Save the World?," *Global Environmental Politics* 1 (2001): 31–52.
17. Ketchum, "The Essence of Cooking Shows."
18. Laurie Ouellette and James Hay, "Makeover Television, Governmentality and the Good Citizen," *Continuum* 22 (2008): 473.
19. Nikolas Rose, *Inventing Ourselves: Psychology, Power and Personhood* (Cambridge: Cambridge University Press, 1998).
20. Angela Byrne, Maureen Whitehead, and Steven Breen, "The Naked Truth of Celebrity Endorsement," *British Food Journal* 105 (2003): 288–296.
21. "Return to Jamie's School Dinners," *Channel 4*, September 18, 2006, accessed May 7, 2010 from http://www.channel4.com/life/microsites/J/jamies_school_dinners/index.html.
22. Asmita Naik, "Did Jamie Oliver Really Put School Dinners on the Agenda? An Examination of the Role of the Media in Policy Making," *The Political Quarterly* 79 (2008): 426.
23. Alex Renton, "Jamie Oliver's Ministry of Food Goes to Rotherham," *The Guardian*, October 1, 2008, accessed August 30, 2011, http://www.guardian.co.uk/lifeandstyle/wordofmouth/2008/oct/01/jamie.oliver.ministry.food.
24. "About Jamie Saves Our Bacon," 2008, accessed May 5, 2010, http://www.channel4.com/food/on-tv/jamie-oliver/jamie-saves-our-bacon/jamie-saves-our-bacon-08-12-12_p_1.html.
25. Alex Witchel, "Putting America's Diet on a Diet," *New York Times Magazine*, October 6, 2009, accessed August 30, 2011, http://www.nytimes.com/2009/10/11/magazine/11Oliver-t.html.

26. Jojo Moyes, "The Naked Truth about Celebrity Endorsements," *The Independent*, August 25, 2000, accessed August 30, 2011, http://www.independent.co.uk/news/uk/this-britain/the-naked-truth-about-celebrity-endorsements-710729.html.
27. "Sainsbury's Gives Jamie Oliver a Ticking Off over School Lunches," *London Evening Standard*, September 14, 2006, accessed August 30, 2011, http://www.thisislondon.co.uk/news/article-23366808-sainsburys-gives-jamie-oliver-a-ticking-off-over-school-lunches.do.
28. Mark Sweney, "Jamie Oliver Endorses Sainsbury's 'Higher Welfare' Chicken," *The Guardian*, October 1, 2008, accessed August 29, 2011, http://www.guardian.co.uk/media/2008/oct/01/advertising.oliver.
29. Bill Gorman, "TV Ratings," *TV by the Numbers*, April 24, 2010, accessed August 28, 2011, http://tvbythenumbers.com/2010/04/24/tv-ratings-date-line-leads-nbc-win-as-the-food-revolution-ends-without-a-bang/49579.
30. Associated Press, "W. Virginia Town Shrugs at Being Fattest City," *MSNBC*, November 17, 2008, accessed August 25, 2011, http://www.msnbc.msn.com/id/27697364.
31. "Jamie Oliver's Food Revolution—Episode 6," *Hulu*, April 23, 2010, Accessed March 5, 2012, http://www.hulu.com/watch/144640/jamie-olivers-food-revolution-episode-6
32. Ibid.
33. Walter Gantz, et al., "Food for Thought: Television Advertising to Children in the United States," Kaiser Family Foundation, 2007, accessed August 25, 2011, http://www.kff.org/entmedia/upload/7618.pdf.
34. Toby Miller, *Cultural Citizenship: Cosmopolitanism, Consumerism, and Television in a Neoliberal Age* (Philadelphia: Temple University Press, 2006), 210.
35. Harvey, *A Brief History of Neoliberalism*, 176.
36. Arun Gupta, "How TV Superchef Jamie Oliver's 'Food Revolution' Flunked Out," *AlterNet*, April 8, 2010, accessed August 26, 2011, http://www.alternet.org/food/146354/how_tv_%20superchef_jamie_oliver%27s%20_%27food_revolution%27_flunked_out/?page=entire.
37. Diane Chapeta, "Jamie Oliver Could Use an Education," *Examiner*, March 8, 2010, accessed August 29, 2011, http://www.examiner.com/x-41514-Bakersfield-School-Food-Examiner~y2010m3d22-Jamie-Oliver-could-use-an-education.
38. Kerry Trueman, in discussion with the author, May 2, 2010.

13 The Man and the Cannibal

A Moral Perspective on Eating the Other

Alexander V. Kozin

A recent upsurge of "cannibal" cases in Europe alerts us to the unsettled character of the behavior that used to be confined to tribal cultures and special circumstances. Recently, mass media began to present cannibalism in a new register, as "recreational" or "erotic."[1] Originating in popular culture, this characterization has been shared by jurisprudence, criminology, and socio-legal studies. Despite much attention given to this phenomenon, its cultural meaning remains elusive. Yet, since popular culture influences all of us through significations of cultural artifacts, decoding significations through culturally significant artifacts can illumine the meaning management process that belies a rhetorical analysis from within popular culture.[2] At the same time, there is little expectation that jurisprudence would be interested in identifying the cultural role and function of cannibalism: Cases of cannibalism are extremely rare, and the perpetrators are usually confined to the margins of society. From a criminological perspective, traditional categories, such as "murder," "crime committed under affect," and "psychiatric intervention," suffice to account for what is considered to be a specific manifestation of cannibalistic behavior. Even the most intensely covered European case of cannibalism, the case of Armin Meiwes, known as "Kannibalen von Rotenburg," failed to turn the act of consuming human flesh into a cultural puzzle. Given the illustrative character of the case, I suggest that we take a closer look at its coverage.[3]

The case develops as follows: Two people meet on the Internet. One wants to eat human flesh. The other wants to die and therefore agrees to be eaten under the condition that his new friend kills him first. The men believe that their actions fall outside of criminal law. They sign a written consent and videotape the entire procedure. Their plan goes wrong, however: When the home-made euthanasia fails, an alleged act of mercy turns into an act of murder. The videotape captures the event and, in the case of the accused, delivers a convincing picture of a man behaving as if overwhelmed by frenzy. After much debate around the notion of consent, the first trial in 2004 in the Kassel district court concluded with a guilty verdict for the reasons of "manslaughter with aggravating circumstances." After the case reopened in the district court in Frankfurt in 2006, the judges decided that killing of a forty-three-year-old engineer was indeed murder and sentenced Armin Meiwes to life in prison. The defense pled guilty for killing on request, which the court judged had not been the case, because the explicit request of the victim had not been the sole motive for his killing. Instead, argued the judges, Meiwes had killed his victim for "selfish purposes."

In this regard, the court identified two characteristics of murder: Meiwes had killed to satisfy his sex drive, and, in addition, he had killed to commit another crime defined by the German Landsgericht (German court of higher instance) as "disturbing the peace of the dead." The court also announced that Meiwes was "undoubtedly psychologically unwell" and therefore in need of psychiatric help. At the same time, warned the court, this recommendation did not have to lead to a mitigation of the sentence, because the murderer had at all times been in control of his actions and aware of their criminal nature. He had shown no remorse after the deed, but had instead started looking on the Internet for new victims right away. The court declared that it was its responsibility to protect potential victims, thus declining the defense's request to lower the extraordinary gravity of the offense only because the victim's consent was given repeatedly and explicitly. Otherwise, Meiwes could have been released on parole after serving fifteen years in prison. An appeal to the Supreme Court is expected.

Similar to a number of the "special circumstances" and "special victim" cases, the "Kannibalen von Rotenburg" case showed continuous tension between the moral and the legal, which here, as in a number of other related cases, results in the moral judgment being subsumed under the legal judgment.[4] The fact of suppression often comes out in the most basic explanation of the motive, or some "prime mover." In this case, the prime mover was the presumption of sexual satisfaction, but also the indication that it was the character of the accused that made the difference between a serial and accidental killer, a murder and manslaughter.

In this chapter, I propose that we examine both components—the presumed eroticism of the act of cannibalism and the presumed moral character of the cannibal—that function rhetorically to construct the cultural meaning of cannibalism for the European context today. My investigation is situated between the psychoanalytic-phenomenological perspective, on one side, and literature, on the other. The relation between the two epistemologies is established by their mutual contamination. The question that motivates this study can therefore be formulated as follows: *What is the cultural meaning of cannibalism as a contemporary phenomenon?* Before confronting this question with a theoretic, I offer a short review of select research on cannibalism. Its purpose is to present main trends in the diverse perspectives on the phenomenon.

Academic literature on cannibalism is largely confined to anthropology, and although other disciplines also tackle this subject, the common ground for the majority of the reviewed research is formed by the anthropological presumption that the cannibal is the exotic other. The exotic other is separated from the non-exotic self by means of attributing the "otherwise" to what is his/her own. The "otherwise" is then defined in exotic terms. Often, in line with contemporary sensibilities, the boundaries for exoticism are set in the critical register that reformulates the critique as self-critique, leading to the representation of cannibalism in an apologist fashion. For example, in a study about the Mianmin of New Guinea, Don Gardner writes about "outsiders" who raid villages, abduct women, and kill and consume some of their captives.[5] Gardner explains their drive to cannibalism by the effects of disconnectedness from the home; as a result, the outsiders are prompted to seek a quasi-home by consuming the other, thus making the other's home their own. In a concrete examination of the New Guinean tribe of the Ambowari, Borut Telban presents the reader with a description of the other who believes that when the hunter kills his enemy, the weapon functions "as a means to transfer certain qualities to the hunter and his *kay*."[6] From this perspective, the other becomes the self prior to his consumption. A hunter who partakes of his kill in fact eats himself, his own strength.

This relationship corresponds to the description by Thomas Ernst about the Onabasulu, an African tribe whose members apparently caught, killed, and consumed *hinane* (witches and outsiders) to redress an imbalance created by their murders.[7] With this emphasis, Ernst strengthens the concept of a pre-existent boundary between the eater and the eaten as the divide set by the insiders. It is sufficient for the other to be designated as consumable when he or she is an outsider who dwells outside of the hunter's normative home. Alan Rumsey, too, stresses that some of the New Guinea tribes actually believed that Europeans themselves were cannibals: "The Ku Waru expressions for foreigner [*kewa*] and cannibal [*kewa nuyl*] are almost synonymous."[8] Seeing the seamen eating lard, the cannibals believed that in fact they were consuming human underbelly.

From the reverse perspective, in the case of the Western cannibal, the phenomenon of cannibalism receives a different account. For instance, William Arens presents several historiographic narratives about those instances of cannibalism that occurred under frontier conditions, for example, at sea or in vast unpopulated areas, and involved Westerners.[9] The case of Alexander Pearce, an escaped Australian felon who killed and ate his companions in the bush, is illustrative in this regard. When caught, Pearce led his captors to the mangled remains of his friends, which, according to his compatriots, "the inhuman wretch declared were the most delicious food."[10] The story of Alfred Parker is similar: When lost in the San Juan Mountains in Colorado in the winter, Parker (presumably, for he never admitted of the actual crime) killed and ate his companions. Arens gives a straightforward explanation for those cases: "In less populous parts of the world, such as the American West, conditions not infrequently become precarious, so that men faced imminent starvation."[11] The non-exotic perspective is intriguing in that it portrays cannibalism as an anomaly caused by either extraordinary circumstances or some psychological dysfunction, very much resembling the most recent case of the French cannibal Nicolas Cocaign, who was convicted of murder with aggravating circumstances at a court in Rouen in 2007.[12]

The foregoing studies, albeit limited in number, are nonetheless representative of certain distinct investigative paths. First, there is a tendency to approach cannibalism through the relationship between the self and the other. Second, it is presumed that the other can be identified by establishing certain behavioral boundaries, or limits. Two such limits become immediately apparent. One is formed by the idea of the exotic, whereas the other is formed by the morally vested notion of abnormality. The former boundary presupposes some kind of separation of the self and the home from the other or the alien. The latter draws the line between the normalized self and the abnormal self. The two boundaries come to embody the metaphor of consuming the other as one's self. The separation of the literal meaning from its symbolic interpretation in a metaphor conceptualizes the issue of the other in a multifaceted theme. In this chapter, I attempt to build on three facets of this theme—the exotic other, the insider other, and the metaphoric other—by investigating the meaning of cannibalism as a cultural metaphor, which is active in the European context, in general, and in the European court of law, in particular. I would like to begin with an inquiry into the origin of cannibalism. In this part, I put a special emphasis on the issue of self-formation.

THE CANNIBAL WITHIN

According to Sigmund Freud, cannibalism is the most primordial form among human drives. It is linked to the first, oral phase of the infantile identity defined specifically as "cannibalistic." Freud arrived at this connection when investigating the case of the "Wolf Man," a neurotic patient fearful of being eaten by his father. "He came to me," wrote Freud, "at the level of cannibalism."[13] Although clearly a metaphor, as all metaphors, the psychological perspective on cannibalism inverses the literal, that is, the normal practice of eating what is not one's own by referring to consuming a part of oneself, as in the infant's activity of thumb-sucking, for example. Cannibalism therefore offers itself simultaneously as a biological given and, at the stage of weaning and social enculturation, a symbol of self- and other-differentiation. Nikolas Royle elaborates: "in making cannibalism a defining concept in the psychoanalytic account of identity and in highlighting 'the devouring affection' of the cannibal, Freud eroticizes both the concept and the discourse of cannibalism."[14] The assignation of sexual pleasure to a cannibalistic act is precisely what prevented the judge in the Armin Meiwes case from accepting the previous manslaughter verdict.

Royle's suggestion that Freud indeed assigned to the cannibalistic drive passive sexuality helps us further characterize the phenomenon of cannibalism as uncanny. In his 1919 essay "The Uncanny" (*Das Unheimliche*), Freud explains the nature of the uncanny as what is "something old and familiar that has undergone repression."[15] The double-sided face of the uncanny can be conflictual and create tension between the primordial and immediately proximal, self and other, illegitimate and legitimate, dormant and expressive. Uncanny phenomena reside in the subconscious; they are therefore the phenomena in flux; they are fantastic in both senses, extraordinary and common. The possibility for this coincidence can be attributed to the Freudian view of consciousness: Prompted by the uncanny, consciousness archives everything unfamiliar in the subconscious.[16] The subconscious holds it safe; yet, obedient to the force of imagination, the uncanny seeps into enunciation, an enactment of the tension. The intimate uncanny is a compulsion, albeit a persistent one. It is not sporadic but rudimentary and indispensable. The extraordinary is neurotic, erotic, homicidal.

Interested in the repressed consciousness, that is, the intimate side of the uncanny, Freud downplays its extraordinary potency to determine the social sphere. In a corrective gesture, Bernhard Waldenfels links the uncanny to the phenomenological concept of the alien, or everything unfamiliar, atypical, abnormal. As a limit phenomenon, the alien dwells in the liminal sphere. Waldenfels takes liminality in the Husserlian sense, as *Zwischen*, or new *logos*, an organization that features connecting nodes but lacks centralization.[17] Unlike the uncanny that belongs to the egoistic consciousness, liminality is an intersubjective structure of the social world. In liminality we experience the alien as "accessible in genuine inaccessibility, in the mode of incomprehensibility."[18] This inaccessibility makes the alien a heterogeneous being who emerges from the tenebrous liminality of incomprehension at the empirical divide between the generatively constituted known—customs, values, morals, and rituals—and the unknown, and therefore potentially shocking and terrifying. In sum, cannibalism is an uncanny phenomenon that belongs to the liminal sphere.

This is the point where the Freudian uncanny and the Husserlian alien converge to assist in an investigation of some cultural aspects of cannibalism: Alienation of the self in consciousness is the co-constitutive part of the other-alienation. The constitution of an identity in the self but with the other is not possible without the participation of the uncanny and the alien; and the latter always already carries the trace of cannibalism. The extreme potency of liminal encounters with the self and the other releases the uncanny into acts of imagined violence. Thus created "mythical narratives attempt to give an account of a genesis that is genetically impossible to know, but generatively possible to experience in the generative density of a cultural tradition."[19] This connection leads us to assume that a work of art will possess not just the potential to reflect but also the capacity to generate cultural artifacts.

From this preliminary examination of the origin of cannibalism, we can also deduce that the phenomenon of cannibalism is primordial, on the one hand, and sociocultural, on the other. In both dimensions, the original and derivative, cannibalism is a phenomenon that deals with the self as it participates in identity (character) constitution as a means of symbolic enculturation. This very reason prompts me to examine the cultural function of cannibalism in a work of imagination, in literature. For the specific artifacts, I suggest Daniel Defoe's *Robinson Crusoe* and Thomas Harris's trilogy, *Red Dragon*, *The Silence of the Lambs*, and *Hannibal*.[20] Closely connected in their treatment of cannibalism, these two works settle on the same semiotic continuum, presenting us with two complementary models of constituting cannibalism in and by a cultural practice. Separated by three hundred years and developing their imaginaries in fundamentally different contexts, Defoe and Harris give us an opportunity of conducting a diachronic analysis of narrative representations of cannibalism. Defoe and Harris also allow us to explore the phenomenon of cannibalism contrastively.[21]

UNMAKING THE CANNIBAL

The story of Robinson Crusoe is well known: As an eighteenth-century English castaway on an uninhabited island somewhere off the coast of Chile in the Pacific, Crusoe spent many years alone before he met another human being. The encounter proved to be dramatic: A footprint left in the sand took Crusoe to a cannibal feast. From this point on, the theme of cannibalism forms the moral pinnacle for the protagonist, who is torn between horror and revenge. In this way, Defoe reflects the aforementioned xenological insights that proffer the traumatic effects of the radical encounter with the alien. The ethical side of that encounter manifests itself in the story-telling: After the moral imperative wins over, Crusoe helps a savage cannibal in his escape. The escapee turns into a friend, a companion, and, after some persuading, a fellow Christian. The name of the rescued savage is Friday. When, at the end of the story, an English frigate saves Crusoe from his captivity, Friday follows Crusoe to the civilized world. This narrative is, very briefly, the story of the encounter and the relationship between a Western man and a savage. Although to the contemporary reader the novel may come across as an adventure, at the time of Defoe it was read primarily in the genre of a morality novel. A morality tale is how I suggest that we read *Robinson Crusoe*, focusing on those means that participated in the moral construction of the cannibal in the eighteenth century.

Let us begin with Defoe's description of cannibalism as a practice: "I saw the shore spread with skulls, hands, feet, and other bones of human bodies."[22] Note the emphasis on the human remains. Presented as the byproduct of the man-eating ritual, the remains give rise to Crusoe's imagination. Shortly after, metonymic signification recedes before the practical orientation, the ways of cooking and eating: "there was a place where there had been a fire made, and a circle dug in the earth, like a cockpit, where it is supposed the savage wretches had sat down to their inhuman feastings upon the bodies of their fellow creatures."[23] Unremarkable in itself, the way of cooking becomes uncanny by referring to the consumed flesh. What is being consumed overrides the normality of cooking and eating. The effect is not just horrifying but incomprehensible, too alien to bear without mitigating it by an explicit judgment: "all my apprehensions were buried in the thoughts of such a pitch of inhuman, hellish brutality, and the horror of the degeneracy of human nature; which though I have heard of often, yet I never had so near a view of before."[24] In the subsequent descriptions, Defoe presents multifold reasoning that is carried out in terms of the Christian discourse that juxtaposes two premises: (a) The savages are who they are because of God's will; (b) they don't know better because they are not Christian.

Crusoe senses the ambiguity; it makes him restless. The moral dilemma exceeds the idea of God's will and spills into the need for action, because inaction condones the savage ways, an unacceptable situation for any true Christian: "for night and day, I could think of nothing but how I might destroy some of these monsters in their cruel bloody entertainment, and if possible, save the victim they bring here to destroy."[25] With this attitude, Crusoe expects to connect to the other, less in the name of his salvation and more as a response to the moral imperative. An opportunity presented itself when, during one of the visits by the savages, a prisoner attempts an escape. He outruns his captors and makes it to the part of the island where Crusoe awaits with two loaded guns. He fires and, at the risk of exposing himself, saves a fellow human being. Yet, he is concerned: "How could I sleep knowing that the savage had a hankering stomach after some of the flesh?"[26] The alienness of the saved other is beyond doubt. It belongs to the wild world and therefore demands another kind of salvation by way of religious conversion, that is, de-alienation.

At first, the intended conversion is presented as if stipulated by the reasons of personal safety. In fact, the transition implies different worlds. Inadvertently evoking the basic psychoanalytic procedure, that is, a transference from one part of the self to the other by way of an abnormal act that, in the process, turns into an acceptable one, Crusoe offers Friday a dietary substitute: "in order to bring Friday off from this horrid way of feeding, and from the relish of a cannibal's stomach, I ought to let him taste other flesh."[27] Crusoe's means may appear mechanical if not crude, but they prove effective. Not only does he offer his "savage" a different kind of flesh; he also associates his offer with a different (civilized) way of cooking: "hanging the meat before the fire in a string, letting the meat turn continually."[28] Once again, the metonymic transference causes a metaphoric reaction: The how of cooking comes to be defined by the product to be consumed. Fortunately for Crusoe, Friday liked goat meat, and after much prodding, "he told me at last that he would never eat man's flesh any more."[29] The second-order transference literalizes the symbolic through the Christian ritual of baptism. Soon after saving Friday, Crusoe introduces God into his life, convincing him that there is a higher value: brotherly love and "thou shall not kill." Friday's conversion takes hold: "no longer my friend and companion yearned for human flesh, he became a more devoted Christian than myself."[30]

The transformations that unmade the allegedly inhuman cannibal and made him into a human person take an intricate path. If we map this path with the help of the Semiotic Square, we might find that the first pair of contraries in Crusoe's narratives about Friday gives us "savage" and "human." The savage is wild and unpredictable. The human is cultured and controlled. Explicitly stated in the text, these terms lead us to the underlying pair of signifiers: "self" and "other," with the corresponding modifiers, "comprehensible" and "incomprehensible." The contradictories produce "not-savage" and "not-human." The relations of implications that unite the terms in the square generate the surface terms "the human flesh-eater" and "the non-eater of human flesh." The modifying descriptions for the first unit in this pair embrace such savage ways of cooking as killing humans, chopping the human body into pieces of flesh, eating it raw or barely cooked, leaving the rest of human remains outside of the space designated as "for the consumption of food." In contrast, the second item indicates a civilized way of cooking: raising your food, killing it humanely, roasting flesh with salt and spices, using garnish, smoking and roasting leftovers for later. Diagrammatically, one can represent this relationship as follows:

SAVAGE ↔ HUMAN

[Other]   [Self]

incomprehensible↓   ↓familiar

NOT-HUMAN ↔ NOT-SAVAGE

(consuming human flesh)

Figure 13.1 Semiotic diagram.

Thus configured, the essence of cannibalism signifies the "how" rather than the "what," that is, how food should be obtained and consumed matters more for the distinction between the wild and the civilized worlds than the fact of eating human flesh. In this model, the transition from the one to the other occurs by way of prohibition on three levels: practical, religious, and social. On the level of praxis, the cannibal becomes civilized once he acquires new practical skills of cooking meat. In turn, a civilized way of cooking is linked to the idea of God, who represents the overreaching normative structure and serves to safeguard the civilized fellowship against certain wild temptations by instituting the murder taboo. The fear is not the only thing that sustains the taboo. On the social level, the cannibal becomes humanized when he leaves the world of the other for the self to become a reflective being connected to the other by empathy. For each of the three distinctions, there is an operation that connects doing with becoming and, then, with being.

Attending to food means becoming human, a man of God, who is being one with the other. In Defoe's model, the operation of religious conversion constructs cannibalism as a cultural phenomenon predicated on the external other and the accompanying *habitus* as a complex of practices. The main function of the savage cannibal for Defoe is the meaning of God for being human. At the actual trial of Armin Meiwes there was no reference to the moral divine. The civilized way took over, and the act of eating human flesh, with or without consent, was not an issue at the trial. Nor was the way of cooking it an issue (in fact, it was reported that some flesh was boiled and some was broiled). It seems that the contemporary Anglo-Saxon culture has introduced a qualitatively different perspective on cannibalism that not only moved from the cultural to the subject-centered practice, but also redefined the sense of cannibalism. I would like to address the new sense in the next section by offering a reading of Thomas Harris's *Hannibal* trilogy, which is taken as an exemplar of the contemporary model that undermines, modifies, and complicates the eighteenth-century perspective.

RE-MAKING THE CANNIBAL

Thomas Harris's first novel, *Red Dragon*, introduces Doctor Hannibal Lecter from the perspective of one of his victims, who also happens to be his capturer, detective Will Graham. Immediately, upon the encounter with the cannibal, the reader is confronted with the difference between madness and evil: "Dr. Lecter is not crazy in any common way we think of being crazy. He did some hideous things because he enjoyed them."[31] The description of Lecter's pathology follows. The attending doctors are perplexed because, for a sociopath, he is too educated, too sensitive, too intelligent, and too functional, making him appear somewhat "normal." One deviation from a regular behavioral pattern stood out: According to Graham, "he has no remorse or guilt at all."[32] In other words, he is not and cannot be marked. He eludes diagnosis. No wonder that Graham chooses to follow up on the previous diagnosis with a distinctly mundane characterization: "Lecter is a monster."[33] But even this definition is quickly circumscribed. In a personal conversation with Lecter, Graham calls him "insane" and names passion as one of Lecter's "disadvantages."

Peculiarly, the first novel does not forward cannibalism as the key manifestation of Lecter's deviance, but puts it as one pathological trait among others. Those others include symbolic torture—piercing with arrows, stabbing, cutting—and seemingly gratuitous attacks on the medical personnel in prison. At the same time, from the standpoint of the plot of the book, this omission is not too surprising, considering the secondary status of Lecter's character in *Red Dragon*. After his brief appearance in the beginning of the novel, Lecter barely shows up in the remainder of the book. His intrigue outlives the plot, however: He comes back as a fully outlined character in Harris's second installment, *The Silence of the Lambs*. In this novel Lecter's cannibalistic drive is not only reintroduced but also brought forward full force.

When FBI special agent Clarice Starling is instructed by her supervisor, Jack Crawford, about how to approach Lecter, she receives two messages. One is a description of Lecter's "inhuman actions"; the other is the repeated characterization of these actions: "he is a monster."[34] Doctor Chilton's description of Hannibal Lecter to Starling is somewhat different at first: "he is a pure sociopath and too sophisticated for standard tests."[35] Curiously, for Chilton, Lecter's monstrosity is reduced to his cannibalistic tendencies. During the first encounter between Starling and Lecter, the latter makes an explicit reference to his cannibalistic practices: "A census taker tried to quantify me once. I ate his liver with some fava beans and a big Amarone."[36] At the same time, he refuses to take his psychopathology for the symptom of eating other men. When Starling proffers an explanation of his abnormality, Lecter objects: "You can't reduce me to a set of influences . . . Can you stand to say I'm evil?"[37] It is hard for the reader to confirm or disconfirm this self-diagnosis. Hannibal's extraordinary, almost superhuman abilities disallow such an interpretation: Drawing Venice from memory, passionately listening to Glenn Gould, quoting Marcus Aurelius—all these cultural indices elevate rather than diminish Lecter. His monstrosity emerges as nothing less than sublime.

In comparison to the savage, who is excessively uncultured, Lecter is excessively civilized and impossibly cultured. He lives for delicacy and taste. In his prison cell, Lecter keeps various cooking books and periodicals—for example, his favorite is *The Joy of Cooking*, a title that clearly eroticizes the activity of eating. When talking to Starling, Lecter continuously gives her lessons in exquisite cuisine: "Dumas tells us that the addition of a crow to bouillon in the fall, when the crow has fattened on juniper berries, greatly improves the color and flavor of stock."[38] The contrast with his inmates and the rest of the psychopaths collected by the Quantico database is startling: If the others kill out of rage, Hannibal may kill out of an excessive sense of politeness. In comparison to the wild savage, who needs the other for sustenance, Lecter kills the other to reinforce the rules of being with the other, or otherness, rather than the other way round, as in isolating the self for the other. For him, the other is but the means to an end that lies outside of his self-interests. It is on this note that the encounter with Hannibal-the-Cannibal in *The Silence of the Lambs* ends.

The third novel reintroduces Hannibal as the main character, along with Starling, who is by now a seasoned FBI operative. In *Hannibal*, Lecter, who earlier escaped from a mental institution, is being hunted by Virgil Mason, a disabled multimillionaire and the sole survivor of Lecter's deeds. In turn, Starling's counterpart is Chief Investigator Pazzi, an Italian detective, who hopes to reap a reward from Mason for Lecter's apprehension. The four characters form an interdependent relationship that expands the previously established theme of cannibalism. All of them are hunters, with Lecter emerging as the super-hunter. Notably, their motivations for hunting differ: While Mason is Lecter's ex-food, that is, he is hunting him for revenge, Pazzi, who is hunting Lecter for money, is his fast food. Starling, however, is neither. Her objective is justice, a higher goal, something Lecter respects and therefore accepts. Personalizing food narrows down the range of symbolic interpretations of cannibalism. The last novel is evolutionary in this respect; it also tends toward a more humanized, i.e., a more medicalized, psychologized, and thus mundane, causal perspective.

In the third novel, Hannibal is no longer a prophet with a grisly past. The evil of his deeds unfolds retroactively. The others continue to view him as both a sociopath and a monster: "there is no consensus in the psychiatric community that Lecter should be termed a man . . . He has long been regarded by his professional peers in psychiatry as something entirely Other. For convenience they term him a 'monster.'"[39] This monstrous Other lives in Florence now. He holds a prestigious scholarly position as the curator at Palazzo Vecchio, which he obtained by eliminating his predecessor and employing his uncanny linguistic ability: He speaks Tuscan, a difficult Italian dialect, virtually without an accent. This ability is one of many that indicate Lecter's superhuman nature. It also points to a new role for the home/alien continuum, the "alien foreigner." In Italy, Lecter feels more at home than in other, less exotic habitats. Here, he no longer needs to attend to the home and its rules. Intriguingly, in contrast to his mission of upholding civilized ways of being with others by killing off deviants, it appears that the means for fulfilling this mission are largely derived from the savage world.

Lecter's relationship to this world is retained through the recovery of the primitive or secondary senses, such as the sense of smell: "he sometimes entertained the illusion that he could smell with his hands, his arms and cheeks, that odor suffused him. That he could smell with his face and his heart."[40] Another connection to the savage world is a symbolic displacement of the actual. Lecter does not just eat people, he devours their traumas: "he eats their confusion, their shame."[41] Lecter claims that the Devil devours a particular kind of sinner: Judases. For an actual example of a Judas, Lecter selects Detective Pazzi. Pazzi, like his ancestors, betrays his master, namely, justice. Working for Virgil Mason, who sees himself as Jesus, makes Pazzi a candidate for the ultimate betrayal because Lecter intends to force him into disclosing the name behind his contract. In the meantime, an avid student of the Bible, Mason takes upon himself the task of the last judgment, an opportunity to kill Lecter and thus atone himself. Years earlier, Lecter had drugged Mason and made him eat his own tongue and cut his own face, leaving Mason to die. However, Mason survived and now lives to avenge his disability in a reversal of justice; he is raising a horde of vicious hogs waiting to devour Lecter alive.

It is not Mason, however, but Starling who catches Lecter. The connection between the two people is not clearly outlined. However, similarly to Lecter, Starling pursues a noble cause. But it is not in the nebulous sphere that she finds Lecter. She finds him in taste: "Taste in all things was a constant for Dr. Lecter."[42] For Lecter, taste is where the symbolic and the metaphoric acts coalesce. Lecter wants to taste Starling (her becoming) and then use her space (the memories of being with her) to reverse time and displace his own childhood trauma. Apparently, Lecter was a son of a noble and wealthy Lithuanian family that dated back to the twelfth century. His parents were killed and their estate was destroyed and pillaged at the end of World War II by the retreating German troops. Only Lecter and a few other children (including his sister) survived. They were hiding in the barn at the estate where, after the Eastern front fell, a few Nazi deserters found them. The soldiers held the children captive and, after they ran out of food, began to eat everything they could find: first a deer shot with an arrow and then the children. Lecter's sister Mischa was among the eaten. This traumatic childhood experience is how Lecter's cannibalism originated.

The transference of his childhood trauma onto Starling completes Lecter's reverse transformation from the inhuman into the human. Saved by Starling from Mason's cannibal hogs, he purifies his own deviance while he is kept captive tied to a ladder inside the hog stall, where Mason's retribution appeared more imminent than ever. Ironically for Lecter, the hogs, who were made cannibals by his enemy, help Lecter regain his human self as they end up devouring Mason. The suppression of his own cannibalistic instinct happens for Lecter in the final act of transference when he literally feeds "impolite" Mr. Krendell from the Justice Department to Starling. In this way, he helps Starling to transfer her anger, and, by saving his muse from her trauma, he reconciles his own conflict. Two ways of healing

Starling are employed simultaneously: through love, a Christian legacy, and through the operation of symbolic displacement, a Freudian legacy. Despite the presence of other kinds of madness, the psychiatric interpretation and the moral theme provide the preferred modes of taking the problematic phenomenon to its resolution. In the background, the remains of the savage consciousness are barely visible. If we construct a semiotic square analogous to the one made for Defoe's *Robinson Crusoe*, we arrive at a distinctly different configuration.

The first pair of contraries for Hannibal Lecter is "monster" and "human." The monster is not just terrifying; he is wildly superhuman. In contrast, the human is emphatically ordinary. The foundational pair of signifiers for monster and human is then not the self and the other but the "ordinary" and the "extraordinary," respectively. The corresponding set of contradictories produces "not-monster" and "not-human." The relations of implications generate a pair similar to the one that we identified with Defoe: "the flesh-eater" and "the non-eater of human flesh." The modifying descriptions for the two units are subtly contrastive, however: In his way of eating, Lecter differs from the savage in that he both eats his victims raw and cooks elaborate meals out of them. Thus, he presents a range of eating practices that Friday does not possess. Another essential difference: Lecter eats his victims alive. The core significance of this difference lies in its motivation. Dr. Lecter eats human flesh because he enjoys what chewing a live human stands for—reinstitution of respect and nobility—so his reasons are not as pragmatic as those of Friday, although Defoe leaves little doubt that the savage enjoyed his human flesh, too. In contrast, a human does not eat human flesh because he doesn't kill humans out of hunger. A taboo and a punishable offense, this outlook becomes a value when it comes to establish and serve the distinction between a monster and a human. The following diagram emphasizes the main connections from the foregoing interpretation:

MONSTER↔ HUMAN

extraordinary↓   ↓ordinary

NOT-HUMAN↔NOT-MONSTER

[evil]   [good]

(murdering a human being)

Figure 13.2   Semiotic diagram.

Furthermore, in Thomas Harris's model of cannibalism, the terms that uphold the "monster-human" distinction are not "God" and "no-God," but "good" and "evil." An evil cannibal differs from the savage cannibal not because of his lack of control over the primordial pleasure drives but by his excess, hence, the superhuman abilities of Hannibal Lecter (strength, intellect, sense). Evil does not need to contain itself; it is the nature of evil to spill out. In comparison to the ungodly ways that can only be transformed, evil can only be reversed. In order for this to happen, evil must refuse its metaphysical origin and become a matter of deviance. In turn, the latter can be attributed to social as well as psychological facts, such as inadequate socialization or psychological instability. In Lecter's case, the origin of cannibalism lies in a deeply residing trauma. It comes from his childhood by way of the regressive transference of empathy. Having witnessed his sister being eaten by the cannibalistic soldiers, he transfers his empathy toward his sister in justice. Other displacements follow. Lecter reverses these displacements by saving Starling, a person he loves, from the metaphorical cannibal. By transferring the origin of his trauma, he redeems and simultaneously re-makes himself. On one level, cannibalism as a cultural phenomenon is constructed on the operation of psychotherapeutic reversal internal to one's self. On another level, childhood trauma may be a more comforting explanation for evil than to conclude that there is no explanation.

CONCLUSION

Cannibalism is a complex social phenomenon. The objective of this study was to capture some of this complexity as it pertains to culture approached from the historical perspective. There are several findings worth being presented at this point. First, as Freud suggests, born at infancy, the phenomenon of cannibalism should be considered as grounded in oral fixation. Only when socialization separates the self from the other can the drive of eating the other be reordered, albeit not completely. The trace of the cannibalistic uncanny persists in the mode of self-alienation that characterizes not only our everyday experience that centers on ourselves but also our relations with others, and, specifically, the alien. It seeps into fictional worlds as well, structuring and defining cultural experiences. An examination of the cultural function of cannibalism in two fictional worlds—Daniel Defoe's *Robinson Crusoe* and Thomas Harris's *Hannibal* trilogy—disclosed the phenomenon of cannibalism in two modalities: (a) as what can be discovered in the other; (b) as what can be reawakened in the self; hence, the uncanny persistence of the theme of cannibalism and its rhetorical effects. In this respect, the practice of eating the other showed itself to be of paramount importance to the rhetorical construction of culture as a normative complex, while culture itself shows itself to be a semiotic manifold that appropriates the phenomenon of cannibalism toward drawing symbolic divisions within, around, and outside of one's cultural home.

NOTES

1. I wish to thank Katharina Draheim, whose expert assistance in collecting materials for this chapter was indispensable for its realization.
2. Barry Brummett, *Rhetoric in Popular Culture*, 2nd ed. (Thousand Oaks, CA: Sage, 2006).
3. All the case-relevant information was collected at http://www.stern.de/politik/deutschland/kannibale-von-rotenburg-meiwes-traeumt-weiter-vom-menschenschlachten-556398.html.
4. The so-called "special circumstances" transpire in a wide variety of cases in which some ritualistic and, at the same time, illegal means or actions have been utilized (e.g., ritualistic castration or stoning). These cases tend to introduce a law within the juridical law by ritualizing an adequate response to a criminal violation in some morally preferential practice.
5. Don Gardner, "Anthropophagy, Myth, and the Subtle Ways of Ethnocentrism," in *The Anthropology of Cannibalism*, ed. Lawrence Goldman (Westport, CT: Bergin and Carvey, 1999), 40.
6. Borut Telban, *Dancing through Time: A Sepik Cosmology* (Oxford: Clarendon, 1998), 676.
7. Thomas Ernst, "Onabasulu Cannibalism and the Moral Agents of Misfortune," in *The Anthropology of Cannibalism*, ed. Lawrence Goldman (Westport, CT: Bergin and Carvey, 1999), 150.
8. Alan Rumsey, "The White Man as Cannibal in the New Guinea Highlands," in *The Anthropology of Cannibalism*, ed. Lawrence Goldman (Westport, CT: Bergin and Carvey, 1999), 107.
9. William Arens, *The Man-Eating Myth: Anthropology and Anthropophagy* (Oxford: Oxford University Press, 1979).
10. Ibid., 149.
11. Ibid., 150.
12. The aggravating circumstances included torturing, brutally killing, and eating his cellmate. See http://www.bbc.co.uk/news/10410286.
13. Sigmund Freud, *Three Case Histories* (New York: Collier Books, 1963), 253.
14. Nikolas Royle, *The Uncanny* (Manchester: Manchester University Press, 2003), 208.
15. Sigmund Freud, *The Uncanny* (London: Penguin Books, 1919/2003), 73.
16. Sigmund Freud, *Group Psychology and the Analysis of the Ego* (New York: Bantam Books, 1960).
17. Bernhard Waldenfels, *Order in the Twilight* (Athens: Ohio University Press, 1996).
18. Edmund Husserl, *Zur Phänomenologie der Intersubjektivität. Texte aus Dem Nachlass. Zweiter Teil: 1921–1928, Husserliana Vol. XV*, ed. Iso Kern (The Hague: Martinus Nijhoff, 1973), 319.
19. Anthony Steinbock, *Home and Beyond: Generative Phenomenology after-Husserl* (Evanston: Northwestern University Press, 1995), 219.
20. I exclude the last book of the tetralogy, *Hannibal Rising* (2007), from the analysis as inessential to the narrative line of the preceding three volumes.
21. Importantly, both fictional worlds are taken as exemplars, or exemplary manifestations of the actual, accessible to a singular consciousness in a modified fashion.

22. Daniel Defoe, *Robinson Crusoe* (1719; London: Penguin Books, 2003), 130.
23. Ibid., 130–31.
24. Ibid., 130–31.
25. Ibid., 133.
26. Ibid., 164.
27. Ibid., 166.
28. Ibid., 168.
29. Ibid., 168.
30. Ibid., 172.
31. Thomas Harris, *Red Dragon* (London: Corgi Books, 1982), 53.
32. Ibid., 53.
33. Ibid., 53.
34. Thomas Harris, *The Silence of the Lambs* (New York: St. Martin's Press, 1988), 6.
35. Ibid., 11.
36. Ibid., 24.
37. Ibid., 21.
38. Ibid., 224–25.
39. Thomas Harris, *Hannibal* (New York: Delacorte Press, 2001), 136–37.
40. Ibid., 187.
41. Ibid., 161.
42. Ibid., 225.

14 On Establishing a More Authentic Relationship with Food

From Heidegger to Oprah on Slowing Down Fast Food

Kara Shultz

WE EAT, THEREFORE WE ARE: THE PHENOMENON OF FOOD IN EVERYDAY LIFE

Without a doubt, food shapes us—our bodies, our well-being, and our minds. Eighteenth-century French gastronome Jean-Anthelme Brillat-Savarin's reputation was revitalized in the twenty-first century when Chairman Kaga, of the reality television competition series *Iron Chef*, resurrected his famous saying: "Tell me what you eat and I'll tell you who you are" ("Dis-moi ce que tu manges, je te dirai ce que tu es").[1] The juxta-positioning illustrated in Kaga's appropriation of Brillat-Savarin's words, popularizes the past in a present hyper-mediated sense and exemplifies a contemporary discursive move toward restructuring our relationship with food in modern life.

Throughout history food has always played a central role in human existence. Reay Tannahill, the author of *Food in History*, argues that food has always been essential to human existence and that an examination of the role of food in human history reveals the political divisiveness of food in human life. "Food remains as essential—and as divisive—as it has ever been, and the comfortable belief that the world's diet is no longer at the mercy of nature and human ignorance is not as solidly founded as it might seem."[2] There can be no question that the food we eat and the way we talk about it play a significant role in constituting who we are and how we relate to one another. In an existentialist move, one might go so far as to say, "We eat and therefore we are."

Ontologically, one might argue that food is essential to being and that to understand the meaning of human life one can simply examine the role food plays in shaping human existence. Carlo Petrini, the founder of the Slow Food movement, asserts the absolute centrality of the role of food, a centrality, he argues, that has been lost and must be reclaimed "if one wishes to interpret—and perhaps influence—the dynamics that underlie our society and our world."[3] In other words, if we understand the role of food in our lives we can consciously seek to change the world through reestablishing what Heidegger would call a more "authentic" relationship with the food we consume.

In 1927 Martin Heidegger wrote his treatise *Being and Time* in an ontological attempt to address the mystery of human existence—to ask questions about the one being who questions the nature of being. Central to Heidegger's thinking on the question of human existence is the concept of *Dasein*, which translates as *being-there*. "*Dasein* is an entity which, in its very being, comports itself understandably towards that being."[4] *Being-there* can be explored only through examining our *average-everydayness*. For Heidegger, one can understand existence by examining the ways in which one engages with the world through everyday existence, thereby "letting that which shows itself from itself show itself from itself."[5]

What is more *average-everydayness* than our consumption of food? To understand the role that food plays in modern life, to let it show itself from itself, one might examine popular discourse about food. In the past ten years there has been an upsurge of interest in the subject of food within the US. Two cable channels (*Food Network* and *Cooking Channel*) feed viewers' desire to consume the subject 24/7 through entertaining food contests and diverting celebrity chefs. Popular documentaries such as Morgan Spurlock's *Supersize Me* and Robert Kenner's *Food, Inc.* expose the devastating consequences of food consumption in an increasingly corporatized food economy. Thousands of books on the subject of food have been published in the past ten years. In addition to the long-standing tradition of publishing guides to cooking, planting and foraging food, and the numerous inducements to diet and get healthy, there has been an explosion of expositions on food safety, explorations of food politics, and interrogations on the sustainability of our current food practices. And then there is the attention paid to food via the mass-mediated, dieting confessions of the iconic Oprah.

In May of 2010 Oprah Winfrey, undoubtedly one of the most influential celebrities of all time,[6] after giving us Dr. Phil (her panacea for mental ills) and Dr. Oz (her remedy for physical ills) unveiled her newest guru to her legions of dedicated fans. "I have come across something so profound that I think [to everyone] who's ever felt [her weight is] a losing battle, here is an opportunity to win," she said. Her discovery was an author by the name of Geneen Roth. Roth has made her living since 1989 selling books—with titles like *Why Weight: A Guide to Ending Compulsive Eating*, *When You Eat at the Refrigerator, Pull Up a Chair*, *Breaking Free from Emotional Eating*—and delivering workshops all echoing the ongoing theme that dieting inevitably leads to binging. Roth and other advocates of the anti-diet, intuitive-eating movement argue that the only way to lose weight long-term is to reconstruct a healthier relationship with food. While Roth has rocketed to popularity as a result of being singled out as Oprah's latest guru, she is clearly one segment of a much wider movement exploring the ways in which, in our industrialized world, humans are increasingly distanced from food.

For Oprah, reading Roth's 2010 *Women, Food and God* had "blown the door off" of her tumultuous relationship with food. Oprah explained that Roth's book allowed her to establish a more authentic relationship with food through calling her to examine the ways in which the temporary substitutions of comfort foods was inhibiting her relationship to God. Roth writes: "Everything we believe about love, fear, transformation, and God is revealed in how, when and what we eat. When we inhale Reese's peanut butter cups when we are not hungry, we are acting out an entire world of hope and hopelessness, of faith and doubt, of love and fear."[7]

Roth is just one example of several prominent authors inviting us to raise our consciousness about eating more mindfully, more slowly, more responsibly, more conscientiously, more cleanly, more sustainably, and more intuitively. Some advocate conscious eating, some mindfulness, some slow food, some prayer, and some clean eating. But all are united in inviting readers to examine their relationship with food as a pathway to connecting with both their inner self and the world around them. Basically, these authors' arguments might be condensed into a single message—we must slow down and pay more attention to the food we eat or we will suffer the terrible consequences of our toxic food environment.

In this chapter I examine four books: (1) Geneen Roth's 2010 *Women, Food and God*, (2) Thich Nhat Hanh and Dr. Lilian Cheung's 2010 *Savor: Mindful Eating, Mindful Life*, (3) Tosca Reno's 2009 *The Eat-Clean Diet Recharged*, and (4) Carlo Petrini's 2007 *Slow Food Nation*, as being connected around a theme of raising our consciousness about what we eat and the impact it has on our bodies and the world around us. Each of these texts clearly attempts what Heidegger terms "a call to conscience."

For Heidegger, history, technicity, and discourse unfolded a machination that caused us to abandon *being*. The only resolution is through coming to know ourselves, which involves a clearing of the machinations in order to reestablish a more authentic relationship through listening to our conscience. In this chapter I examine the proselytizations of these self-help, anti-diet, conscious-eating lifestyle authors through the phenomenological thinking of Martin Heidegger and his philosophy of self-mindfulness.

Heidegger's notion of *Dasein* (being-there) is complicated by the possibility of different modes or ways of being. *Dasein* can be (1) unaware and undifferentiated or (2) aware but uncaring and therefore inauthentic or (3) mindfully embracing potential in anticipatory authenticity. According to Heidegger *Dasein* is the condition that makes authenticity and inauthenticity possible. Each individual has the choice to define themselves in terms of the ideological commitments of the mass culture or to embrace a more unique and ultimately more authentic self. "The Self of everyday Dasein is the *they-self*, which we distinguish from the *authentic* Self—that is, from the Self which has been taken hold of in its own way."[8] In this chapter I interrogate the potential of these rhetorical texts to solicit, perhaps even liberate, authenticity in our relationship to food in contemporary life.

DAS MAN: MODERNITY, INDUSTRIALIZATION, AND THE AGRI-ECONOMY

A vast majority of the non-cookbook food publications on the market today decry the "toxic food environment" manufactured by the corporate food industry. Tosca Reno warns her readers that "Food corporations see people like me and you as a free-for-all market of hungry consumers upon whose backs they would like very much to profit."[9] Carlo Petrini presages that industrial farming and globalization are perpetuating an "ecological bankruptcy," which is in effect "mortgaging the future." Reno discloses the "chemical warfare" on our food, decrying that "our food has literally been doused with chemicals at every stage of its life from seed to consumption."[10] Pollution, soil death, scarring of landscape, reducing energy sources, loss of biological and cultural diversity, and greenhouse gases are, they argue, the ultimate and inevitable consequences of our continuing on the mindless path we are blindly following.

Wynne Wright and Gerad Middendorf examine the challenges of our changing global food systems: "As we migrated away from the farm and the dinner table through the twentieth century, our consciousness of food likewise migrated away from the biological and social basis of production."[11] Utilizing efficient but unsustainable practices, the corporate food industry manufactures and markets "artificial," "counterfeit," "anti-foods," which are so homogenized and far removed from their "natural" state that they are but a simulacrum of "genuine food" placed on the shelves of "the soul-destroying supermarkets."[12]

However, in recent years with the threat of global warming looming, there is a growing awareness that we are paying the price for a diet of affluence, not just economically but in terms of both our personal and our planet's health. What makes writing and thinking about food so difficult is that food is omnipresent in our daily lives, not just as sustenance for life but as a reflection of our identity. Yet the food we eat is inextricably connected to political and economic realities. "Food influences our lives as a relevant marker of power, cultural capitol, class, gender, ethnic and religious identities."[13] Recent books on food attempt to raise readers' consciousness about the moral repercussions of eating animals,[14] the health consequences of genetically engineered foods,[15] and the dilemmas inherent in the abundant and convenient diet marketed in advanced industrialized society and its contributions to catastrophic climate change.[16]

One might argue that the corporate food industry, with its commitments to production in spite of the costs to human well-being and ecological and cultural diversity, represents the nameless, faceless *They* described in Heidegger's theory of being. *Das Man*, which has been translated as *the One* or *the They*, refers to the authority the collective society wields in pro-scribing, shaping, and dominating public opinion. "We take pleasure and enjoy ourselves as *they* take pleasure; we read, see, and judge about litera-ture and art as *they* see and judge."[17] Beings are necessarily, according to Heidegger, "Beingamongst-one-other."[18] The influence of *das Man* to con-stitute reality, to frame and shape *being*, results in what Heidegger terms "*thrown-ness.*" When we unquestioningly submit our individual sense of being to *das Man* we are condemned to live an undifferentiated life.

FAST FOOD AND FEEDING THE UNDIFFERENTIATED MASSES

We live modern life at a hectic pace often resulting in mindlessness. A fast-food nation,[19] we eat on the run, grabbing, microwaving, and pop-ping open cans. The convenience, speed, and availability of these homog-enized foods, which bear little resemblance to their origins (a Chicken McNugget has very little in common with the chicken it is meant to simulate), produce unknowledgeable, uninformed, and undifferentiated beings. Petrini warns "The obliteration of gastronomic knowledge in the United States has been total, and its effects on public health are rapidly making themselves felt."[20]

In a Heideggerian sense the undifferentiated person is unaware of the influence that others have upon their behavior, their choices. The undif-ferentiated being moves through life as an automaton, a puppet—uncon-sciously responding to the ideological commitments of *das Man*. Mindless individuals, what Heidegger calls the "*undifferentiated*," are unaffected, unquestioning, and unaware of the effect others (*das Man*) have upon his or her life. The *undifferentiated* being fails to recognize his or her *thrown-ness*, fails to take responsibility for his or her existence, and thereby ulti-mately fails to listen to his or her conscience.

The effortlessness by which we receive the bountiful foods marketed in the industrialized world has resulted, the four authors argue, in a distinc-tive lack of appreciation for the life, the work, the sacrifice of the food we consume. For these advocates of conscious eating our attitudes toward fast food exemplify the *undifferentiated* individual exemplifying her own *thrown-ness* as she purchases prepared, supersized foods preserved by a lengthy list of ingredients she cannot pronounce and that her grandmother would not recognize, and then ingests them automatically with overly sim-plified hand-to-bag and food-to-mouth repetitive and thoughtless motions without care as she drives her car down the road.[21] The undifferentiated masses imbibe the fatty, sugary, salty, addictive fast foods produced by the corporate food industry, forgoing the growing, chopping, and slow cook-ing of food.

FAT OF THE LAND: DIETING AND INAUTHENTICITY

The authors of a multitude of popular texts point to our omnivore's dilemma and warn that the corporate food industry is quite literally killing us.[22] The world's perilous state of health is due to the systems by which food is produced and consumed. Eating the overly homogenized, chemically doused, artificially flavored food of the corporate food industry is responsible for a multitude of health problems, including, they argue, obesity.

Food is increasingly constructed in popular discourse as a problem. One cannot turn on the television, open a magazine, surf the net, or listen to the radio without hearing something connected to the "obesity epidemic." According to the World Health Organization website "Obesity has reached epidemic proportions globally, with more than 1 billion adults overweight—at least 300 million of them clinically obese—and is a major contributor to the global burden of chronic disease and disability." Too much food is not necessarily a good thing. Hanh and Cheung refer to the crisis of the modern "obseigenic" food environment,[23] where we are bombarded with messages encouraging us to eat more and move less.

Citizens of industrialized nations living in the land of plenty find themselves caught up in a never-ending battle to lose weight. Consider Weight Watchers, Jenny Craig, Nutrisystem, Slim Fast, the Atkins diet, the Zone diet, Susan Powter, Richard Simmons, the cabbage soup diet, the grapefruit diet, the rotation diet, Fen-phen, Redux, Meridia, Aspartame, Splenda, Xilotol, Olestra—the list of the methods that Americans have tried to lose the excess pounds goes on and on.

The *inauthentic*, unlike the *undifferentiated*, recognizes his or her own *thrown-ness* but reacts by only substituting another type of thrown-ness. The inauthentic self cares about things because others proscribe it. "Normally, we treat things in the world as imposing their meanings upon us: this is important *because it is a job* or *because it is cold* or *because it is what my family wants* or *because it is a law*." [24] However, a consequence of living according to the dictates of *the They* is a disowning of one's own self.

As a nation we are obsessed with our bodies. The ideal of slenderness and the subsequent anti-fat ideology, conditioned by and reinforced in the mass marketplace, shape our desires. In spite of (and some might argue somewhat as a result of) our growing obsession with weight and the shrinking standards for bodily perfection, the average body has continued to become progressively heavier—producing a contradictory and paradoxical state between our slim ideals and heavy realities. These contradictions create for many an unrelenting discomfort with their bodies and a desperate need to conform to the normalizing constraints so very much a part of the dominant symbolic landscape.

According to the recently revised, if somewhat arbitrarily selected, federal height and weight standards, ninety-seven million Americans (55 percent of the population) are now deemed to be "overweight." Perpetuating the widespread and institutionalized belief that fat is bad, both in terms of aesthetics and health, a recent article in *Harper's* laments "obesity" as a national "epidemic," which is "spinning out of control," suggesting an estimated cost to the US in the hundreds of billions by 2020, "making HIV look, economically, like a bad case of the flu."[25] Within American society eating had become a shameful experience, physical activity a monotonous chore, and dieting a cultural rite of passage. A powerful stigma, directed both inward in the form of self-loathing ("I hate my thighs") and self-flag-ellation ("I can't have that, it looks fattening") and directed outward in the form of prejudice ("No more fat chicks!") and ridicule ("Did you hear the one about the fat guy . . ."), has become firmly entrenched in American cultural discourse. Fat, therefore, must be reviled, worked off, and atoned for. Prejudice against fat people is persistently justified by the notion that if the fat person just tried harder, just indulged less, he or she might become a thin person. Fat people are pushed to the margins of mainstream society. Longing to be thin while becoming increasingly fat, the American society is caught in what cultural critic Laura Kipnis argues is a site of deep social contradiction. "Fat is something a significant percentage of the American public bears not only undisguised contempt for but also, in many cases, an intense, unexamined, visceral disgust."[26] Roth explains her own experience with the roller coaster of dieting:

> Since adolescence, I'd gained and lost over a thousand pounds. I'd been addicted to amphetamines for four years and to laxatives for two years. I'd thrown up, spit up, fasted and tried every diet possible, from the All-Grape-Nuts diet to the One-Hot-Fudge-Sundae-a-Day diet to Atkins, Stillman and Weight Watchers. I'd been anorexic—spending almost two years weighing eighty pounds—and I'd been quite overweight. Mostly overweight. My closet was stuffed with eight different sizes of pants, dresses and blouses. Crazed with self-loathing and shame . . . [27]

In spite of considerable financial and emotional investment, it is estimated that most diets fail, with 98 percent of dieters either not losing weight or not maintaining weight loss.

Moreover, Americans continue to gain weight: In the past decade, the average American adult has gained eight pounds. Failing to lose time and again, many have come to view food as something they love and something they hate. Conflicted and struggling to lose weight, many morbidly obese Americans underwent Roux-en-Y gastric bypass surgery. The surgical pro-cedure separates the stomach into two sections, creating a new small pouch the size of a thumb, and bypasses the small intestines. The result is that patients are restricted in the quantity of food they eat, do not experience hunger as a result of the restricted eating, and do not absorb calories as before. RNY patients initially lose 80 percent of their excess weight and maintain 50 percent of the weight loss over time. As a result, the number of gastric bypass surgeries have been steadily increasing, up more than 600 percent between 1993 and 2003.[28] Weight loss surgery is part of a perhaps inevitable progression to control our bodies in the out-of-bounds context created by the industrialization, transportation, and commercialization of the food supply, which provides an abundance of fatty, sugary, and salty foods that are often stripped of nutrients during factory processing.

The works by Hanh and Cheung, Petrini, Roth, and Reno are part of a spate of new books encouraging Americans to change their lifestyles by rethinking their relationship with food. The argument is that processed foods are nutrient-deficient and highly caloric, while plant-based, unprocessed foods such as whole grains, legumes, and fresh produce, which are rich in fiber and nutrients needed for a healthy body, are increasingly difficult and expensive to obtain. Their argument is not a new one. Brillat-Savarin in 1826 explored the connection between food and health in general and food and obesity in particular, writing: "The second of the chief causes of obesity is the floury and starchy substances which man makes the prime ingredients of his daily nourishment. As we have said already, all animals that live on farinaceous food grow fat willy-nilly; and man is no exception to the universal law."[29] However, the vast number of books being marketed today that encourage "conscious eating" as a way to lose weight is astonishing. A quick search of Amazon.com produces 786 hits for mindful eating and 1,293 hits for clean eating.

THE CALL TO CONSCIENCE: ANXIETY, AUTHENTICITY, AND THE ROLE OF INVITATIONAL RHETORIC

Individuals fed up with a toxic food environment and the soul-destroying inevitability of failing at dieting experience anxiety. According to Heidegger anxiety makes authenticity or mattering possible. An individual can become resolute in his or her own concerns separated from the normative concerns mandated by *the They*. The act of authenticity is ultimately a resolve to hold oneself open to value, to meaning. In his essay, "The Self as Resolution: Heidegger, Derrida and the Intimacy of the Question of the Meaning of Being," John Russon investigates the nature of authentic selfhood, specifically addressing the notion of authenticity as "anticipatory resoluteness" in order to demonstrate that the question of the meaning of being is the most intimate question in human life.

> Authenticity becomes possible here, because this mood of anxiety has a unique capacity to disclose something about our existence. In this anxiety where nothing matters, what is on display is precisely that "mattering" matters; i.e., it is how we care about the world that lets things be significant. Anxiety, in other words, discloses "care" as the fundamental meaning of our reality, and in so doing, it discloses the

way in which my reality and the reality of my world are interwoven. Authenticity is the distinctive stance in which I own up to this, my role as "caregiver," so to speak, of my world: it is uniquely *up to me* to take my world up in a meaningful way.[30]

The individual can then quite literally listen to his or her own conscience as a way of resolving to be one's own self.

The authentic self accepts both being and nothing-ness, recognizing that we exist and therefore we will also cease to exist. According to Heidegger we are always *beingtowards-death*. The ability to recognize this ultimate possibility opens up the potential for a transformation of the authentic self—a process of being true to one's own self, of living life according to one's own being.

Should one pay attention to the discourse on the hazards of our current food practices one cannot help but feel extreme anxiety personally and politically. Thus the timing and conditions are "ripe" for change. In response the group of authors examined in this chapter, whom I will label collectively as "conscious eating advocates," argue that we must slow down, eat clean, and stop, calm, and rest the mind. We must become more mindful through practices such as meditation, shamatha, and prayer. Petrini presents a compelling and eloquent argument for the kind of radical action required: "Food and its production must regain the central place that they deserve among human activities, and we must reexamine the criteria that guide our action . . . This situation demands much more than simple change, of course: it demands a radical change in mentality, more complexity of thought, and more humility and a greater sense of responsibility toward nature."[31] This anxiety, according to Heidegger, ruptures a space, a potential for opening ourselves to the transformative possibilities of authenticity. However, the role of rhetoric in the formulation of authenticity remains a matter of some disagreement.

In Heidegger's major work—*Being and Time*—his exploration of rhetoric is limited to a single sentence. In 2007 Susan Zickmund explored a recent translation of Heidegger's 1925 Winter Semester course on *Plato's Sophist* in attempting to understand the possibility for rhetoric to play a positive role in fostering authenticity. According to Zickmund, Heidegger uses the term "deliberation" as synonymous with rhetoric.[32] For Heidegger deliberation is the way in which the phronetic or prudent nature of *Dasein*'s insight is made manifest. Deliberation can lead one to being resolved to act according to an individual conscience. Deliberation as the foundation for decision-making involves one in the act of *being-together-as-speaking-together*. Thus the role of rhetoric in *being* lies in its constitutive potential. Rhetoric can be utilized to reinforce the status quo or to invite one to explore a range of other potential meanings about what matters most. Zickmund argues that for Heidegger the role of rhetoric in *being* is to encourage responsible or prudent action (phronesis) via the act of conscientious deliberation. The individual through rhetoric can thereby choose to act beyond the unrecognized authority of the ideology of the They and consciously commit to a more ethical course of action.

Authentic *Dasein* can "co-disclose this potentiality in the solicitude which leaps forth and liberates."[33] Michael J. Hyde's scholarship has blended Heidegger's phenomenology into the study of rhetoric. Rhetoric, according to Hyde, provides an impetus, a call to conscience, a space for a resolute *Dasein* to guide others. For Hyde, Heidegger's concept of conscience is central as a term that identifies "our 'projective' involvement with the temporal process of becoming and understanding that which we are: our possibilities."[34] However, habit is the central weapon of *das Man*. Habits reinforce our complacency to remain inauthentic, mindless automatons, going through the motions of life without ever really engaging ourselves in possibilities beyond our routines. Rhetoric, according to Hyde, can serve to interrupt the undifferentiated influence of *das Man*, "the call of conscience brings us face to face with the fact that we are creatures whose desire of the 'good life' requires us to assume the personal and ethical responsibility of affirming our freedom through resolute choice."[35] Rhetoric, produced by an authentic self, can serve as an exigence calling others to recognize their own conscience.

Within rhetorical action is the potential for the creation of a counterpublic committed to awakening others to their authentic selves. The role of rhetoric lies not in constructing the possibilities for being but in opening up and inviting others to open themselves to the possibilities. Rhetoric, used by an authentic *Dasein* who is "'communicating' and 'struggling' with others, can bring about a 'modification' of our publicness.'" In doing so, rhetoric "can sound a call that interprets the complacency of our everyday world of common sense and common praxis and thereby summons us to choose, to act, and perhaps to change our lives for the 'better.'"[36]

If rhetoric plays the central role of opening up possibilities for authentic being then perhaps an understanding of rhetoric as something "beyond persuasion" is necessary. Sonja K. Foss and Cindy L. Griffin's theory of invitational rhetoric illuminates the potential contributions of rhetoric to authentic being. Because invitational rhetoric welcomes the inclusion of a variety of perspectives and the sharing of alternative viewpoints and rejects the imposition of the speaker's perspective, rhetoric can potentially serve *Dasein* by releasing the possibilities of a situation rather than dictating a response.

> Absent are efforts to dominate another because the goal is understanding and appreciation of another's perspective rather than the denigration of it simply because it is different from the rhetor's own . . . Invitational rhetoric is characterized, then, by the openness with which rhetors are able to approach their audiences . . . [R]esistance is not anticipated, and rhetors do not adapt their communication to expected resistance in the audience.[37]

Invitational rhetoric is unique in that it invites the auditor to engage in the deliberative process. The rhetoric acts as an offering, an opening, an availability. The outcome is not planned, nor predetermined. However, the potential for transformation exists within the interaction between the rhetor and the auditor. Invitational rhetoric engages the participants in a conversational process of discovering, questioning, and re-thinking the situation. The process potentially encourages new ways of thinking and acting to emerge.

The four authors examined in this chapter are each inviting their readers to change the way they eat. These four authors are representative of the discourse currently being propagated about food. Carlo Petrini is the eloquent, self-proclaimed gastronome who founded the Slow Food movement in an attempt to reclaim traditional food ways in his Italian homeland.[38] Thich Nhat Hanh and Dr. Lilian Cheung, the eminent spiritual leader and a renowned nutritionist, combine Buddhist philosophy with the science of nutrition as a path to learning to eat and live mindfully in order to achieve health and peace in our everyday lives.[39] Former bodybuilder Tosca Reno began writing about clean eating in the fitness magazine *Oxygen*. She is the body and face of her own stylized clean eating "phenomenon" popularized in her *Eat-Clean* books and the *Clean Eating* magazine aimed at helping you "reclaim your life, your health and your well-being."[40] Geneen Roth, the Oprah-endorsed reformed compulsive eater, promotes a set of seven eating guidelines grounded in her philosophy that "our relationship to food is an exact microcosm of our relationship to life itself."[41]

All four, and indeed the whole genre of conscious eating literature, articulate the connection between the pleasures of eating and the politics of food. For these authors the pleasure and the politics of food are inseparable. Pleasure and politics are enacted in our choice of commitments: "*Choosing to make this choice*—deciding for a potentiality-for-Being, and making this decision from one's own Self. In choosing to make this choice, Dasein *makes possible*, first and foremost, its authentic potentiality-for-Being."[42] Through our choices we communicate our commitments. Petrini explains the significance of our food choices: "Our choice of food . . . is the most powerful communicative tool that we possess. Our decision about what to buy and consume, in a world where everything is geared to profit, it is the first significant political act we make in our lives."[43] What we eat, when we eat, with whom we eat are powerful choices about our commitments.

We must, they insist, choose our food with care. The authors suggest that we learn to more mindfully appreciate the possibilities of our food. Russon explains the response is not predetermined, not required, but is in Heidegger's sense an *undecidable call*. "It does not offer a prefabricated answer (a decision): it precisely puts one in the position of having to originate a way of taking up the call."[44]

Hanh and Cheung, Petrini, Reno, and Roth advocate *mindfulness*. For Heidegger to be mindful is to anticipate possibilities. They argue that our compulsions with fast food have necessitated a counter-balance. Petrini argues that: "When fast food became universal, Slow Food found its raison d'etre; when globalization exercised its homogenizing power over taste, at once reactions sprang up which regarded localism and diversity as a value."[45]

Consider the potential pleasure and politics in the seemingly simple act of eating an apple. Hahn and Cheung describe the way to more mindfully eat an apple as an illustration of the kind of transformative relationship with food they advocate. First, you must slow down and really focus on the apple you are eating. Next, notice the particulars of kind, color, smell, and so on, recognizing that the apple is more complex than just being a snack— it is a "part of the greater whole." Then you must take a bite and chew consciously (twenty to thirty times for each bite), becoming fully engaged in the act of appreciating the apple you are eating.[46]

However, the four books are not all equally successful as invitational rhetoric designed to encourage and liberate their auditor's *Dasein*. Tosca Reno's *Eat-Clean* diet book series in a final analysis fails to fulfill the liberatory potential of clean eating. Although her books combine the philosophy of clean eating with instructions for eating clean in the form of recipes, grocery lists, and menus as impetus to action, in the end, her appeals fail to release other possibilities of meaning within the situation. Although Reno recognizes the need to change, she in the end supports the ideological commitments of *das Man*. She argues that one should eat clean because: "You are tired of being sick, fat, grumpy, depressed, over-looked, drained of energy, uninterested in sex and a list of other symptoms too long to mention."[47] Reno's books and magazine are marketed and ulti-mately can be reduced to another diet book aimed at selling books to encourage women to lose weight and thus obtain the "lean" bodies desir-able in popular culture.

Geneen Roth's books take the form of personal testimonials as she uti-lizes the story of her own journey to frame transformative possibilities for her readers. After making the connection between food and God, recog-nizing a hunger for comfort rather than a hunger for comfort foods, Roth stopped dieting and reached what she calls her "natural weight," which she has successfully maintained for over three decades. "But more than the new body size, it was the lightness of being that enthralled me."[48] While this quote would seem to imply that the journey is about achieving the "light-ness of being," indicating a call to a more authentic way of being, Roth's invitation is limited in opening up only a singular path to transformation rather than articulating the undecidability of transformative possibilities.

Hanh and Cheung, the Buddhist and the nutritionist, use all the right vocabulary to tap into the notion of mindfulness as a path to a more peace-ful and happy existence. However, in the final analysis their book sub-scribes to an inauthentically limiting version of happiness. Happiness for Hanh and Cheung is not about living a healthier life, but taking control and ending one's struggle with weight.

The authentic self must move beyond "going along" with the preoccupations of the masses. The prevailing assumption behind the "obesity epidemic" is that fat is unhealthy, unattractive, and avoidable. Yet in spite of the millions of dollars spent, the incalculable psychic and physical energy expended, and the extreme deprivation diets undertaken, both the medical community and the popular press continue to warn of a rising global "obesity epidemic." The term "epidemic" is utilized to suggest a looming disaster, a contagious disease that authorizes and indeed requires drastic measures be taken to intervene in order to save us from our "'effortless' Western lifestyle which has become progressively hostile toward physical activity and dietary restraint."[49] The "quiet shift in America's worries" about fat, "the advent of systematic concern about dieting," and movement toward slimness via dieting as an ideal represents a significant and enduring shift in our collective cultural consciousness.[50] "Dieting, weight consciousness, and widespread hostility to obesity form one of the fundamental themes in modern life."[51]

Authenticity involves making the decision to let things matter, to accept the role we play but to make the commitment to more consciously and carefully enact that role as we recognize the undecidability evidenced in the possibilities of our responses to the call to conscience. Then Carlo Petrini provides the most compelling invitation to transformation.

Petrini invites us to consider the quality of the food we eat. The three principles he articulates are deceptively simplistic. Food, Petrini argues, should be good, clean, and fair.

Food is good when it is pleasing to the palate and to the mind. The methods of production and transportation should be clean, i.e., socially equitable, environmentally healthy, economically affordable, and culturally sensitive. And the food we eat should be justifiably fair to the communities that have produced it. To ensure this quality of care for ourselves and our planet we must realign our role from consumers to co-producers as we answer Petrini's call to conscience by embracing the principles of eco-gastronomy toward strengthening our food communities.

> The quest for slowness, which begins as a simple rebellion against the impoverishment of taste in our lives, makes it possible to rediscover taste. By living slowly, you understand some things, too; by slowing down in comparison to the world, you soon come into contact with what the world regards as its "dumps" of knowledge, which have been deemed slow and therefore marginalized. By exploring the "margins" of slowness, you encounter those pockets of supposedly "minor" culture that are alive in the memories of old people, typical of civilizations that have not yet become frantic—traditions that guide the vital work of good, clean and fair producers and that are handed down after centuries of empiricism and practical skills.[52]

Petrini's book is at once an eloquent treatise on the importance of slowness, an exploration of the "worrying picture" of the landscape of food today, and an appeal for auditors to undertake change. Petrini's expressed aim "to develop ideas, raise awareness, and arouse passion" succeeds in his refusal to dictate a single solution. Rather the text entreats the reader to follow his or her own conscience by remaining open to the possibilities of meaning in our food situation.

NOTES

1. Jean-Anthelme Brillat-Savarin, *The Physiology of Taste: Or, Meditations on Transcendental Gastronomy* (1826; Washington, DC: Counterpoint, 2000).
2. Reay Tannahill, *Food in History* (1972; New York: Crown Publishers, Inc., 1988), xvi.
3. Carlo Petrini, *Slow Food Nation: Why Our Food Should Be Good, Clean and Fair* (New York: Rizzoli Ex Libris, 2005), 36.
4. Martin Heidegger, *Being and Time*, rev. ed. (New York: Harper and Row Publishers, 1962), 78.
5. Ibid., 58.
6. Kimberly Springer, "Introduction: Delineating the Contours of the Oprah Culture Industry," in *Stories of Oprah: The Oprahfication of American Culture*, ed. Trystan T. Cotton and Kimberly Springer Jackson (University Press of Mississippi, 2010), vii–xix. "Oprah Winfrey's embodiment, her cultural productions, her actions, and her ideology constitute The Oprah Culture Industry (TOCI). The sheer number of productions and enterprises indicates TPCI's extensive reach into American lives, media and culture."
7. Geneen Roth, *Women, Food and God: An Unexpected Path to Almost Everything* (New York: Scribner, 2010), 2.
8. Heidegger, *Being and Time*, 157.
9. Tosca Reno, *The Eat-Clean Diet Recharged* (Mississauga, Ontario: Robert Kennedy, 2009), 17.
10. Reno, *The Eat-Clean Diet Recharged*, 18.
11. Wynne Wright and Gerad Middendorf, eds., *The Fight over Food: Producers, Consumers, and Activists Challenge the Global Food System* (University Park: The Pennsylvania State University Press, 2008), 4.
12. Petrini, *Slow Food Nation*, 41.
13. Fabio Parasecoli, *Bite Me: Food in Popular Culture* (New York: Berg, 2008), 2.
14. Jonathon Safran Foer, *Eating Animals* (New York: Little, Bend and Company, 2009).
15. Karl Weber, ed., *Food, Inc.: How Industrial Food Is Making Us Sicker, Fatter, and Poorer—and What You Can Do About It* (New York: Public Affairs, 2009).
16. Christopher D. Cook, *Diet for a Dead Planet: How the Food Industry Is Killing Us* (New York: The New Press, 2004).
17. Heidegger, *Being and Time*, 164.
18. Ibid, 166.
19. Eric Schlosser, *Fast Food Nation: The Dark Side of the All-American Meal* (New York: HarperCollins Publishers, 2005).
20. Petrini, *Slow Food Nation*, 47.

21. Reno, *The Eat-Clean Diet Recharged*, 17–18, laments our "fast food, drive-thru, get-it-quick, super size it, pull-up-to-the-buffet-and-stuff-yourself attitude toward food"; Tich Nhat Hanh and Lilian Cheung, *Savor: Mindful Eating, and Mindful Life* (New York: HarperCollins, 2010), 41, examine the ways in which the fast pace of our high-tech living is contributing to mindless eating and mindless living. Food corporations seek to make food as convenient, accessible, and addictive as possible.
22. Cook, *Diet for a Dead Planet*; Foer, *Eating Animals*; Michael Pollan, *In Defense of Food: An Eater's Manifesto* (New York: Penguin, 2008); Michael Pollan, *The Omnivore's Dilemma: A Natural History of Four Meals* (New York: Penguin, 2006); Wright and Middendorf, *The Fight Over Food*, 2008.
23. Hanh and Cheung, *Savor*, 12.
24. John Russon, "The Self as Resolution: Heidegger, Derrida and the Intimacy of the Question of the Meaning of Being," *Research in Phenomenology* 38 (2008): 99.
25. Greg Crister, "Let Them Eat Fat," *Harper's* 300 (2000): 41–42.
26. Laura Kipnis, "Fat and Culture," in *Near Ruins: Cultural Theory at the End of the Century*, ed. Nicholas B. Dirks (Minneapolis: University of Minnesota Press, 1998), 203.
27. Roth, *Women, Food and God*, 13.
28. Barbara Thompson, *Weight Loss Surgery: Finding the Thin Person Hiding Inside You* (Pittsburgh: Word Association, 2008).
29. Jean-Anthelme Brillat-Savarin, *The Physiology of Taste: Or, Meditations on Transcendental Gastronomy*, trans. M. F. K. Fisher (1826; Washington, DC: Counterpoint, 2000), 209.
30. Russon, "The Self as Resolution," 99.
31. Petrini, *Slow Food Nation*, 23.
32. Susan Zickmund, "Deliberation, Phronesis, and Authenticity: Heidegger's Early Conception of Rhetoric," *Philosophy and Rhetoric* 40 (2007): 406–15.
33. Heidegger, *Being and Time*, 344.
34. Michael J. Hyde, *The Call of Conscience: Heidegger and Levinas, Rhetoric and the Euthanasia Debate* (Columbia: University of South Carolina Press, 2001), 25.
35. Ibid., 25.
36. Michael J. Hyde, "The Call of Conscience: Heidegger and the Question of Rhetoric," *Philosophy and Rhetoric* 27 (1994): 382.
37. Sonia K. Foss and Cindy L. Griffin, "Beyond Persuasion: A Proposal for an Invitational Rhetoric," *Communication Monographs* 62 (1995): 6.
38. Petrini, *Slow Food Nation*.
39. Hanh and Cheung, *Savor*.
40. Reno, *The Eat-Clean Diet Recharged*, 10.
41. Roth, *Women, Food and God*, 2.
42. Heidegger, *Being and Time*, 312–13.
43. Petrini, *Slow Food Nation*, 87.
44. Russon, "The Self as Resolution," 100.
45. Petrini, *Slow Food Nation*, 102.
46. "Take an apple out of your refrigerator. Any apple will do. Wash it. Dry it. Before taking a bite, pause a moment. Look at the apple in your palm and ask yourself: When I eat an apple, am I really enjoying eating it? Or am I so preoccupied with other thoughts that I miss the delights that the apple offers me? . . . When you eat the apple, just concentrate on eating the apple. Don't do anything else. And most important, be still . . . Being focused and slowing down will allow you to truly savor all the qualities the apple offers: its sweetness, aroma, freshness, juiciness, and crispness. Next, pick up the apple

from the palm of your hand and take a moment to look at it again. Breathe in and out a few times consciously to help yourself focus and become more in touch with how you feel about the apple. Most of the time, we barely look at the apple we are eating. We grab it, take a bite, chew it quickly, and then swallow. This time, take note: What kind of apple is it? What color is it? How does it feel in your hand? What does it smell like? . . . Look deeply at the apple in your hand and you see the farmer who tended the apple tree; the blossom that became the fruit; the fertile earth, the organic material from decayed remains of prehistoric marine animals and algae, and the hydrocarbons themselves; the sunshine, the clouds, and the rain. Without the combination of these far-reaching elements and without the help of many people, the apple would simply not exist. At its most essential, the apple you hold is a manifestation of the wonderful presence of life. It is interconnected with all that is. It contains the whole universe . . . It feeds your body, and if we eat it mindfully, it also feeds our soul and recharges our spirit" (Hanh and Cheung, *Savor*, 39–42).

47. Reno, *The Eat-Clean Diet Recharged*, 10.
48. Roth, *Women, Food and God*, 4.
49. Michael Gard and Jan Wright, *The Obesity Epidemic: Science, Morality and Ideology* (New York: Routledge, 2005), 2.
50. Peter N. Stearns, *Fat History: Bodies and Beauty in the Modern West* (New York: New York University Press, 1997), 3–4.
51. Ibid, vii.
52. Petrini, *Slow Food Nation*, 180.

15 Narratives of Hunger
Voices at the Margins of Neoliberal Development

Mohan J. Dutta

In the backdrop of the neoliberal framework of globalization that articulates development in terms of structural adjustment programs (SAPs) in the global South, this chapter takes a culture-centered approach to co-construct stories of hunger at the material margins of neoliberal governmentality in contemporary India. The erasure of the subaltern sectors from global discursive spaces is intrinsically tied to top-down frames of development under neoliberalism that enforce state-based policies to support the agendas of transnational corporations (TNCs).[1] Interconnected with the absence of subaltern voices from policy platforms is the implementation of neoliberal policies that carry out corporate agendas under the veneer of state-based projects of development.[2] Because development becomes the framework through which neoliberal policies get instituted in the global South, the discursive engagement with subaltern communities who experience these development policies and their effects directly becomes an entry point for imagining possibilities of structural transformation. The culture-centered approach therefore is positioned as a meta-theoretical framework that interrogates the erasure of subaltern voices in development policymaking, and resists this erasure through the foregrounding of subaltern voices in the co-constructions of knowledge claims about development.[3]

The chapter begins with an overview of the culture-centered, meta-theoretical framework for understanding neoliberalism as the context for situating hunger, particularly as it relates to the development and dissemination of top-down development interventions carried out by state-based policymakers and program planners that define the agendas of the neoliberal nation-state. Drawing upon postcolonial and subaltern studies theories, I engage with the (im)possibilities of representing subaltern narratives in dialogues with rural community members in India who negotiate their everyday struggles with hunger amidst the narratives of development that promise to meet the needs of the poor through economic development. The culture-centered reading of hunger re-presented in this chapter talks back to the dominant narratives of development under liberalization by questioning the fundamentally unequal nature of state policies that undermine local capacities in agrarian communities in the global South. The voices of the poor re-presented within the discursive spaces of knowledge production in mainstream academe (as reflected in this chapter) rupture the altruistic notions of development that serve as the façade for state-based agendas of supporting TNCs at the cost of the poor.[4]

The culture-centered approach emphasizes the necessity for listening to narratives in the subaltern sectors through subaltern deconstructions of mainstream development logics that typically go unchallenged. This deconstruction happens predominantly through subaltern conversations about everyday lived experiences, juxtaposed in the backdrop of the grand narratives of state claims and specific policies that are supposedly directed at addressing the needs of subaltern communities. Therefore, when subaltern communities talk back to the dominant epistemic structures, the taken-for-granted assumptions within these structures are brought into question.[5] In other words, listening to the voices of subaltern sectors becomes a strategy for disrupting the hegemony of the neoliberal narrative of development. The stories narrated through dialogues with local community members render visible the structural violence carried out by development programs framed within the agendas of trade liberalization and privatization of agrarian resources in the global South.[6] Within the specific context of this chapter, the aesthetic of neoliberal representations of an economically burgeoning India is interrupted by the stories of hunger that speak to the violence written into the political and economic configurations of the neoliberal nation-state.[7]

Localized narratives of hunger talk back to the dominant epistemic structures in the mainstream by sharing with us the multitudes of ways in which individuals, communities, and families enact their agency as they seek access to food within specific policy contexts where access to food becomes more and more scarce. The stories of oppression written into the dominant structures are juxtaposed in the backdrop of local articulations of subaltern agency that work within and against these hegemonic structures to imagine possibilities of resistance and social change in the backdrop of neoliberalism. The rhetorical journey presented in this chapter weaves together stories, performances, poetry, and songs drawn from my decade-long fieldwork in West Bengal, India, as well as the narratives of hunger collected from public discourses and public policy documents about agrarian issues in India, where hunger emerges as a key thematic in the articulations of local meanings of development.

CULTURE-CENTERED APPROACH TO SOCIAL CHANGE

The meta-theoretical commitment of the culture-centered approach engages with the erasure of the subaltern sectors from the spaces of development policymaking and intervention planning, noting the ways in which this symbolic erasure is tied to the perpetuation of material oppression of the poor in the nation-state.[8] As a critique of neoliberal governmentality, the culture-centered approach attends to the idea that systematic erasure of the voices of poor communities in development planning and implementation lies at the heart of the perpetuation of material practices and policies that disenfranchise the poor. Noting this erasure, then, the basic commitment of the culture-centered approach is on co-creating spaces for dialogue where voices of subaltern communities may be heard.[9]

With an emphasis on listening, it is noted that the de-centering of Euro-centric universals of development planning offers an entry point for theorizing from the margins.[10] In this sense, then, dialogues with voices at the margins offer the entry points for rendering impure the conceptual categories of the neoliberal logic based on the values of privatization, trade liberalization, and the minimization of state-based subsidies and social services for the poor.[11] When the poor indeed do talk back, they offer alternative rationalities that question the taken-for-granted ideas of development and its assumptions of trickle-down economics under the broader umbrella of structural adjustment programs (SAPs).[12] In the rest of the chapter, we listen to stories from the subaltern sectors of India to offer entry points for social change and structural transformation. The taken-for-granted assumptions of neoliberalism are interrogated through the presence of subaltern narratives constituted around hunger. In setting up the contexts for the stories that articulate alternative narratives of development, I will first walk through a discussion of neoliberal policies and development.

Agriculture, Neoliberalism, and Development in India

Neoliberal ideology, as framed within the "new policy agenda" or "Washington Consensus," builds upon the fundamental notion of privatization of resources and promotion of a global free market through the minimization of trade-related tariffs.[13] Loans channeled through the international financial institutions (IFIs) were utilized to impose specific trade liberalization policies on the global South that seek to restructure these economies in the South.[14] The economic principles of neoliberalism work hand-in-hand with the political force that is exerted by IFIs and key northern nation-states to push through a set of economic reforms or policies that usually include cutting tariffs and other trade barriers; reducing government intervention in the economy; cuts in social spending; reducing or eliminating subsidies that provide important benefits for the poor; privatizing public enterprises and services; usurping large sectors of public resources such as land in the global South to promote specific trade configurations; and emphasizing exports as the engine of growth.[15] Highlighting the inherent superiority of economic liberalism, including the design of an international economic order based on free markets, private property, individual incentive, and a minimal role for the state, the neoliberal ideology is framed within the language of development and modernization, and is furthermore carried out through global trade policies and agreements, constituted under the framework of the General Agreement on Tariffs and Trade (GATT), and its later version, the World Trade Organization (WTO).[16] Structural adjustment programs (SAPs) and trade-related intellectual property rights (TRIPS) have played key roles in the context of the question of hunger in rural communities of the global South.[17]

Structural Adjustment Programs

Under SAPs, Third World countries have been required to open up their doors to transnational seed companies, thus shifting peasant-based forms of agriculture that depended on local circulation of seeds for subsistence to dependence on commoditized terminator seeds that needed to be purchased by farmers from season to season.[18] As opposed to the locally grown seeds, the genetically modified (GM) seeds are chemical-intensive and water-intensive, thus creating additional cycles of dependence on global agro-corporations. In this shift from peasant-based systems of agriculture to systems of agriculture that were largely dependent on agro-chemical and seed corporations, the World Bank has played a major role through its loan programs that were directed at making the national seed industries more market-responsive.[19] As a result, the seed sector was privatized; the locally circulated, government-subsidized, and community-based circulations of seeds have been replaced by commoditized purchase of genetically modified seeds manufactured by transnational corporations.[20] Government-sponsored extension programs have on one hand stopped offering government-subsidized seeds to farmers and, on the other hand, have started offering GM seeds to farmers.[21]

Under the structural adjustment programs, specific varieties of GM seeds have been promoted by the government under the premise that these seeds would increase efficiency, optimize pest resistance, and generate maximum yield.[22] These GM seeds respond to fertilizers and pesticides, which are also manufactured by the TNCs, thus leading to an external input-driven system as opposed to the traditional system, which was driven by locally available resources. Also, farmer's cropping patterns have shifted from mixed cultivations to monocultures of hybrids that are fueled by external inputs. The emphasis on privatization has also influenced the types of loans available to farmers, shifting from public sector, low-interest loans and extensions to high-interest, private sector loans.[23] Overall, then, the political economy of agriculture has shifted away from traditionally sustainable, local forms of agriculture.

Simultaneously, the emphasis on external liberalization of agriculture has dictated that agricultural subsidies be reduced, which has resulted in the price rise of food grains supplied through the Public Distribution System (PDS).[24] The price rise of the food grains supplied through the PDS then led to the rise in market prices of food grains.[25] In order to then address the underserved sectors, the government introduced a specifically subsidized PDS.[26] However, the subsidized products typically do not reach the underserved markets and get leaked into other areas because of corruptions that exist within state structures.[27] In addition, given the distant locations of the underserved areas and the lack of literacy among tribal populations, even when subsidized food grains do reach these underserved areas, community members pay prices higher than the stipulated prices. As the government shifted its subsidies from the PDS to subsidies for exporting grain, the PDS prices were quite similar to market prices, thus making food grains fairly inaccessible to the laboring masses.[28] In the case of the Indian states of Maharashtra and Andhra Pradesh, the prices of food grains very quickly made them out of the reach of the poorer sectors.

Agreement on Trade-Related Aspects of Intellectual Property Rights (TRIPS)

The Agreement on Trade-Related Aspects of Intellectual Property Rights (TRIPS) came into effect in 1995 as a result of the 1986–94 Uruguay Round of the General Agreement on Tariffs and Trade (GATT), and was seen as a pivotal element in fostering international trade.[29] According to the WTO, governments need to ensure that innovators have the right to prevent others from using their innovations and the right to negotiate payment from others in return for using their innovations. However, because the extent of protection and enforcement of these rights varied widely across geographical boundaries, causing much tension, the "new internationally agreed trade rules for intellectual property rights (i.e., TRIPS) were seen as a way to introduce more order and predictability, and for disputes to be settled more systematically."[30] The TRIPS Agreement covers the following areas of intellectual property: copyright and related rights (the rights of performers; producers of sound recordings and broadcasting organizations); trademarks; geographical indications including appellations of origin; industrial designs; patents including the protection of new varieties of plants; the layout designs of integrated circuits; and undisclosed information.[31] The agreement stresses fair and equitable action against infringement of intellectual property rights, and the need to make corrective action procedures less complicated, less costly, and less time-consuming.

The repercussions of TRIPS can most clearly be seen in the case of basmati rice in South Asia. The TRIPS Agreement threatens food security by (a) not recognizing indigenous communities' rights over their resources and (b) by enabling biopiracy or the appropriation of local biological resources without consulting the local community or representative state actors. Constituted in the realm of questions of legitimacy of knowledge structures and the political economy of these structures, TRIPs treats indigenous knowledge as common property because it is not patented; the idea here is that if knowledge is not patented, it is not owned and therefore is open to technological modifications, which can then be patented.[32] Woods notes that the TRIPS Agreement does not extend either patent or geographic protection to the traditional knowledge of indigenous people; for example, the patent laws under TRIPS do not adequately recognize traditional forms of breeding as "prior art" (i.e., the entire body of knowledge available to the public before a given filing or priority date for any patent, utility model, or industrial design). This has thus led to multinational, biotechnological corporations successfully seeking patents on food grains, which in turn negatively impacts local economies.[33] In addition, TRIPS enables biopiracy to take place with relative ease, especially in lesser-developed countries that are rich in genetic resources and low in technology. Access to technology in developed countries allows richer countries to harness and reproduce genetic material for patenting, thereby enabling the expropriation of local resources and bringing them under the instruments of control of TNCs to generate greater global profit.

The case of RiceTec, a Texas-based multinational agri-business company that sought to patent basmati rice, is a case in point. Basmati rice is traditional to India and Pakistan, and in 1997 comprised 4 percent of India's export earnings, garnering premium prices in the international market. In September 1997, RiceTec successfully applied for several patents on the basmati rice and grain lines. The Pakistani and Indian governments refuted the patents, stating that the plant varieties and grains already exist as a staple in India, and that neither variety of rice can be grown in the US. The US Patent and Trademark Office rescinded fifteen of the twenty patents granted. However, the five remaining patents continue to permit RiceTec to exclude others from making, using, and selling its patented basmati rice in the US until September 2017. What this means is that the rice-producing nations in South Asia will have a smaller (and perhaps non-existent) international market in the coming years. In addition to marginalizing access that developing countries have to international markets, TRIPs also enables biopiracy. For example, the RiceTec's US patent claimed the invention of "novel rice lines with plants that are semi-dwarf in stature, substantially photoperiod-insensitive and high-yielding, and that produce rice grains having characteristics similar or superior to those of good quality basmati rice grains produced in India and Pakistan."[34] However, what the policy does not take into account is that the patent takes ownership of genetic material originally developed by South Asian farmers; the germplasm from these varieties was initially collected in the Indian subcontinent and later deposited and processed in the US and other places. In addition, TRIPS allows the patent holder to usurp the "basmati" name, which itself could jeopardize the sale of basmati from South Asia due to confusion.[35]

The patenting of food grains can have major implications for the economy and food security in the least developed countries (LDC). In many of the LDCs, food grains such as rice form a vital part of people's diet.[36] Asian rice provides up to 85 percent of the calories in the daily diet of 2.7 billion people. According to the Trade & Environment Database (TED, 2005), with the basmati patent rights, RiceTec will be able not only to call its aromatic rice "Basmati" within the US, but also to label it "basmati" for its exports. This means farmers that depend on basmati cultivation and export in India and Pakistan will lose out not only on the 45,000-tonne US import market, which forms 10 percent of the total basmati exports, but also on its position in markets like the European Union, the United Kingdom, Middle East, and West Asia. This would certainly hit the local economy in rice-growing regions of India and Pakistan. As farmers lose markets for their crops, their incomes will be hit hard, leading to increased inability to spend on a basic necessity like food. Thus, the very resources that are a part of the day-to-day life of indigenous groups have to be purchased at a price from the technologically advanced countries and from transnational corporations, creating the scenario for continuous exploitation.

The combination of TRIPS and SAPs in the context of the Third World has resulted in the large-scale co-optation of agricultural spaces as the markets for the seeds and chemicals manufactured by TNCs. Furthermore, TRIPS emerges as a disciplinary site of control for enacting the hegemony of global agri-businesses such as Monsanto. With 94 percent of the global acreage for genetically modified food in 2000 under the control of Monsanto, large sectors of agricultural land come under the purviews of Monsanto, thus ensuring that the TNC uses the articulations of intellectual property rights to bring additional acres of land under its domain and further establish its dominance in global markets. As local farmers are surrounded by more and more genetically modified seeds in their agricultural lands, the chances of contamination with genetically modified seeds increase, and so do threats of being litigated by the agri-business giants for the violation of property rights.

Stories of Pain

Pain
In the silent moment
In the long pause
Between our exchange
The shame
In your eyes
In the story you shared
Of not
Making enough money
From begging
From door to door
The shame in sharing with me
That they went hungry
For the whole day.

In my fieldwork in West Bengal over the last decade, hunger marks the narratives that I have co-constructed with men and women who often share their pain in not being able to offer food to their children. Hunger is storied as a bodily response, reflected in the pain felt in the stomach, often storied in the experiences of parents seeking to offer the basic resource of food to their children. The pain of hunger is felt physically, but it also leaves its mark much deeper in the emotional responses attached to going without food, and particularly so in not being able to feed one's children. Participants refer to this emotional response in the framework of *lajja*, especially as it relates to their sense of self in securing access to food for their families. *Lajja*, a Bengali word, stands for the loss of face and dignity. Although similar to "shame," it goes much deeper than the English usage of shame in terms of the deep-seated sense of failure that it carries. In the stories in the poor households of Bengal narrated through in-depth interviews, *lajja* is felt because of the threat to the fundamental identity as a parent in not being able to carry out one's fundamental responsibility as a parent. It is in this backdrop of shame and pain that parents experiencing hunger over months commit suicide along with the children, sometimes feeding poison to the entire family. There were multiple stories that circulated during my fieldwork that narrated the death of families because of the inability to secure access to food.

The foregoing excerpt from the poetry I jotted down during one of my field visits in 2004 was a reflection of an interaction with a mother, *Lata*, who was sharing her pain at not being able to offer the basic necessity of life to her children: food. Her pain as a mother was intrinsically tied to the pain her children felt physically, having to go hungry night after night, because there was no money to be made during the monsoon season and there were no sources of income. This was the month of July, and it had been pouring constantly for the past ten days or so, and in the midst of the rains, *Lata* had difficulty finding a paying job. Business overall was slow and the merchants at the local shops did not sell much of their products, and therefore, had no economic resources really to employ anyone. Unable to find a job, she let go of her sense of dignity to go begging for money, and did not have any luck. She talked about going to middle- and upper-middle-class homes in search of jobs as a domestic worker, but had no luck. Her pain embodies a sense of loss as a mother in not being able to provide food for her children. Even as tears rolled down her cheeks as she shared the stories of her struggles with food, she noted how she needed to share this story so that other people could hear the story and work toward changing local and national policies. She noted:

> It does not make any meaning that food is so expensive these days. Even to buy a little bit of rice or little bit of oil, you will need a lot of money. Even if I find a job, almost all my money from the day's work will be gone in trying to purchase food, and still then, it will not last me

for many days. The prices of rice, *daal*, vegetables, these things keep increasing and there is no one to put a stop to these rising prices.

The story of pain in not being able to offer food to one's children then is constituted within the broader story of structural lack of access to food because of food policies. The rising price of food is noted as the most important aspect of food insecurity. Furthermore, participants such as *Lata* also questioned the basic assumptions in the logic that food for children has to be bought at a price and is not available in nature like it's supposed to be.

This narrative of loss at not being able to offer food for the children is noted in the story of *Becharam*:

> When they are in pain (referring to his children), it is hard for me to watch it as their father. I can't stand the shame of not being able to provide for them. As their father, that is my duty. Who will provide for them if I don't.

Becharam's shame at not being able to carry out his duty as a father is negotiated amidst his inability to provide food for his children. He points out that he is unable to carry out his duties as a father. This familial responsibility for providing food often falls on the father and mother in the household, who are physically capable of earning money. Similarly, *Kanti* voices that it is her responsibility as a mother that her children have enough to eat:

> I have to ensure that they have the food. For that, even if my husband and I have to go hungry for many days, that is OK, because the children need to eat.

In their negotiation with the circumstance of not having enough food then, *Kanti* and her husband *Kebla* discuss the ways in which they ration resources in order to make sure that their children have enough to eat. In this instance, Kanti observes that she often goes hungry in order to ensure that the children have enough to eat and that they are getting adequate nutrients.

When initiating conversations about meanings of health, community members from rural Bengal often discuss hunger as central to their understanding of health. The experience of hunger in these stories is embodied in the backdrop of the narratives of development and modernization of Bengal, the building of new industries, and the cleaning up of forest areas in order to bring about development in the region. Rural community members often draw our attention to the displacement of the rural way of life as being tied to the lure of development that is offered to them by politicians; and their subsequent disappointments as promises of economic solvency and development remain undelivered in local communities. *Ram* shares that "all the politicians come and go, but nothing happens to us."

Similarly, *Shilpi* points to the idea that "no one really cared for the poor." Therefore, the life of the poor is often focused on simply trying to keep afloat, to just make enough resources so that one could get by. *Subodh*, a thirty-four-year-old fisherman from the nearby fishing village that is right next to *Dutta Bari*, my home, says:

> Food is not really there. The search for food can be a difficult one this time of year because nobody has much to offer. I think everyone is struggling and trying just hard to make a living. So I can go to catch some fish and then hope that I will sell the fish in the market, and then bring some food home for my wife to cook. But sometimes finding the fish is the challenge. It is all luck, whether you have the fish for the day or not.

Worth noting in this narrative is the everyday struggle with resources and the day-to-day uncertainty that is faced by rural community members. This everyday uncertainty gets played out most fundamentally in the daily struggle for food resources for households in rural Bengal.

Food as Ownership

When discussing their struggles with hunger, participants often discuss the notion that although they are the ones who do the physical work on the agricultural farms to produce the food crops, the food remains inaccessible to them. Therefore, being situated in agricultural communities and often working directly on the paddy fields, it comes across as quite paradoxical to the participants that in spite of putting their labor into the fields, they are not guaranteed access to food. Noting the paradox in this situation, they question why it is that their labor is often not adequate to fetch them the resources for buying basic food that is central to their ability to live. *Shontu* eloquently points this out:

> I had been working during the harvesting season every day but the babu had not sold his crop yet and he did not have any money to give me. So here I had worked to harvest the paddy, but I did not have any rice to take home with me. The children were waiting each day hoping that I would bring money home and I didn't have anything to bring.

Foregrounded in this narrative of *Shontu* is the irony of the immediate context; although he had done the physical work to harvest the paddy, he did not have any money to buy the rice. The question of ownership of food becomes foregrounded in this logic. Because food is mediated through the market, landless farmers such as *Shontu* and their families remain deprived of the basic food that they believe should be their rightful possession. *Kanu* notes similarly:

It surprises me that even when I work hard, I don't have enough for the year round to feed my children. The money that comes in is very little and it goes the same day often. So even working hard does not mean that I will have the money that I could assure that my family will have something to eat. When it rains a lot, and I don't have work, we go hungry because there is no money left over.

Although *Kanu* points out that he works very hard all year round, that is not enough for him to be able to ensure that the family has something to eat all year round. For him, money is spent on a daily basis, and the living of the family for the day depends upon what he is able to bring in at the end of the day. Along these lines, *Jonardon* talks about the rising prices of food ingredients:

Food is so expensive that you can hardly buy anything these days. You simply can't afford to buy rice or your basic vegetables, and here I am not talking about anything special, just the basic things to get by. For example, rice, some *daal* [referring to legumes], onion, potatoes, and some vegetables occasionally. I am not talking about things like meat and fish. I am just talking about cheap things that are the basic necessities. They are not cheap anymore.

The story that is shared by *Jonardon* narrates the entry of food into the logic of the market. Through this process of commoditization, food has been rendered inaccessible to the subaltern sectors of the globe, even to those members of agrarian communities who work hard year-round trying to grow food. Rather than being abundantly present in nature that served as the source of food, food has to be purchased in exchange of labor in the marketplace. Therefore, community members such as *Jonardon* in the global South spend their days looking for ways to make a living so that they could purchase the foods from the marketplace. Landless laborers such as *Jogot* also point out that labor does not always equate to having food at the table. He says, "I can work very hard for the day, put in a lot of work in the Sun, and still not have enough money to buy anything much at all to feed the whole family. Sometimes the prices of rice and vegetables are very high, and there is no control on the price."

Parbati eloquently points this out:

You tell me. It used to be that everything was available in nature. The fruits and vegetables are supposed to be in nature, aren't they? Every child should have fruits and vegetables to eat, and they should be able to just go to the forest like we used to do as children and pick the fruit and then eat it. But you can't do that anymore. Much of the forest is gone; and even in the parts where there are still trees like the mango trees, the children can't go pick the mangoes because the government has guards now that oversee the forest.

In *Parbati*'s questions, the taken-for-granted assumptions surrounding the commoditization of food become evident. That food should be a commodity to be purchased at the marketplace does not make any sense to her. That children should not be able to just go into the forest to pick fruits to eat them does not seem natural to her. In fact, she notes that nature wanted food to be available in plenty and that it is unnatural for fruits to be sold in the marketplace so that sellers could profit from them. She suggests that the fruits were meant to be for children to enjoy. She points to her own childhood and notes how she along with her friends would go to the jungle to pick the fruits and then eat them. *Korimana* elaborates on this very same point about the ownership of fruits and vegetables:

> The *babus* own the trees so that fruits from the trees belong to them. They cleaned up the forests that belonged to us. There used to be plenty of forests around here, and those forests had plenty of trees that gave plenty of fruits. Sometimes there would be so much fruit that you didn't even have to climb the trees. You could just go into the forest and pick the fruits. But they have been clearing up the forests to build more and more houses. And now the babus own the trees that fall within their land. So when our children go to get these fruits, they are chased away by the guards being called thieves.

Korimana interrogates the meaning of ownership within the backdrop of stealing. She asks whether it is really the act of stealing when children go into the gardens of the *babus* to pick fruits that should be rightfully theirs. She also interrogates the notion of property by suggesting that the forests that were owned by the village communities have now been cleaned up to make room for the houses that are being built by the middle- and upper-middle-class babus. This question of ownership as it relates to access to food returns the gaze at the dominant structures of neoliberal governance in contemporary India by questioning fundamentally the logic of urbanization and land grab that have punctuated the narratives of development.

Logics of Land

As indicated in the previous section, these stories of hunger are interconnected with the stories of land grab within the context of development. As cities have increasingly expanded and more and more agrarian lands have been taken over under the logic of development, it has also meant that less and less land is available for growing food, and for feeding the hungry. *Labonyo* notes this by saying, "Where are you going to find the spinach leaves in the rainy season? It used to be that you could walk out and pick leaves. Not any more, as more houses have taken up the land." Intrinsically tied to food are logics of ownership of land because land is the source of food. Land in this sense of the collective is a property of the collective; however, participants point out that this collective property has been usurped from the poor and turned into private property for profits. *Shome* points out, "Land is what you need to grow food. The land now is being sold out by the government to the Tata people (Tata is one of the largest India-based corporations and was recently involved in displacement-based politics in Singur because of its desire to build a car manufacturing unit in the area). This point is elucidated by *Sona*:

> Food comes from the soil. The land is our mother. She provides for food and takes care of our hunger. When she is happy, there is abundance. There is more than enough for everyone to eat. In good seasons when she blesses us all, we used to have more food.

In noting soil as the source of food, *Sona* points to the interconnection between land and food. In articulating the idea that land as a part of nature provides abundantly for everyone, she points to the central role of land in addressing hunger in the rural areas of West Bengal. The happiness of the soil here is related to the idea of treating it well and respecting it. However, as more and more industrial projects have been built by the state, the opportunities for growing food for local communities have dramatically reduced. *Kanti* states the following, "There is nothing we can do? If we don't stand up like the farmers in Nadigram, everything will be taken over by the government."

Nimai discusses the story of Singur and Nadigram in West Bengal, where farming communities were displaced from their land by the arrival of a development project that sought to build a car manufacturing factory in the area:

> In deciding what to do with the land, our land, no one talks to us. We don't matter. Look at what the government did in Nandigram and Singur. This was fertile land, land that was giving a lot of food. The families were happy because they had abundance from the land. And then the government came in, and tried to fool the people. When they didn't still give in, it tried to put them in jail.

In pointing out the story of Singur and Nadigram, *Nimai* notes that the poor had very little say about what happened with their land. The government just came in and tried to manipulate the poor. He further notes that when manipulation tactics such as offering bribes did not work, the government then resorted to the use of violence. For the participants, the increasing spread of development projects in the area has also meant increasing threats of displacement from land resources.

In these local stories of participants, what becomes evident is the absence of the poor from platforms of policymaking and implementation where development policies are configured. It is through this absence then that the poor don't get to have a say on policies and programs that displace them from their land. This point is noted by *Ballu*:

Who gets to decide what happens with our land? Not us. We are never consulted. Nobody asks us anything about what should be done with things that belong to us. They just take these things. They rob them from us, and then use some big language and some big promise as they are doing the robbing. Because we are poor, it does not matter. They can do what they want to. They can come in here and steal. They can take away things that rightfully belong to us. This goes on for year after year.

Being poor here then is connected with not being able to have access to resources to seek out justice. Because one is poor, when injustice is carried out, there are no spaces or systems to turn to. Notice also here the labeling of state-wide land grab as an act of stealing. In this sense, then, development in the form of urbanization, mining, and rapid industrialization of the rural sectors is carried out through the stealing of land from the poor. As I started attending to this story that was being shared by community participants in my fieldwork, this is what I noted:

For year after year, this township has grown. There are ever more houses. The places that used to be greenery and paddy fields all around are now cement and concrete buildings that fulfill the middle-class dreams of urban areas. What I have been hearing in the last couple of weeks makes me wonder about the hypocrisy in the story of development that I see in the newspapers that set these projects up as projects of growth. The stories of *Ram* and *Kona* make me wonder about the real intent of this development game: Development for whom? For whose purposes? Who gains from these development projects? Because certainly from looking at the pain and agony of the poor it does not seem like the story of trickle-down growth is working.

My co-constructions with the participants further build on questioning the narrative of development that turns collective resources into private resources that can be utilized for generating profit. Development then has emerged as a trope within the framework of neoliberalism to further contribute to the problem of hunger in the rural communities of West Bengal.

SUBALTERN RATIONALITIES, HUNGER, AND NEOLIBERALISM

Subaltern rationalities co-constructed through this chapter re-present alternative rationalities for organizing global food systems, bringing into question the logic of neoliberal modes of organizing global food systems. The stories re-presented through our dialogic co-constructions articulate the subaltern understanding of food as a natural resource, embedded freely within nature and accessible naturally to be picked up, outside of the discourses of private ownership that are central to neoliberalism. When participants discuss fruits and vegetables being freely available in forests for picking, they note the concept that food is meant to be naturally available in plenty, as a part of the "natural" relationship of human beings with nature. In this articulation of food being available in abundance and freely in nature, the subaltern narratives interrogate the commoditization and privatization of food resources, noting the structural violence embedded in these forms of privatization of food resources. When food becomes a commodity in the market to be sold and traded by private sellers, it becomes inaccessible from the subaltern communities in the global South who have minimal access to these economic resources. The commoditization of food therefore is seen as an unnatural state, one that enacts its violence through the disenfranchisement of the poor from the mainstream systems of food production, distribution, and consumption.

The violence of neoliberalism is rendered visible through the stories of pain and death constituted within the framework of hunger in the global South, in the stories of parents not being able to offer food to their children. Everyday struggles of the poor for a source of living is juxtaposed amidst the relationship of food to participation of the poor as sources of labor in the neoliberal marketplace. The only way that food can be accessed among the communities I worked with is through the participation of community members in the neoliberal economy as sources of labor. The increasing deforestation of local spaces in the global South and the urbanization projects that have displaced the poor from their natural spaces of living and their lands are tied to the disenfranchisement of the poor from the natural sources of food. Co-participants articulate a subaltern rationality that frames these urbanization, privatization, industrialization, and development projects as acts of stealing, built on the backbone of land grab. Turning the neoliberal concept of private ownership on its head, subaltern rationalities articulate the notion that the project of private ownership of natural resources is accomplished through the stealing of the resources of the poor. In this context, participants note that in the politics and economics of contemporary India, this is accomplished through the disenfranchisement of the poor from policy platforms that push neoliberal policies under the rubric of development.

NOTES

1. David Harvey, *A Brief History of Neoliberalism* (London: Oxford University Press, 2005).
2. Mohan Dutta and Mahuya Pal, "Dialog Theory in Marginalized Spaces: A Subaltern Studies Approach," *Communication Theory* 40 (2010): 363–86.
3. Mohan Dutta, *Communicating Social Change: Structure, Culture, Agency* (New York: Routledge, 2011).
4. Dutta, *Communicating Social Change*, 8.

5. Dutta and Pal, "Dialog Theory," 363–64.
6. Dutta, *Communicating Social Change*, 60–61.
7. Ibid., 195–96.
8. Ibid, 58.
9. Ibid, 58–61.
10. Ibid, 19–25.
11. Dutta and Pal, "Dialog Theory," 370.
12. Vandana Shiva and Gitanjali Bedi, eds., *Sustainable Agriculture and Food Security: The Impact of Globalisation* (New Delhi: Sage Publications, 2002), 34–38.
13. Ibid, 26.
14. David Korten, *The Post-Corporate World* (San Francisco, CA: Kumarian, 1999), 28.
15. David Korten, *When Corporations Rule the World* (Bloomfield, CT: Kumarian, 1995), 3–36.
16. Ronald Labonte, "Globalization and Reform of the World Trade Organization," *Canadian Journal of Public Health* 92 (2001): 248–49.
17. Dutta, *Communicating Social Change*, 54.
18. Timothy Edward Josling, Stefan Tangermann, and T. K. Warley, *Agriculture in the GATT* (London: Macmillan, 1996), 9–13.
19. Vandana Shiva, *Staying Alive: Women, Ecology, and Development* (London: Zed, 1989), 4–18.
20. Vandana Shiva, *Stolen Harvest: The Hijacking of the Global Food Supply* (Cambridge, MA: South End Press, 2005), 22–32.
21. Ibid., 8.
22. Vandana Shiva, *The Violence of the Green Revolution: Third World Agriculture, Ecology, and Politics* (London: Zed, 1991), 40–48.
23. Shiva and Bedi, *Sustainable Agriculture*, 22–26.
24. Ibid., 4.
25. Vandana Shiva, *Earth Democracy: Justice, Sustainability, and Peace* (London: Zed, 2005).
26. Vandana Shiva et al., *Seeds of Suicide: The Ecological and Human Costs of Globalization of Agriculture* (New Delhi: Research Foundation for Science, Technology and Ecology, 1997).
27. Shiva, *Earth Democracy*, 13.
28. Shiva, *Stolen Harvest*, 18.
29. "World Trade Agreement 1994," *World Trade Organization (WTO)*, accessed August 29, 2011, http://www.wto.org.
30. Ibid.
31. Ibid.
32. M. Woods, "Food for Thought: The Biopiracy of Jasmine and Basmati Rice," *Albany Law Journal of Science and Technology* 13 (2002): 123–43.
33. Ibid., 127.
34. "Basmati: TED Case Study," *American University*, accessed August 29, 2011, www1.american.edu/ted/basmati.htm.
35. Ibid.
36. Shiva, *Stolen Harvest*.

Contributors

Garrett M. Broad is a doctoral student at the University of Southern California's Annenberg School for Communication & Journalism. His work focuses on the role of communication and media in the promotion of community-level social change, with a particular interest in food system issues.

Michael S. Bruner earned his PhD at the University of Pittsburgh, where he began his academic career as a teaching fellow. He went on to teach at the University of Maryland's European Division and at the University of North Texas. He now is a professor in the Department of Communication at Humboldt State University. He has published essays from a critical and a rhetorical perspective in a variety of journals, such as *Argumentation and Advocacy*, *Communication Quarterly*, and *Environmental Ethics*. His book chapters are published in several edited volumes, including *Food as Communication* (2011), *Contemporary Media Ethics* (2006), *Enviropop: Studies in Environmental Rhetoric and Popular Culture* (2002), *Worldview Flux: Perplexed Values among Postmodern Peoples* (2000), and *Landmark Essays on Rhetoric and the Environment* (1998). In addition, his conference papers on food issues have addressed the following topics: "Anti-Organic Rhetoric," "Learning, Knowing, and Deciding About Food: The Case of the Center for Science in the Public Interest," and "Fear Appeals in Public Argument about Genetically Modified Foods."

Donovan Conley is an associate professor of communication studies at the University of Nevada, Las Vegas. He received his PhD from the Department of Speech Communication at the University of Illinois, Urbana-Champaign, in 2004. Conley's research falls at the intersection of rhetoric and cultural studies. He studies the ways everyday citizenship is rhetorically produced, examining the rituals, aesthetics, affects, and material conditions that shape up our patterns of belonging. Conley's recent project explores the relationship between food and citizenship, focusing on the political dynamics of the concepts "taste" and "communion."

Mohan J. Dutta is a professor of communication in the Brian Lamb School of Communication and the associate dean for Research and Graduate Education in the College of Liberal Arts at Purdue University. He teaches and conducts research in critical theory, poverty and social change, performance for social change, community-based social change interventions, critical health communication, and activism for social change. His work on culture-centered approaches to social change engages with subaltern communities at global margins to configure a politics of social change and social justice.

Justin Eckstein received his MA in communication studies at the University of Nevada, Las Vegas. He is currently a doctoral student at the University of Denver. His research investigates the intersection of materiality, affect, and argumentation.

Carrie Packwood Freeman is an assistant professor of communication at Georgia State University in Atlanta. As a critical/cultural studies media scholar, her research publications encompass critical animal studies, environmental communication, media ethics, and strategic communication for social change, with a specialty in vegan advocacy and farmed animal protection. As a volunteer, Freeman has run animal activist/vegetarian grassroots groups in Georgia, Florida, and Oregon and now co-hosts an animal rights radio show and an environmental show on WRFG-Atlanta's community radio.

Joshua J. Frye holds a PhD from Purdue University. He is an assistant professor in the Department of Communication Arts at the State University of New York at Oneonta. His primary research interest is in the production, dissemination, and uptake of persuasive messages, especially of an environmental and political nature. He has published numerous scholarly articles pertaining to environmental communication, the rhetoric of sustainable agriculture, organizational and social movement leadership, and a book, *The Origin, Diffusion, and Transformation of Organic Agriculture*. He served as a sustainable agriculture extension agent with the US Peace Corps in Honduras during 1997–99. He is a Speakers Bureau member for the New York Council for the Humanities. He has also provided communication consulting to various clients, including leadership communication training to the American Red Cross and strategic public communication to the sustainable agriculture industry.

Laura K. Hahn earned her PhD at The Ohio State University. She now is a professor in the Department of Communication at Humboldt State University, where she specializes in social advocacy, rhetorical theory/criticism, and gender communication. Her relevant published work includes: "I'm Too Sexy for Your Movement: An Analysis of the Failure of the Animal Rights Movement to Promote Vegetarianism," in *Arguments about Animal Ethics*, ed. Greg Goodale and Jason E. Black (Lexington Books, 2010); "Cultural Expressions through Food," in *Agriculture, Food and Society Syllabi and Course Materials Collection*, a publication of the Association for the Study of Food and Society and the Agriculture, Food and Human Values Society (2010); and "Accessible Artifact for Community Discussion about Anarchy and Education," in *Contemporary Anarchist Studies: An Introductory Anthology of Anarchy in the Academy*, ed. Randall Amster et al. (Routledge Press, 2009).

Alison Henderson is a senior lecturer in the Department of Management Communication in the Waikato Management School at the University of Waikato, New Zealand, where she teaches and researches in organizational communication and public relations. Her research interests focus on the changes associated with new technologies, particularly in relation to food, health, and the environment. She currently holds a Marsden grant administered by the Royal Society of New Zealand, examining innovative food technologies and "healthy" food. She has published articles in *Discourse Studies* and the *Journal of Public Relations Research*, and was a guest editor for a recent special issue of the *Journal of Communication Management*.

Vanessa Johnson recently completed her master's thesis, with a full scholarship funded by a Marsden grant, examining innovative food technologies and "healthy" food, and graduated in 2011 with a master's degree in management studies. She has previously worked as a communication adviser for a medical practitioners' professional association, a small communications firm, and a secondary school. She also teaches group exercise classes part-time, having done so since 2001.

Alexander V. Kozin (PhD in speech communication) is an international research fellow at the Free University in Berlin, Germany. His interests reside at the juncture of phenomenology, semiotics, and cultural studies. He has published in the areas of phenomenology, semiotics, psychology, sociology, cultural studies, discourse analysis, linguistics, and communication studies. His recent work has been situated in the field of law-and-action. Currently, he is involved in a pilot project on law, emotion, and culture conducted under the auspices of the Institute for Philosophy at FU Berlin.

Oana Leventi-Perez is an MA student at Georgia State University in the Communication Department. Her research interests include environmental communication and communication strategies for advancing animal rights. Her research thesis examines the way in which Disney's animated films depict the human-animal relationship and promote animal rights in a market of anthropocentric consumers. On a professional level, Leventi-Perez has acquired extensive experience working in the public relations field, experience which has culminated in a communications assistant position with the David Ogilvy Department of Communication and Public Relations in Romania. She is actively involved with several animal rights groups, such as People for the Ethical Treatment of Animals and the Humane Society of the United States.

Raymie E. McKerrow is the C. E. Zumkehr Professor in the School of Communication Studies at Ohio University in Athens. He is past president of the National Communication Association, and current editor of the *Quarterly Journal of Speech*. His research reflects contemporary, critical approaches to rhetorical theory and criticism.

Jean Retzinger is a lecturer and the assistant director of Media Studies at the University of California, Berkeley. For the past two decades, her research has examined environmental implications of agriculture and food production practices as well as popular culture representations of food and farming. Recent essays and articles have appeared in *Edible Ideologies: Representing Food and Meaning* (SUNY Press, 2008) and *Environmental Communication: A Journal of Nature and Culture.*

Maxwell Schnurer earned his Ph.D. at the University of Pittsburgh, taught at Marist College, and now serves as an Associate Professor in the Department of Communication at Humboldt State University. His emphases are Rhetoric, Social Movements, Gender, Critical Theory, and Freedom. His publications include his book, *Many Sides*, and a wide range of articles and chapters on activism, animal rights, argumentation, and grass roots movements.

Natasha Seegert is a doctoral student in the Department of Communication at the University of Utah. She worked for two years as the youth gardening coordinator at Wasatch Community Gardens, where she taught organic gardening to youth, and she is the former associate director of the Environmental Studies Program at the University of Utah. She occasionally finds time to weed her own garden.

Abigail Seiler is a graduate student at the University of Maryland, College Park, in the Department of Communication. She also holds an MA in the anthropology of food from the School of Oriental and African Studies, University of London. Her research interests include food justice in American cities, the global effort for food sovereignty, gender and domesticity, and fair food.

Kara Shultz earned her PhD in speech communication from the University of Denver and joined the faculty at Bloomsburg University in 1991. With a focus on leadership and public advocacy, her teaching and research interests include the analysis of the role of rhetoric in constructing representations of diverse cultural identities. Her latest research projects examine the controversy over the growing popularity of the use of technological innovations to perfect "disabled" bodies through cochlear implant surgery, bariatric surgery, and limb lengthening surgery. She has received a National Endowment for the Humanities grant to study and has published several essays on the rhetoric of persons with disabilities, appearing in the national journals the *Quarterly Journal of Speech* and *The Howard Journal of Communications* and in the edited volumes *Conflict and Diversity* and *Handbook of Communication and People with Disabilities*.

John R. Thompson is a PhD candidate at the University of Texas at Austin, writing his dissertation on the topic of food and the rhetoric of globalization. Thompson's research agenda is shaped by globalization and its impact on rhetorics of constitution, identity, and political economy. He also asks questions of how underlying constructs of rhetorical theory—e.g., audience, ethos, topoi—might change when the landscape is global. In addition to studying food and teaching speech and business and managerial communication at St. Edward's University in Austin, Thompson is a home chef, cooking for his wife and two children.

Index

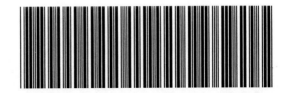